# Concise Guide to Sports Injuries

**For Elsevier:**

Commissioning Editor: *Claire Wilson*
Project Manager: *Morven Dean*
Designer: *Stewart Larking*
Illustration Manager: *Merlyn Harvey*
Illustrator: *Graeme Chambers*

# Concise Guide to Sports Injuries

Malcolm T F **Read** MA (Cantab) MRCGP DRCOG DM-Smed FISM FFSEM (UK) FFSEM (Irl)

Sir Roger Bannister Award

Specialist in Orthopaedic and Sport and Exercise Medicine, London, UK

Foreword by
**Bryan English** MB ChB DO Dip Sports Medicine FISM FFSEM (Irl) FFSEM (UK)
Chief Medical Officer, Chelsea Football Club, London, UK

SECOND EDITION

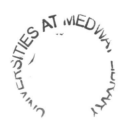

**CHURCHILL LIVINGSTONE**

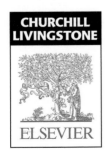

ELSEVIER

Edinburgh London New York Oxford Philadelphia St Louis Sydney Toronto 2008

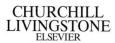

## CHURCHILL LIVINGSTONE
### ELSEVIER

An imprint of Elsevier Limited

First edition 2000 © Reed Educational and Professional Publishing Ltd
Second edition 2008

ISBN: 978 0443068737

**British Library Cataloguing in Publication Data**
A catalogue record for this book is available from the British Library

**Library of Congress Cataloging in Publication Data**
A catalog record for this book is available from the Library of Congress

**Notice**
Neither the Publisher nor the Author assume any responsibility for any loss or injury and/or damage to persons or property arising out of or related to any use of the material contained in this book. It is the responsibility of the treating practitioner, relying on independent expertise and knowledge of the patient, to determine the best treatment and method of application for the patient.

*The Publisher*

Printed in China

# Contents

# Acknowledgements

The practice of Sport and Exercise Medicine requires a team approach. I have had the privilege of working with a top team, my family. Romy, my wife, has been a constant support, my daughter Stephanie and her husband Alan have provided the action photographs, whilst my son Jeremy and daughter-in-law Emma have given their experience as an orthopaedic surgeon and children's nurse to broaden the approach of this physician. To all at BUPA Wellness, musculoskeletal clinic, and particularly the clinical team whose knowledge I have purloined, and especially Dr Philip Bell, my student and now close colleague, my grateful thanks.

# Preface

This book is not a textbook of sports medicine but a concise, practical guide to the problems that can face a doctor or physiotherapist with a sports team or in a sports clinic.

## General

The book can be used by selecting the area of interest from the index, or by turning to the relevant *anatomical area* concerned, such as the knee. Here a diagram of the pain distribution may help the clinician to consult the various differential diagnoses covered, or, if the differential diagnoses are known, to consult a list of *differential diagnoses* (e.g. medial knee pain, medial meniscus). In some areas, such as the knee, this is then divided into elements of the history that group them together, for instance swollen or non-swollen, and medial or lateral areas of pain reference. These are then further subdivided as follows.

## Findings

Findings include the history and signs and symptoms that are specific to the problem. Many sports injuries have a primary injury, which may have a pure, complete diagnostic picture, but many have a combination of injuries; for example, elbow pain may stem from a lateral epicondylitis together with a radiohumeral joint arthropathy. The findings deal only with the particular injury under discussion and not the combinations created by associated injuries. However, the reader is referred on to the relevant associated injuries so that the whole diagnostic picture can be completed. Perhaps the most important principle of orthopaedic medicine is to realize that many patients develop a trick move to protect the primary injury, and when this trick move becomes over-strained then pain appears elsewhere, and may in fact be the presenting feature. Thus a knee may be protected by 'rolling round' the hip, producing a trochanteric bursitis, or the hamstring insertion become flared whilst protecting a weak knee.

## Cause

The cause covers the mechanism of the injury and the tissues damaged. No treatment can be considered to be complete, and the injury will recur if the cause has not been dealt with.

## Investigations

These do not include investigations to exclude the differential diagnoses, unless they are watershed investigations. It is not cost-effective to carry out investigations if the clinical diagnosis is clear and the patient is improving; therefore these situations are defined as 'none are clinically required'. As magnetic resonance imaging (MRI) improves, so its role may develop even further. It is still an expensive investigation and does not give clear pictures of all injuries, though, combined with an arthrogram, it is hugely effective. At present, MRI is not as reliable as computed tomography (CT) for cortical bone, but is certainly better for soft tissue injuries. Whether MRI or SPECT scanning can pick up the earliest bone lesions may depend upon whether the lesion is medullary or cortical. Bone scanning is a good watershed investigation if there is a wide anatomical area to be covered in one investigation, or if the specific anatomical location cannot be well defined by clinical examination. X-ray may still be the best and cheapest investigation for myositis ossificans, calcific tendinitis, loose bodies and joint instability, as well as fractures. Real-time diagnostic ultrasound does rely on the skill of the ultrasonographer, who can provide a huge range of information about the soft tissues. In fact, clinicians are well advised to gain some skill with this investigation, which can also help with the accurate placement of injections.

## Treatment

Treatment is not covered in detail, but in principle. Details of the pulse rate and fluctuations of ultrasound, or the wavelength of laser, are for other books, as are the techniques and doses of injections. The aim of treatment in sports injuries, indeed all locomotor problems, is to return the patient to locomotor efficiency, and a series of *rehabilitation ladders* are included that may be used to guide recovery. Patients left to manage their own recovery will rest until pain-free and then return to full activity, break down again, rest and return to full activity, ad nauseam, until advised properly. The body responds to incremental loads, and these loads must be within the tolerance of the injured structure or the injury will recur. The ladder principles develop a rehabilitation rate which is dependent upon the individual's progress, not some arbitrary healing rate. These are expanded in the chapter on Rehabilitation (see Chapter 20). *Proprioceptive training*, balance and coordination cannot be trained by 30 minutes of physiotherapy twice a week, but require regular exercises that can be done every hour over the day, including, for amateurs, the working day. Thus, for example, balancing on one leg whilst cleaning one's teeth, or adding a half knee bend whilst answering the telephone, plus walking up stairs without using the calf, will all aid a weak uncoordinated knee more effectively than 20 minutes on a wobble board twice a week. *Cross-training* is the ideal way to maintain cardiovascular fitness, using other exercise programmes to maintain fitness whilst resting the injured part, and these regimens are referred to in the chapter on Rehabilitation. Rhythm, which controls technique by not allowing a trick move, must be encouraged. Athletes are goal achievers who will cheat to reach their goals by using other techniques, which will function at lower skills or speed but break down at high speed or higher skill levels. It is better to progress correctly, even if more slowly. All athletes, if left to themselves, will practise what they are good at, rather than their weaknesses. Thus injury can sometimes be the best time to work on poor skills. Use the injury lay-off time as a friend and not an enemy.

## Caveats

These are problem areas, where it is easy to overlook a totally different diagnosis or complication, and can remind the reader to think wider and further.

## Sports

This section deals with those sports which have technical problems that either cause the injury or require a particular type of rehabilitation or training technique. Reference will be to a right-handed player.

## Comments

Comments are made as observations and thoughts of the author, reflecting over three decades of experience.

## Rehabilitation

This includes cross-training advice to maintain aerobic fitness, standard advice on incremental training, and rehabilitation ladders which can be given to the patient for guidance on training with an injury. Some ladders are for technical problems, such as tennis elbow, and others for the muscles and coordination (for example for the knee), where there are two or more ladders that can be used. Patients who jump the ladder steps often produce a recurrence of the injury. If a new problem develops during rehabilitation, it suggests that the old injury is being protected by a trick movement, which is now also suffering from overuse and becoming injured. This trick movement must be recognized and corrected before it becomes 'patterned' into the rehabilitation. Be pedantic about skill, not rapidity, of return to competition.

## Team doctor

The section on team doctoring is to introduce those who go with teams, or advise on exercise, about some of the physiological and practical problems that might be encountered. Not every variant or problem can be covered, but a working idea of what might be expected if the reader were to travel with a team is presented. Large textbooks are written on the physiology of exercise, and this chapter is to afford a brief insight and understanding of the problems that affect the exercising patient.

## Glossary

Some specialist letters refer only to eponyms, so many of these, and other technical terms, are explained in more detail in this chapter. Eponyms have been used in the diagnostic section so that this section can be used as a quick reference for those familiar with the terms. Others, who may be less familiar with a particular diagnostic technique, are referred on to the Glossary, and this chapter will give the reader a brief idea of the 'how, what and why' of the test.

Malcolm TF Read
2008

# Foreword

It is a privilege to be asked to write the foreword for the long-awaited 2nd edition of Malcolm Read's *Concise Guide to Sports Injuries*. The 1st edition, published in 2000, was a best seller of its kind and the 2nd edition provides more insight into the workings and thoughts of the author. Malcolm's own Preface summarises the aims and objectives of the book, which is clearly aimed at the pragmatists working in the field. Carefully read his Preface more than once before you venture into the main text. He describes how sports injuries should be approached by those who want to work 'hands on' in this field. This book impresses in that it is what it says it is: a concise guide. Most importantly, it is one of the most readable books to be produced in the areas of sports and exercise medicine (SEM) and musculoskeletal medicine combined.

A firm strong point in this book is the coverage of the problems concerning the spine and the lower leg down (covering approximately 50 and 110 pages respectively, i.e. well over half the book). The approach of these chapters shows a strong musculoskeletal focus that has long been the mainstay of the author's work and experience. The areas of differential diagnosis in this text are the most common disorders and not, as can be the case in other texts, a collection of rare pathologies that one may not see in a working lifetime. These chapters allow the reader to peruse the factual differential of problems at the anatomical site, alongside the useful caveats that Malcolm has placed amongst the text. Indeed, his Preface may modestly say that there is no 'evidence' behind these caveats; however, Malcolm's personal experience is evidence in itself and should be read in such a way. The sports medicine practitioner should also note the strength of these chapters is that of solid musculoskeletal medicine and realise that a sports practitioner should have a heavy base of musculoskeletal training in order to practice as a specialist in this area. In fact, this level of bias in training is now mandatory. In the past the sports medicine practitioner had a training that was far too weak in the area of musculoskeletal basics and this was, and is, evidenced by the fact that most 'sports medicine' texts have been limited in this area, the very one that should be the foundation of the specialist working in sport.

The chapters on the ankle and foot (approximately one-sixth of the book) are particularly informative and show the author's depth of knowledge and understanding. The radiological images are used with full effect, as they are in the chapters on the spine. It is also in the area of the foot where the sections of the book entitled 'sports' and 'comment' are most enjoyable. To Malcolm these may be, at times, throw-away areas pieced together in a conversational manner, but to the reader these are gems that should be highlighted and absorbed. Malcolm Read gives the reader an insight into his decades of experience and lets us in on some of the secrets of his success.

The chapter on rehabilitation and training with an injury is the most unique and is, for me, the highlight of the book. The ladders that Malcolm uses provide clarity in an area that is poorly covered in the majority of similar publications by other authors. This method of understanding rehabilitation pathways should become standard for those working with athletes. Even if one analyses a particular ladder and disagrees with certain steps, what Malcolm Read is trying to get across is the important principles of rehabilitation and to get the reader to think in a systematic way. He produces a framework upon which to work, thus enabling any reader to expand the process to adapt the rehabilitation plan to the individual athlete. This is how this clever and unique chapter should be read.

The final chapter, prior to an extensive glossary, is on team doctoring. This is another gem of a chapter that is full of useful information for the doctor that travels with sports people. Perhaps these pages will find themselves in the travelling bags of the doctor on his/her journey. They would, indeed, be a useful companion.

In summary, this book is exceptional. It is easy to read and well presented. The book achieves exactly what it sets out to achieve and, once again, I refer the reader to Dr Read's own Preface. The author is an Olympian after competing for his country in the Olympics with the hockey team of Great

Britain. This is probably one of the reasons why this text reads from an athlete's perspective, as well as from that of someone who has worked with athletes at all levels. The text sets out to help the reader help the athlete. The impressive nature of the book is in its honesty, from someone who has been there, seen it and done it.

Malcolm Read is one of the rare breed of authors/lecturers who have the ability to combine evidence-based material with the good advice and anecdote, sourced from years of experience and from a mind that has always continued to ask questions and to learn.

Malcolm retired from his medical practice in 2007. Was it by coincidence that in his home country of the United Kingdom the specialty of sports and exercise medicine was finally recognised by the government as a specialty in its own right? Probably not, as his contribution to the specialty has been immense. To the many of us who were lucky enough to be his students, he is the godfather of SEM in the UK.

Bryan English
2008

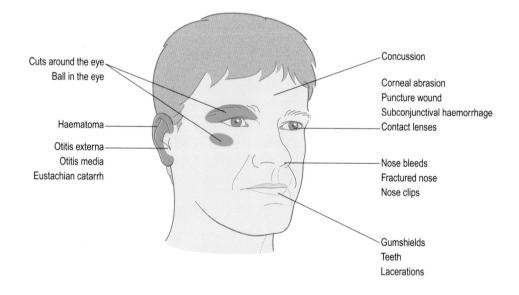

Cuts around the eye
Ball in the eye

Haematoma

Otitis externa
Otitis media
Eustachian catarrh

Concussion

Corneal abrasion
Puncture wound
Subconjunctival haemorrhage
Contact lenses

Nose bleeds
Fractured nose
Nose clips

Gumshields
Teeth
Lacerations

# Chapter One

# Head injuries

It is important to learn and maintain advanced life-saving techniques. This book is a guide and not a substitute for books or courses directed to that end.

## Concussion

In many sports serious head injury is an unlikely event, but when it happens and no one knows where any of the medical equipment is stored then disaster looms; so thorough preparation at the venue is important. Even if the venue is foreign, it is important to know the whereabouts of the stretchers, preferably a scoop stretcher, and semi-rigid, lock-on, cervical collars. Clinicians should find out the whereabouts of the resuscitation equipment, either from the venue or attending paramedics at the site, and ensure that it is working, or take their own. The telephone number of the nearest hospital competent to handle emergencies should be recorded in the medical area, and the medical organizer of an event should inform the management of that hospital of the time and date it will take place.

## Airway or neck protection

The airway is vital, and its restoration must take precedence, even in the presence of spinal injury. Concussion and cervical spine injuries often coexist, and the possibility of cervical spine injury in an unconscious patient must never be overlooked.

## Signs of concussion are present if:

(a) there has been even the shortest time of unresponsiveness

(b) the patient fails the Maddocks' questions [1] (see Suspected Concussion chart, p. 3)

(c) there is post-traumatic amnesia (this may begin 30 s or so after the injury)

(d) the patient is unsteady walking heel to toe, or unable to hold the ball

(e) the patient complains of giddiness, double vision, or is vomiting

(f) the patient has been unconscious, has spasms, or convulsions.

## Off the pitch check

AVPU: record a base line and monitor at 5 minute intervals.

A Alertness
V responds to Verbal commands
P responds to Pain
U Unconscious

## Check for possible complications

(a) Lacerations, scalp tenderness, haematoma, and blood or cerebral spinal fluid from nose or ears for underlying fractures. A small skin wound can hide a fracture.
(b) Subconjunctival haemorrhage.
(c) Signs of neck injury such as paraesthesia [2].

## Transfer to hospital

(a) Record the Glasgow coma score [3] (see Glossary), and send this with the patient (tape the chart to the inside of the medical case so it can be remembered).
(b) Note rising blood pressure or falling pulse, head down position may aggravate the blood pressure.
(c) Treat with continuous oxygen.
(d) Label the patient with name, and birth date if it is known.

## Instructions to friends or relatives of an athlete sent home

Advise them, write down the head injury instructions and emphasize that the overriding principle is that any deterioration warrants transfer to hospital for medical attention. Supervision should continue for 24 hours.

## Return to competition or training

This should not occur until the athlete has passed a full neurological examination, has no headache and no headache after exercise [4]. Some sports have an arbitrary time to match fitness; for example rugby is 3 weeks, and boxing 28 days first time, 84 days second time and 1 year third time. Elite sports arrange pre-season neuropsychological testing (see www.cogsport.com/cms), and the athlete is permitted to return to sport only when a repeat test has returned to, or is better than, baseline recordings. This may be earlier or later than the above arbitrary times.

### Caveat

**Although concussion is common in contact sports, one major source of head injuries in children comes from swinging golf clubs, where the back swing or the follow through strikes another player who is standing close by. Coaches, parents and children must be aware of this potential risk.**

## Punch-drunk syndrome

Appropriate application of guidelines to concussion [5] should prevent the punch-drunk syndrome, which can occur years later and shows signs and symptoms of slight mental confusion, slowness of thought, personality change, memory impairment, hand tremor, nodding head movements, unsteady gait and dysarthria [6].

## Protective helmets

No helmet can prevent all head and neck injuries. The helmet does not prevent contrecoup injury [4], nor violent rotation of the head, but it is an effective prevention from lacerations and haematomata. The hard outer shell dissipates incidental blows, but the crumpling of the polystyrene inner shell absorbs most of the energy. Any crash helmet that has been subject to damage should be changed, as the integrity of the inner shell cannot be guaranteed (see Mouth, below).

# Eyes

Prevention is better than cure! Snow blindness has occurred in those removing sunglasses or goggles to take photographs, and water may reflect the sun's rays, causing similar problems. Prescription glasses may be made with polarized, or photochromic material, and polarized shields may clip onto normal lenses. Cages or helmets worn during cricket or American football, and motorcycle helmets, protect the face and eyes from trauma, whilst sparring helmets for martial arts functionally deepen the orbit. However, specially designed squash and badminton eye guards are often ignored, although both the squash ball and shuttlecock 'fit' the orbit, and a 'blow out' fracture of the orbit can cause total loss of an eye. During squash games the calling of 'lets' and 'penalty points' should be encouraged. Players with less skill, who tend to hit the ball regardless of the danger to the opponent, cause many unnecessary injuries.

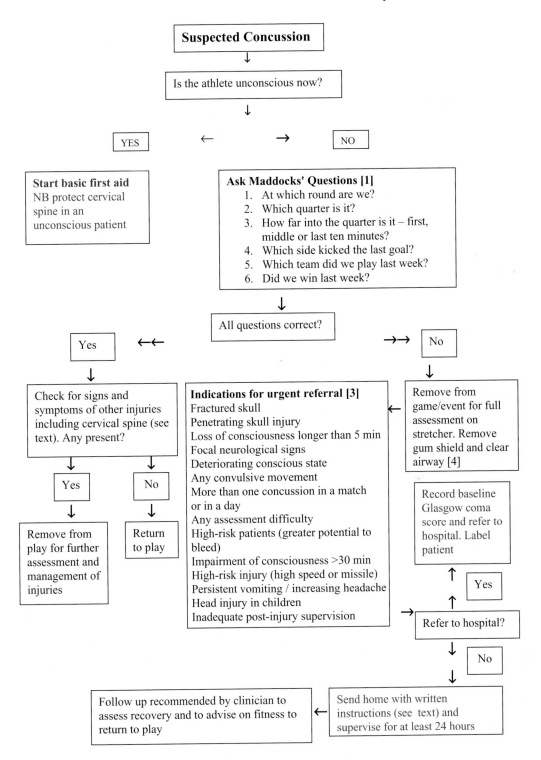

**Suspected Concussion**

↓

Is the athlete unconscious now?

↓

YES ← → NO

**Start basic first aid**
NB protect cervical spine in an unconscious patient

**Ask Maddocks' Questions [1]**
1. At which round are we?
2. Which quarter is it?
3. How far into the quarter is it – first, middle or last ten minutes?
4. Which side kicked the last goal?
5. Which team did we play last week?
6. Did we win last week?

↓

All questions correct?

Yes ←← →→ No

Check for signs and symptoms of other injuries including cervical spine (see text). Any present?

Remove from game/event for full assessment on stretcher. Remove gum shield and clear airway [4]

**Indications for urgent referral [3]**
Fractured skull
Penetrating skull injury
Loss of consciousness longer than 5 min
Focal neurological signs
Deteriorating conscious state
Any convulsive movement
More than one concussion in a match or in a day
Any assessment difficulty
High-risk patients (greater potential to bleed)
Impairment of consciousness >30 min
High-risk injury (high speed or missile)
Persistent vomiting / increasing headache
Head injury in children
Inadequate post-injury supervision

Yes   No

Remove from play for further assessment and management of injuries

Return to play

Record baseline Glasgow coma score and refer to hospital. Label patient

↑ Yes

↑

Refer to hospital?

↓ No

↓

Follow up recommended by clinician to assess recovery and to advise on fitness to return to play

Send home with written instructions (see text) and supervise for at least 24 hours

## Medical 'eye injury kit'

(a) Small mirror.
(b) Pencil torch.
(c) Ophthalmoscope.
(d) Sterile washout fluid.
(e) Local anaesthetic eye drops (amethocaine).
(f) Fluorescein.
(g) Antibiotic drops or ointment – check expiry dates regularly.
(h) Eye patches, and micropore or clear tape.
(i) Visual acuity chart.
(j) Contact lens fluid.

## Cuts around the eye

Allow 3–4 weeks for adequate soft tissue healing.

(a) Acute – remove from the field of play, 1:1000 adrenaline swabs, steristrips, cyanoacrylate or embucrylate (superglue) and/or suturing. Cover the wound.
(b) Subacute – subcuticular suturing and enzyme creams.

Caveat

Eyelids or medial epicanthic folds, which may involve the tear duct, require specialist referral.

## Corneal abrasion

Application of amethocaine and fluorescein will allow adequate examination of the eye where corneal abrasion or a foreign body is suspected. An antibiotic cream or drops can be applied. Remove loose foreign bodies. Close the eyelid and keep the eye shut by covering with an eye patch for 24–48 hours.

Caveat

The findings of an embedded foreign body, penetrating injury, hyphaemia (blood in anterior chamber) or dendritic ulcer require urgent referral for an ophthalmic opinion.

## Puncture wound of the eye

Note any history of a penetrating wound. Signs of hyphaemia, pear-shaped iris, enlarged or poorly reacting pupil, cloudy vision and impaired visual acuity should be referred for an ophthalmic opinion.

Caveat

A late sequela of a puncture wound of the eye may be a sympathetic response in the other eye.

## Blow to the eye

(a) Large (e.g. cricket ball plus in size, elbow, fist). Check for hyphaemia and orbital fractures, especially of the inferior orbit. Note diplopia may also occur as a late sequela, when the inferior rectus muscle is tied into the healing inferior orbital fracture. If in doubt, refer for ophthalmic opinion.
(b) Small (e.g. squash ball, shuttlecock, knuckle, point of elbow). A small ball striking the eye will 'fit the orbit' and may be catastrophic, causing a blow-out fracture of the orbit and loss of an eye [7]. However, one-third of orbital blow-out fractures are sustained in sport. Though visual acuity recovery is complete, almost universal loss of binocular vision occurs [7]. Check for hyphaemia and a posterior chamber bleed if the fundus and retina cannot be visualized. If in doubt, refer for ophthalmic opinion.

## Subconjunctival haemorrhage

If the haemorrhage appears segmental and in the anterior aspect of the sclera, it is probably of no consequence; however, if the posterior aspect cannot be visualized, then consider major trauma to the eye, a fractured skull and cerebral contusion, and refer for a further opinion. If visual problems, or a possible penetrating injury have occurred, refer for ophthalmic opinion.

## Contact lenses

These should be soft, and a spare pair should be available. They are usually displaced around the eye, but are occasionally lost outside the eye, when the replacement lens is required.

## Glasses

These should be (plastic) polycarbonate, have sprung ear clips, and have a nose bridge that holds the glasses away from the face to prevent misting up.

## Eyes at risk from trauma

In a patient with only one functioning eye, check for previous retinal detachment or Marfan syndrome. Unfortunately, the risk of possible retinal detachment in severe myopia is not altered by laser surgery to correct the myopia.

## Vision

Visual training in sport is becoming commonplace, particularly for the non-dominant eye. Defective vision may be remediable, and a full ophthalmic assessment is advised, even in people with apparently good vision [8].

# Ears

Prevention is better than cure. Scrum caps, or taping of the ears, prevents damage to the pinna, and ear muffs and ear plugs should reduce acoustic trauma.

## Haematoma of the pinna (cauliflower ear)

(a) Acute – aspirate and apply a compression bandage. The aspiration must be aseptic and will probably require repeating on several occasions.

(b) Chronic – no effective treatment is available until cosmetic surgery can be advised, when the playing days are over. Perichondral tears should be well aligned, sutured and covered by antibiotics. This may require referral to a plastic surgeon.

## Otitis externa

This is common in swimmers. However, soft moulded earplugs may help, though they have been known to cause the problem during insertion. Dry the ears, but do not use cotton wool buds on sticks, which excoriate the external auditory meatus. Warm olive oil drops pre-swimming, and 5% acetic acid in isopropyl alcohol drops after swimming [9], may help. Swab for *Staphylococcus* or *Candida* spp, if troublesome, and treat as required.

## Otitis media

Participation in sport is permitted if athletes are non-toxic (temperature or pulse rate not raised; see Chapter 21: Head colds), but diving, especially scuba, should be avoided. Swimming should cease with a perforated drum, but ear, nose and throat (ENT) surgeons may vary as to whether they consider grommets to be a contraindication to swimming.

## Eustachian and sinus catarrh

In the acute stage this may be relieved by menthol inhalations, and dope test-negative nasal decongestants, but great care should be taken to avoid medicines with ephedrine, pseudoephedrine, phenylpropanolamine, or any other banned substance. The label of contents should be read carefully, as proprietary preparations with the same name may differ in content between countries. The allergic element may be controlled with steroid insufflation, cromoglyconates, and non-sedative antihistamines, but parenteral steroids are banned without a Therapeutic Use Extension (TUE; see Chapter 21). Surprisingly, once scuba divers learn to re-pressurize their ears, diving is said to help the condition.

# Mouth

Gumshields should be cast made, to allow maximum compression thickness over the teeth cusps but cause the least interference with the palate, which enables easy mouth breathing. They should be worn in all sports where potential impact may occur, including squash, where blows from the racket can occur. Gumshields do not prevent concussion but protect the teeth [10,11]. Displaced teeth should be replaced and splinted. Avulsed teeth and crown fragments should be kept, but handled only by the crown. In an alert patient they should be replaced within 60 minutes, or stored in the buccal sulcus, until a dentist can be reached. However, if the athlete is not fully alert, the tooth should be stored in a sterile solution (saline), or milk, and a dentist consulted within 2 hours. It should not be assumed that missing teeth or fragments are still 'on the park' if they have not been found, and the patient should be X-rayed to check the fragments have not been inhaled or swallowed. Fractured teeth involving dentine are painful on air sufflation and require a dental review [6]. Sometimes a tooth may discolour and die some years after it has been traumatized. Underlying fractures of the jaws should be excluded. Lacerations in the tongue and mucosa often heal well without sutures.

## Nose

### Nose bleeds

The patient should be sat up and the head tipped forwards, and compression applied externally over Little's area, preferably for 5 minutes, by a person other than the patient. 1:1000 adrenaline packs may be used, but with continued bleeding, or posterior nasal cavity bleed, a referral to the ENT department should be made.

**Caveat**

**The presence of clear cerebrospinal fluid from the nose is diagnostic of a cranial fracture.**

### Fractured nose

(a) Undisplaced – may be treated by managing the bleeding and soft tissue injury.

(b) Displaced – should be reduced, especially in the young, as a fracture may reduce the size of the nasal passage and increase the likelihood of sinusitis.

**Caveat**

**A septal haematoma may be diagnosed by increasing pain, fever and localized redness and swelling of the septum, which requires evacuation and aspiration. Refer to an ENT department.**

### Nose clips

(a) Sprung – the idea is to close the external nares; used for synchronized swimming.

(b) Strips – the idea is to open the nares and ease respiration. There is an effect at rest but they do little or nothing to aid respiration during exercise, as this is predominantly by mouth breathing. However, nose strips during the recovery phase produce a feeling of more controlled and easy respiration.

## References

1 Maddocks DL, Dicker GD, Saling MM. The assessment of orientation following concussion in athletes. Clin J Sports Med 1995;5(1):32–35

2 National Health and Medical Research Council. Head and neck injuries in football. Canberra: Australian Government Publishing Service; 1995

3 Teasdale G, Jennett B. Assesment of coma and impaired consciousness. Lancet 1974;2:81–84

4 Ryan AJ. Protecting the sportsman's brain (concussion in sport). Br J Sports Med 1991;25:81–86

5 McCrory PR. Were you knocked out? A team physician's approach to initial concussion management. Med Sci Sports Exerc 1997;29 (7 Suppl):S207–212

6 Reid D. Sports injury assessment and rehabilitation. Edinburgh: Churchill Livingstone; 1992

7 Jones NP. Orbital blow out fractures in sport. Br J Sports Med 1994;28:272–275

8 Loran DF, MacEwan CJ. Sports vision. Oxford: Butterworth-Heinemann; 1995

9 Bruckner P, Khan K. Clinical sports medicine, 3rd edn. New York: McGraw-Hill; 2006

10 Chapman PJ. Orofacial injuries and international rugby players' attitudes to mouth guards. Br J Sports Med 1990;24:156–158

11 Jennings DC. Injuries sustained by users and non users of gum shields in local rugby union. Br J Sports Med 1990;24:159–165

### Further reading

Bruckner P, Khan K. Clinical sports medicine. 3rd edn. New York: McGraw-Hill; 2006

Reid D. Sports injury assessment and rehabilitation. Edinburgh: Churchill Livingstone; 1992

UKADIS diagnosis of concussion in sport. Ukadis laminate UKADIS/PDJ 2004

# Chapter Two

# Chapter Two

2

# Axial skeleton

The axial skeleton is dealt with in some detail, as analysis of the areas of injury seen by sports physicians, physiotherapists and osteopaths showed that 75 to 80% of problems were spinal [1].

## Part 1 **Functional anatomy**

### The disc

Each disc has a central nucleus pulposus, a surrounding annulus fibrosis and the limiting cartilage end plates.

### Nucleus pulposus

The nucleus pulposus is a soft hydrophilic substance contained within the centre of the disc. The nucleus pulposus can move within the confines of the annulus fibrosis (Fig. 2.1).

### Annulus fibrosis

The annulus is at its weakest in the posterolateral region, where the cellular structure is less well organized. Therefore, the nucleus pulposus most commonly herniates in a posterior or posterolateral direction, and less commonly in a lateral direction, towards the spinal canal.

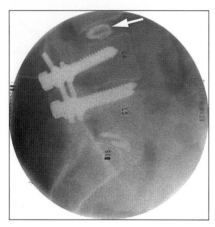

**Figure 2.1** • The discogram clearly outlines a normal nucleus pulposus at L3/4. L4/5 vertebrae are surgically stabilized.

## Cartilage end plate

This represents the anatomical limit of the disc. The annular epiphyses of the vertebral body develop in the marginal part of this thin end plate. Stress changes across this area, in the teenager, produce pain and diagnostic X-ray changes of Scheuermann's epiphysitis (Fig. 2.2). Rarely, trauma may produce an avulsion of the disc's bony attachment, creating a posterior marginal node, or limbus fracture, in teenagers where there is a small avulsion fracture of the vertebral end plate that can protrude into the spinal canal [2,3] (Fig. 2.3).

## Ligaments

- The *anterior longitudinal ligament* supports the anterior aspect of the vertebral bodies, including the discs.

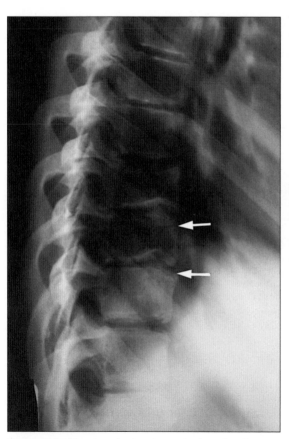

**Figure 2.2** • The dorsal spine shows the irregular disc spaces and end plates of Scheuermann's epiphysitis.

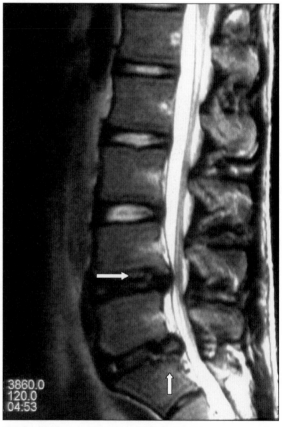

**Figure 2.3** • A posterior marginal node at L4 and L5 where the posterior ring epiphysis of S1 is fractured and at L4 the cartilage end plate is protruding into the spinal canal.

- The *posterior longitudinal ligament* is attached to the posterior aspect of the vertebral bodies, but creates the anterior wall of the spinal canal. It is not as strong as the anterior ligament.
- The *ligamentum flavum* forms the posterior aspect of the spinal canal. It is an elastic ligament that helps maintain the upright posture and the return of the spinal column to its erect position after bending.
- The *supraspinous ligament* runs over the tips of the spines and connects with the *interspinous ligament* that joins the spinous processes. The ligaments are strongest at the lumbar level.

## Facet joints

The vertebral arches are joined at their bases by the synovial, zygapophyseal joints, whose shape will control the range of movement between the concomitant vertebrae. The thoracic vertebrae favour lateral bending and rotation, whilst the lumbar facets favour flexion, extension, and lateral bending, at the higher lumbar levels (Fig. 2.4).

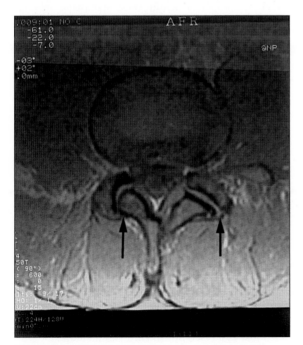

**Figure 2.4** • MRI scan showing zygapophyseal (facet) joints. The ones shown here are abnormally asymmetric and as such may produce an unstable movement pattern.

## Innervation

The innervation of the disc, posterior longitudinal ligament, periosteum, venous sinuses and spinal dura is from the sinuvertebral nerve and contains spinal and sympathetic branches. The nerve may also provide fibres to the facet joints. (This nerve is surgically sectioned, or destroyed by cryo- or radiorhizotomy, which is one form of treatment for chronic facetal pain.)

## Spinal cord and meninges

The spinal cord ends at the level of L1/2. The nerves that exit below this level are contained in meningeal coverings to the level of S2, the cauda equina, and the filum terminale connects the meninges to their eventual insertion. A median raphe tethers the meninges to the spinal canal and can be responsible for a caudal epidural flowing only to the left or the right side. Arachnoid cysts between the pia mater and the arachnoid mater may be seen on magnetic resonance imaging (MRI), especially in the sacrum (Fig. 2.5). They are thought to have no clinical significance, apart from the Tarlov cyst, in which the nerves pass through the cyst as opposed to around it. Surgery is best avoided. A caudal epidural given with a long needle may penetrate a cyst and result in a spinal anaesthetic being administered. The technique should employ a short needle passed through the caudal hiatus, but not up the canal.

## Function of the vertebral column

The major function of the vertebral column is to support and protect the spinal cord from physical trauma. The spinal ligaments support the vertebral column so that less muscle energy is required to maintain its erect posture. During movement the large mass of posterior vertebral muscles, particularly multifidus, is primarily responsible for intrinsic stability. However, with increased dynamic loading, both intra-abdominal and intrathoracic pressure increases. The increased intra-abdominal pressure can be harnessed to support the vertebral column by contracting transversus abdominis muscles. This action produces a pneumatic cushion (tyre effect), which will support the anterior aspect of the vertebral column. Core stability exercises and skills use this principle for functional muscle control of the back.

In the lumbar spine the movements of flexion, extension and side flexion compress the disc on one

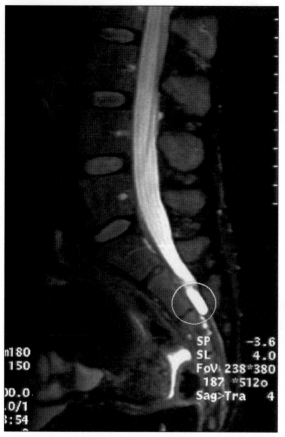

Figure 2.5 • An asymptomatic sacral arachnoid cyst.

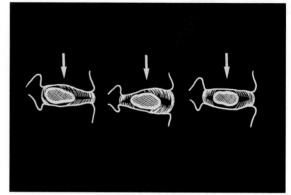

Figure 2.6 • The nucleus pulposus moves in relation to back position.

edge and stretch the other, and this movement pushes the nucleus pulposus towards the stretched surface so that, in flexion, the nucleus pulposus will move posteriorly, towards the weakest area of the annulus (Fig. 2.6).

Flexion of the spine is limited by the elasticity of the ligamentum flavum, the inter- and supraspinous ligaments, the posterior part of the disc and the posterior longitudinal ligament. The range of extension is limited by the anterior longitudinal ligament, the anterior part of the disc, plus the close packing of the facet joints and spinous processes against one another.

Thus, the vertebral column may be balanced in the vertical position, but it is more stable in extension, when the facet joints interlock. During forward flexion the body performs like a crane, with the pelvis and the legs becoming the tower, and the spine the side arm. In this position the spinal segments will destabilize.

The side arm can be stabilized by a pressure bag running along its length. This pressure bag is created by raised intra-abdominal pressure, and the walls of the bag consist of the abdominal muscles, diaphragm, pelvic floor and the paravertebral muscles. The transversus abdominis and the multifidus muscles seem most important. Similarly, walking, jumping, running, and so on, produce pelvic displacement that will produce spinal instability, unless stabilized. Core stability techniques are designed to train these stabilizing muscles, both local and global [4], to reduce excessive lumbar segmental instability. Various methods, such as the Alexander technique [5] and active alert [6], have been around for many years, and the early 21st century clinicians prefer the early 20th century Pilates techniques.

A dam wall is unable to resist the water pressure if the wall is built straight or with a concave surface to the water. The water pressure is resisted by a convex surface. This principle must also be employed during the times that intra-abdominal pressure is raised, when the lumbar spine should be held in some degree of extension. The over straight, splinted spine with increased intra-abdominal pressure ('sergeant major's back') shows a high L1/2, L2/3 discal pathology. The unsplinted or flexed spine encourages posterior disc creep.

## Arachnoid cyst

The spinal meninges may pocket spinal fluid to form arachnoid cysts (see Spinal cord and meninges).

# Part 2 Clinical application

## PART CONTENTS

## Referred pain

Damage to the lumbar spine may cause localized pain, or referred pain to the groin, buttock, thigh, shin, calf, ankle or foot, with or without accompanying local back pain. It is therefore essential to include examination of the back when assessing a patient who presents with pain in the lower limbs. Equally, upper limb pain examinations should exclude referral from the cervical spine.

### Leg pain

There are certain clues in the history that suggest pain is referred from the nerve root or dura:

(a) Night pain that wakes the patient from sleep, as opposed to pain created by the movement of turning in bed. The former suggests that movement is not the cause.

(b) 'Pins and needles' or paraesthaesia in the leg. The distribution may give a clue as to the root level involved.

(c) The pain may be worse on coughing, or blowing the nose, which produces a Valsalva effect, increasing intraspinal pressure.

(d) Radiation of pain into the foot is usually from the nerve, not facet or sacroiliac joint.

(e) Descriptions of the pain include hyperaesthesia, burning, lancinating, electric shock, water-flowing sensation in the limb. However, burning, relentless pain in a stocking distribution, is more diagnostic of a possible regional pain syndrome or peripheral neuropathy.

(f) The intensity of pain description, with a VAS (visual analogue pain scale) up at the 8–10 level. In these cases there may be few clinical findings, apart from, perhaps, a positive slump test.

## Bone pain

All the usual causes of bone pain must be considered when examining patients with sports injuries. Patients with tumours (Fig. 2.7) and infections of the spine give a history of a continuous pain, usually with an insidious onset, that may or may not be affected by biomechanical movement. Locomotor problems are affected by normal biomechanical movement patterns, which alter the pain intensity, and may at times be pain-free. In young patients it is important to consider the possibility of ankylosing spondylitis and the other spondylarthropathies.

## Non-mechanical back pain

The possibility of a non-mechanical cause of back pain should be considered with a presentation of just one of the following:

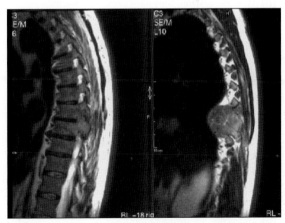

**Figure 2.7 •** A myeloma that presented with diaphragmatic pain. X-rays were normal. Localized facetal tenderness was found, but needling the area elicited no bony resistance and subsequent MRI findings are shown.

(a) Night pain, without movement, that wakes the patient.

(b) Unremitting pain.

(c) Pain not made worse by movement.

(d) Loss of weight.

(e) Systemically unwell.

(f) Raised temperature.

(g) Generalized aches and pains; myalgia.

(h) Other joints are painful.

(i) Flitting joint pains; arthralgia.

(j) Dysuria.

(k) Eye symptoms: iritis, uveitis, conjunctivitis.

(l) Urethral discharge, sexually transmitted disease, human immunodeficiency virus (HIV).

(m) Skin problems – rash, psoriasis.

(n) Known primary carcinoma.

(o) Hypo/hyperthyroidism.

(p) Family history of spondylarthropathy.

## Mechanical back pain

There is no black and white method of diagnosing mechanical back problems. The pointers to diagnosis and management are obtained from the patient's history, examination, and investigations that include blood tests, MRI, computed tomography (CT), discography and intradiscal injections. Disc probing involves an injection of the disc, facet joints and sacroiliac joints, under narcoanaesthesia, to see which reproduces the patient's pain. Common biomechanical problems include:

(a) disc herniation, annular tears, and nucleus pulposus pressure on the annulus. Damaged discs also have a chemical element to the pain. High levels of phospholipids have been found in damaged, painful discs [7,8]

(b) facet joint arthrosis, or arthritis

(c) pars interarticularis fractures (spondylolysis and its unstable bilateral form spondylolisthesis)

(d) wedge fractures of the vertebral body

(e) Scheuermann's vertebral ring epiphysitis, and the rare posterior marginal node (see in Part 1: Cartilage end plate)

(f) sacroiliac dysfunction

(g) ligamentous strain

(h) interspinous impingement

(i) spinal stenosis and lateral canal entrapment

(j) myofascial and muscle pains, and spasm, are usually secondary to the underlying cause.

## Coccygeal pain

A fall on the base of the spine may damage the sacrococcygeal ligaments. Sitting and full flexion are painful. A ring cushion, occasionally posterior mobilization of the coccyx, and steroid injections around the inflamed sacrococcygeal ligaments will help. Dural pain may refer to the sacrum and coccyx and have no obvious mechanical signs. If the coccyx is tender to palpation, both externally and per rectum, then a trial of sacrococcygeal ligament injection should be given. If not, then a trial of an epidural is worthwhile. Coccygeal resection seems to have ongoing postoperative problems.

## Management of back pain

### The history

The history may be diagnostic and will help define management. Non-traumatic, mechanical, lumbar back lesions may be divided into flexion-orientated, extension-orientated or mixed. It must always be remembered that, when one element of the spine is dysfunctional, there will be some degree of stretch of the adjacent ligaments and alteration in the mechanics of the surrounding joints. For example, a disc displacement will have its main component of flexion-orientated pain, but there will be some consequent disturbance of the facet joints and stretch of the surrounding ligaments, with secondary spasm of the muscles, producing additional pain patterns.

### Localized muscle injuries

Localized muscle injuries do occur in the back, but there is almost always a history of direct trauma; without this, an underlying lesion should always be suspected. Visualization of the muscle damage can be achieved with real-time ultrasound or an MRI scan.

### Nerve root damage

There may be signs of a nerve root palsy, with motor signs relevant to the damaged nerve root. The degree of sensory disturbance, except perineal, does not alter the treatment and need not be tested. The distribution of sensory symptoms is a sufficient guide to the root level. If invasive, accurate, localized treatment is planned, then MRI is a reasonably accurate indicator of the disc and root level. Nerve root involvement is suggested by 'pins and needles', numbness, hyperaesthesia and night pain, in a radicular distribution.

### Caveat

**There are some patients who are desperate to convince the clinician that their pain is really severe. They appear slightly hysterical over their history and there may be very few clinical signs, even a negative slump test. These patients invariably have dural pain, and a trial of an epidural is usually successful in relieving their pain.**

The distribution of the symptoms indicates the level; for example groin, T12/L1; front of thigh, L2/3; front of thigh, knee and anterior shin, L3/4; back of leg to calf, shin or foot, L4/5 S1; sole of foot, S1; perineal or perianal, S3/4. The signs of nerve involvement of the sciatic nerve are: straight leg raise reduced, Lasègue's and/or slump tests positive. The femoral stretch test is positive for the femoral nerve involvement; the Valsalva and Kernig's tests are positive if the dura itself is involved (see Glossary for these tests, also Lhermitte, Dural stress tests and Adverse neural tensioning).

## Weakness from nerve root palsy

### Caveat

**Note that the oblique exit of the lumbar spinal nerves from the spine can permit one disc to involve two nerves and therefore create multiradicular signs and symptoms, but a disc hernia does not damage more than two nerves, so, if more than two roots are involved, the diagnosis is likely to be diabetes, nerve disease or a space-occupying lesion.**

### Lumbar spine nerve root signs [9]

L1/2   Weak psoas.

L3/4   Weak quadriceps and diminished or absent knee jerk.

L4   Weak tibialis anterior and diminished or absent knee jerk.

L5   Weak extensor hallucis longus, extensor digitorum longus, extensor digitorum brevis, peroneals. Peroneal weakness can present with either L4 or L5 root involvement.

S1   Weak calf, hamstring and diminished or absent ankle jerk.

S1/2   Weak gluteals.

S3/4   Loss of control of the anal sphincter or micturition. Loss of perineal sensation and reduced or absent anal/perineal reflex.

### Caveat

**S3/4 root involvement requires emergency surgery.**

## Rectal and vaginal examination

Any clinical suggestion of an intrapelvic lesion warrants a vaginal or rectal examination.

## Rest

The accepted, evidence-based wisdom is that simple back pain should not be rested in bed. However, in the acute phase of a disc lesion, the dura may be so painful and irritable that even slight movement exacerbates the pain. In this case rest is helpful. Certainly, patients who are better in the morning, and know they get better with rest, should be actively persuaded to take time off to rest as it will hasten the healing process. Sometimes, moving a patient by car for treatment flares the problem more than the treatment improves it, and in these cases it is better for the patient to be rested rather than travel for treatment.

Those patients not made worse by extension should try lying prone, and then gradually increase the lumbar lordosis with pillows under their chest. Extension McKenzie exercises may be added, but both exercises should be stopped if there is an exacerbation or peripheralization of leg pain. L2/3 and L3/4 discs are often helped by flexion McKenzie exercises, and with pillows under the knees when lying supine and under the hips when lying prone [10]. These postures will help to encourage flexion. Once the acute sensitivity has settled, then activity should be encouraged. An epidural can relieve this acute sensitivity more rapidly.

### Caveat

**The mattress should be appropriate to the problem. So beware the standard 'orthopaedic' mattress, for, as a rule, hard mattresses encourage extension, soft mattresses encourage flexion, and 'one size may not fit all'.**

# Posture

> ## Caveat
>
> Individualized, postural re-education creates a mechanism for successful self-management in most cases of back pain.

Perhaps 80% of the management of painful backs is the correct adjustment of the individual's posture, and this may cure and prevent recurrences. Not every back responds to the same postural correction. Thus a flexion-orientated problem (annular disc bulge) requires extensions to improve and prevent disc creep (see Chapter 5: Lumbar spine). Facet joints, and L5/S1 collar stud discs (Fig. 2.8), will require pelvic tilting to flatten the lordosis. However, the latter may require pelvic tilting (flexion) initially and, as the disc regresses and loses its collar stud formation, will then require the extension manoeuvres typical of an annular disc. A thoracolumbar kyphosis may have a compensatory low lumbar lordosis, so that the adjustment of posture in this case will be extension at the thoracolumbar junction but pelvic tilt at the lumbosacral junction. Too much postural advice is given in general terms, without taking into account the variations within and between backs. Some backs may have to be used in a neutral position, emphasizing neither extension nor flexion.

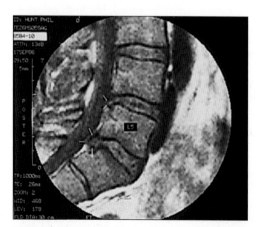

**Figure 2.8 •** A retrolisthesis of L5 on S1 shows on X-ray by a bulging of the disc space into the body of L5. A 'collar stud' prolapse of the disc is seen on MRI and extension will nip this 'collar stud' (*arrows*).

The individual correct posture should then be stabilized by muscle control (see Glossary: Core stability).

## Correcting the posture

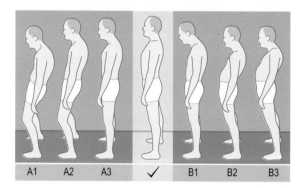

### Group A: Rounded back (A1, A2 and A3)

The pain is worse bending over, sitting, driving and getting out of a chair, when the back feels a little stuck and is eased by leaning backwards. The pain is reduced when lying face down, and arching backward. More lumbar lordosis is required.

**A1** Straighten the knees, and stand with the weight on the balls of the feet, to allow increased lumbar lordosis. Straighten the dorsal spine, standing tall. Draw back the head on the shoulders.

**A2** Allow lumbar lordosis, but flatten the stomach muscles, particularly the transversus abdominis. Stand tall through the upper spine, and straighten the head on the shoulders.

**A3** Standing too straight produces long-term stress in the upper lumbar vertebrae. Allow a thoracolumbar lordosis to occur and reduce pelvic tilt. These people invariably stand with their weight on their heels, so move the balance to the balls of the feet.

*To increase extension:*

**(a)** Sleep on a hard mattress/floor/futon.

**(b)** Sit on a low chair, with a high desk, and raise the computer screen.

**(c)** Sit with one foot drawn under the chair, or the knee pointing to the ground.

**(d)** Use a 'wedge' cushion on the chair, 'kneel on' chairs, or tilt the front of the chair downwards.

Use a cushion in the small of the back, or a lumbar roll. Try tying a towel around the waist at night.

**(e)** Drive sitting upright and closer to the steering wheel, with bent arms. This relaxes the back.

**(f)** Stand with the centre of gravity towards the balls of feet. Sit and stand tall, using the core stabilizers.

**(g)** If slumping in an easy chair, slump with the lumbar spine in extension.

**(h)** When leaning over a solid object, stand with legs wide apart, to lose height, brace the pelvis against the solid object and maintain the forward lean, with an extended spine.

**(i)** Lock the back in extension whilst bending or lifting, and splint the spine with a core stability technique.

### The neutral position

The neutral position is the ideal posture but varies between individuals, so the following description has degrees of tolerance. The patient should stand with the weight balanced over the middle of the feet, with a slight lordosis, stomach muscles (transversus) gently tightened and braced by multifidus. The thorax is raised to straighten the dorsal spine. The chin and head are drawn back, not up. The arms and scapulae should hang naturally without tension, and not be forced backwards.

### Group B: Hollowed (sway) back (B1, B2 and B3)

The pain experienced by these patients is worse whilst standing relaxed, with a lumbar lordosis, leaning backwards, and lying face down. The Alexander technique [5] helps this group of patients (see Glossary: Core stability).

**B1** Stand taller through the dorsal spine, straighten any rounded back, and straighten the head and neck.

**B2** Flatten the stomach (transversus) to support and splint the spine against the back muscles (multifidus).

**B3** Tilt the pelvis to flatten the lower back, and shift centre of gravity towards the heels.

*To decrease extension:*

**(a)** Sleep on a soft mattress.

**(b)** Instead of standing, reduce the lumbar lordosis by perching or half sitting on the edge of a table. Use a bar stool, even at the kitchen sink. Use a shooting stick when sightseeing.

**(c)** Stand with one foot resting on an object raised 15–20 cm; e.g. the foot rail in a pub.

**(d)** Stand with the body's centre of gravity towards the heels.

**(e)** Use a core stability technique to lock the back in neutral position when bending or lifting.

## Bending

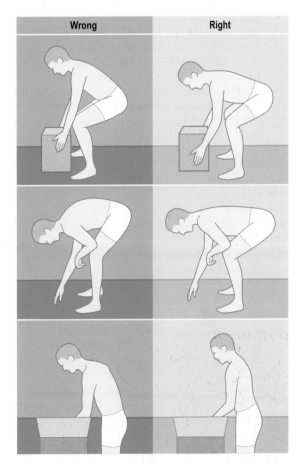

The nucleus pulposus moves posteriorly during flexion of the spine (see Fig. 2.6), so when compression of the disc is increased, as in lifting, then the forces on the posterior aspect of the annulus may cause a tear or herniation/prolapse. Lifting or bending with a slight lordosis helps to prevent this prolapse. Many diagrams show people lifting with a straight back, and knees bent, but with the lumbar lordosis reduced by a pelvic tilt. This position is difficult to hold whilst lifting. When one watches weightlifters and people bending over working in the fields, these people stand with their legs wide apart and stick their bottom out whilst maintaining a neutral back and a tense abdomen to lift.

## Training

(a) Weights – the back must be stabilized to lock into neutral, preferably extension, even when sitting. The moment this back position cannot be held, the exercise should be stopped. If the back has to be bent to aid the exercise, then the target muscles that are being trained will have fatigued sufficiently for the back muscles to be recruited in to help with the exercise. At this stage the back is liable to damage and the target muscles are no longer being trained correctly. If lumbar extension cannot be held, then the weight is too heavy, or the wrong technical position for the exercise is being used.

(b) Sit-ups – 'neutral back' abdominals should be used (Figs 2.9–2.11). Sit-ups with a twist (crunches) manipulate the spine and can cause problems.

(c) Rowing – upright rowing risks losing lumbar neutral or extension. The rowing ergo should provide the same effect if used with a hard pull, and it does not risk the back as much. On the ergo, the back should be locked into neutral or extension and the exercise performed in the mid-range to prevent overreaching or 'lying back' too far.

(d) Gymnastics – walkovers should not be done by hyperextending at L5/S1 but rather by spreading the spinal extension up and through the whole lumbar spine.

(e) Swimming – produces extension and thus is excellent for flexion-orientated problems but poor for extension-orientated problems, which tolerate backstroke better. Running in a floatation jacket may be tolerated.

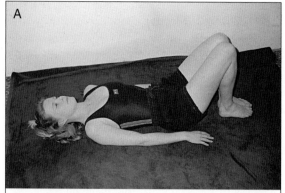

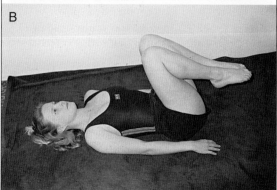

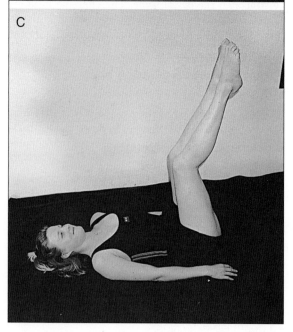

**Figure 2.9 •** Exercise for lower abdominals. **(A)** Lie supine with bent knees. **(B)** Bend the hips to flatten the back into spinal neutral. Tighten transversus abdominis and multifidus. **(C)** Straighten the knees so there is no tension on the back and then lower the legs until the back starts to extend, at which stage re-flex the hips until the back is neutral again, then hold the transversus and multifidus tight, either for a count of 7 or for as long as possible.

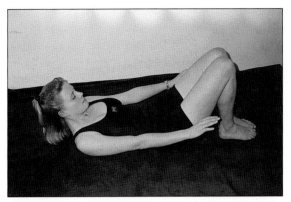

**Figure 2.10** • Exercise for the upper abdominals. Lie as for Fig. 2.9A then flex the neck and shoulders and hold.

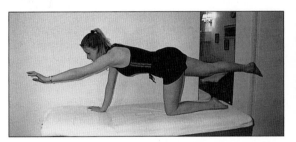

**Figure 2.11** • Super (wo)man. Hold a neutral back position, raise the opposite leg and arm but do not lose body tension. This exercise and those using the 'Swedish ball' work the pelvic and back muscle stabilizers.

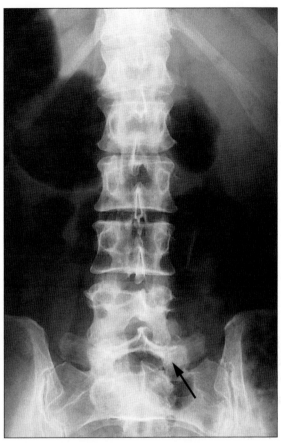

**Figure 2.12** • Hemilumbarization. The old East German regime would not accept a congenitally abnormal spine for elite training because these abnormalities produced too many problems.

(f) Cycling – is good for extension-orientated problems, but the patient needs to sit upright with raised handlebars for flexion-orientated problems. The frame may have to be lengthened.

(g) Running – should be avoided until symptoms have disappeared, as the impact compresses the disc and facet joints. On resuming exercise it is better if the runner tries to run 'tall' and 'core stabilize' the pelvis and back (see Figs 2.11, 20.11, 20.12). Figures 2.12 and 2.13 illustrate some back problems.

## Home and workplace

The back and neck cause most problems, whether sitting at a desk, bending over in the garden or during household tasks. Many of these problems can be avoided if the patient observes the following guidance:

(a) Do not wedge the telephone between the head and shoulder because this twists the neck sideways, producing facet and disc problems. The use of an earpiece or headset is recommended.

(b) Adjust the computer and chair to the correct height. If the computer terminal is set too low on the desk and the chair is too high, or if the patient wears bifocals, he or she may sit slumped with a rounded back whilst at the same time hyperextending the neck for long periods to look at the computer screen. Glasses should be adjusted to focus on the screen – 'computer glasses'.

(c) The computer screen should be about 15–30° below eye level, and the keyboard and mouse should be operated with relaxed shoulders and

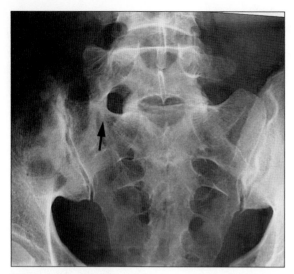

**Figure 2.13** • Hemisacralization.

bent elbows. If the screen and keyboard are positioned to one side, then the twist to use the keyboard will cause dorsal problems. Most people sit too slumped during a long day, and the lumbar and dorsal spine need to be straightened so that the head is balanced – not looking up or down and not pushed forward.

(d) Office chairs should be fully adjustable – the tilt of the seat, the lumbar curve, and the back and height – to each individual's use.

(e) A kneel-on chair, seat wedge (thinner at the front) and lumbar rolls will help pain produced by sitting with a rounded back. This is particularly so for patients whose back is eased by stretching their back into extension when standing up from sitting a while (see Posture).

(f) Lumbar supports in cars are useless, unless they adjust up and down to fit the lumbar curve of the patient in question. Car seats, despite all the adjustments available, often leave the arms too far from the steering wheel and the head against the roof. Those with back problems need to sit nearer the steering wheel, with bent arms, in order to take the tension out of the back. Many cars do not have enough headroom to 'sit tall', and a poor driving position may result in consequent back pain.

(g) In the home, sit to the front of the chair, or sideways on a sofa, resting the back against the arm and pointing one knee towards the floor;

this will tilt the pelvis and increase lordosis in a comfortable, relaxed way.

(h) No one goes out and runs for 2–3 hours without any training, yet people will go into the garden and do 2 hours of weeding and digging and then wonder why they have back problems. It is important to learn to bend with a neutral to lordotic back, buttocks out, hips and knees bent, and weight over the middle of the feet (see this chapter: Bending).

(i) Plan 5–10 minutes of bending jobs around the house and garden, and alternate with 5–10 minutes of standing and reaching jobs.

(j) Try vacuuming to the side, and slightly behind the hips.

(k) Standing half bent over a sink, ironing board, etc., is a killer for the back. Standing with legs wide apart drops the height without bending the back or straining the knees. Leaning the front of the thighs into the side of the sink enables a neutral back position to be held whilst reaching into the sink.

(l) Use the 'bottom out' position for all half bent positions, from brushing the teeth to making the bed and emptying the car boot or oven.

# References

1 BUPA Wellness musculoskeletal clinic internal audit; 2005

2 Leroux JL, Fuentes JM, Baixas P, Benezech J, Chertok P, Blotman F. Lumbar posterior marginal node (LPMN) in adults. Report of 15 cases. Spine 1992;17(12):1505–1508

3 Larado J-D, Bard M, Chretien J, Kahn MF. Lumbar posterior marginal intra osseous cartilaginous node. Skeletal Radiol 1986;15(3):201–208

4 Mottram S, Comerford M. Exercise therapy: spine. In: Hutson M, Ellis R (eds) Textbook of musculoskeletal medicine. Oxford: Oxford University Press; 2006. Ch. 4.3.12

5 STAT and PAAT. Society of Teachers of Alexander Technique and Professional Association of Alexander Teachers. www.stat.org.uk; www.paat.org.uk

6 Tucker WE, Armstrong JR. Injury in sport. London: Staples Press; 1964

7 Saal JS, Goldthwaite N, Saal JA, et al. Cellular response to lumbar disc herniation: and immunohistologic study. J Orthop Med 1990;12(3):73

8 Saal JS, Franson RC, Reynolds JB, Saal JA, White AH. Comparison of inflammatory enzyme activity in normal

lumbar discs and degenerative discs. J Orthop Med 1990;12(3):74

9 Cyriax JH, Cyriax PJ (eds). Lumbar nerve roots. In: Cyriax's illustrated manual of orthopaedic medicine, 2nd edn. Oxford: Butterworth-Heinemann; 1993. pp 236–239

10 McKenzie RA. Treat your own back, 6th edn. New Zealand: Spinal Publications; 2006

## Further reading

Cyriax JH, Cyriax PJ (eds). Cyriax's illustrated manual of orthopaedic medicine, 2nd edn. Oxford: Butterworth-Heinemann; 1993

Hutson M, Ellis R (eds). Textbook of musculoskeletal medicine. Oxford: Oxford University Press; 2006

Palastanga N, Field D, Soames R. Anatomy and human movement: structure and function. London: Heinemann Medical; 1989

Watkins R (ed.). The spine in sports. St Louis: Mosby; 1996

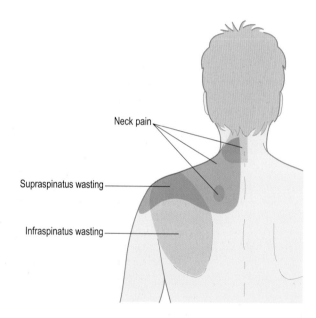

Neck pain

Supraspinatus wasting

Infraspinatus wasting

# Chapter **Three**

3

# Neck

This book is not a first aid or advanced life-saving instruction book and should be used only as a guideline – formal training is recommended for all pitch-side support staff.

 Caveat

**Vertebrobasilar insufficiency risk factors should be assessed before manipulation of the cervical spine [1].**

## Injury on the pitch

Damage to the neck may be acute, traumatic and disastrous, and all pitch-side doctors must be trained in the use of semi-rigid lock-on collars and log-roll techniques, which should be utilized for any player with a head and neck injury, who has 'pins and needles', numbness, motor weakness, or who is suspected of a neck injury. Five people must be involved with 'log-rolling' and stretchering the patient, feet first, off the pitch. The senior physician should control the head. Scoop stretchers are effective and the neck should be supported not only in a semi-rigid support to prevent flexion of the neck but also by pads (which are best attached to the stretcher) to prevent side flexion. The airway is still the primary consideration; it must be guaranteed to be clear, and then supplemental oxygen administered. A neurological assessment should be recorded and the patient removed to hospital, preferably, in the case of a severe injury, to a neurosurgical unit. It is better to be safe than sorry [2,3].

## Whiplash injuries

Perhaps, the whiplash effect can best be appreciated by considering the possible consequences to various tissues. Muscles around the neck that try and decelerate the flexion/extension moments will suffer a severe eccentric load, which may tear some of the fibres or produce delayed-onset muscle soreness (DOMS) (see Glossary). The onset of pain is not immediate but tends to come on 24–48 hours after injury and can last up to 3 months. Anti-inflammatories and Rest, Ice, Compression, Elevation (RICE) (see Glossary) will help in the first place, followed by the usual electrotherapeutic modalities to control inflammation, such as ultrasound and interferential, plus gentle stretching and exercises to regain muscle function and calm the injury.

If there is displacement of the vertebral column, the pain may present at the time of the accident and can represent facetal dysfunction. This is helped by corrective manipulation or mobilization [4]. The displacement may also affect the cervical disc, causing disc displacement, dural irritation and root compression. Wearing a cervical collar, neck traction and cervical root-blocks may be of benefit in these cases.

The intravertebral and dural suspensory ligaments may be torn, often leaving an acutely sensitive neck where all movements hurt; however, MRI scans show little wrong, probably because the scans are often taken long after the acute inflammatory phase and only in the chronic adhesive phase. This cause of pain, again, needs a more conservative approach, with rest, neck support and gradual rehabilitation, even cervical epidurals. Finally, the spinal cord may be affected, producing:

(a) a central cord syndrome – this can result in pain but also affects the bladder and bowel, temperature, and motor control in the upper limb

(b) an anterior spinal artery syndrome – in this there is immediate distal paralysis and transection of the cord with no residual distal function.

The above range of problems can all exist together, and each tissue element must be treated not only on its own merit but also as a whole, with respect to its effect on the other elements. It is this combination of injuries that makes management of whiplash a problem. Secondary protective muscle spasm is often provoked, and, if allowed to establish, produces myofascial pain, best treated with massage, needling or spray and stretch techniques. The most common long-term effects are degenerative facetal changes, which may produce pain and may also narrow the lateral canal and irritate the nerve root. Some 30% of whiplash injuries still cause pain many years later, even when their legal issues have been settled to satisfaction. Because ageing also produces facetal wear and tear, argument exists as to the long-term effects of whiplash [4–7].

## Cervical disc

### Findings

See MRI scan in Figure 3.1:

(a) Mild – an asymmetrical pattern of neck pain, with a soft end feel to the passive neck range of

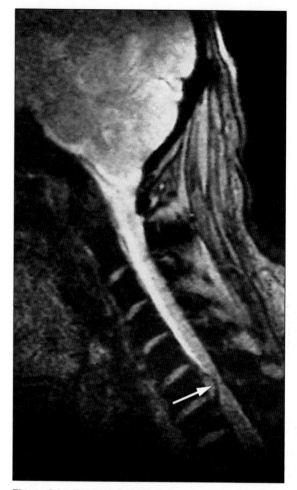

**Figure 3.1 •** T1-weighted MRI shows a cervical disc causing dural compression and a root palsy, but no cord compression. Conservative management was successful.

movement. Flexion may produce pain lower down the dorsal spine and, if root compression is present, pain to the appropriate dermatome, flared by neck movement. Brachial nerve tensioning tests and Adson's manoeuvre may be positive (see Glossary).

(b) Severe – cervical root symptoms and signs may be present; these include:

C1    (Rare, there is no disc between C1 and C2), parietal pain; weak, painful and limited neck rotation; think cancer.

C2    Occipitofrontal pain, sympathetic signs of altered facial sweating may be present; think facet joint or cancer.

C3    Numb cheek; rarely, weaker scapular elevation but disc prolapse is rare.

C4    Numb point of the shoulder, trapezial and anterior chest pain and hyperaesthesia. A weak scapular elevation is uncommon.

C5    Altered sensation over the lateral deltoid. Weak deltoid, supraspinatus, biceps and infraspinatus. Biceps and brachioradialis jerk are diminished.

C6    Altered sensation over the shoulder to the lateral forearm and thumb. Weak extensor carpi radialis; brachialis, biceps, subscapularis and pronation may be weaker and biceps jerk is diminished.

C7    Altered sensation in the fingers. Weak latissimus dorsi, triceps, common flexors of wrist, and triceps jerk diminished.

C8/T1 Altered sensation, radiating to the ulnar aspect of the arm, in the fourth and fifth digits. Weak intrinsic muscles of the hand [8,9].

(c)  Cord compression shows symptoms and signs in the back and the leg that do not seem to fit with the appropriate lumbar or dorsal back examination. Lhermitte's sign (Fig. 3.2) and Valsalva may be positive (see Glossary).

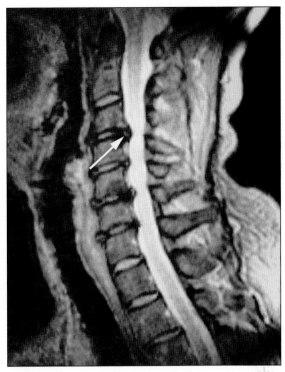

**Figure 3.2 •** Lhermitte's sign was positive, suggesting cord compression, and surgery was required.

## Cause

The cervical disc may be prolapsed or herniated or, less commonly, suffer an annular tear.

## Investigations

X-ray shows chronic disc space narrowing, whereas MRI and CT will display the disc lesion and its cervical level, whilst excluding other intraspinal causes. MRI alone displays the annular tear.

## Treatment

(a) Mild – mobilization techniques, such as Maitland's manipulation, Mulligan's 'nags and snags', and traction to the neck. Avoid a 'head-hanging' posture into flexion whilst working at a desk, or whilst lying in bed reading with the head flexed forward on the chest. Specially designed neck pillows may help, but often switching between two ordinary pillows whilst lying on the side and one pillow when lying prone or supine, may be adequate, as may tying a cord around the pillow to form a butterfly wing shape, which supports the neck from side flexions.

(b) With root signs – support the neck and limit the range of movement with a cervical collar. Try traction (this may be too painful). Most of these disc lesions tend to settle by themselves over 6–12 weeks and the pain can be eased by avoiding neural tensioning caused by neck movement in specific directions and by stretching the arms up or outwards, which pulls on the neurovascular structures that are inflamed. A paravertebral or X-ray controlled root-block, and if needed a cervical epidural, will settle inflammation and ease pain. Sometimes, trigger-point injection or acupuncture will help the presumed myofascial element of the pain caused by muscle spasm. Failure to progress may require surgical decompression of the disc.

(c) Cord compression with signs and symptoms spreading towards the legs requires surgical decompression.

## Sports

Cervical discs should not be twisted or stressed. Even axial compression and impaction from running is painful so that, most times, the pain will not let the patient play games. Once reduced and stable, running may be commenced and neck movements progressed to extensions, such as a serve at tennis and badminton; however, rugby scrums and impact sport should be avoided for 6–9 months or until the neck is totally symptomless.

## Comment

Thank goodness most cure themselves over time. Most treatments are directed to controlling the pain whilst the disc settles, usually over 6–12 weeks. Paravertebral root-blocks, which can be administered in the clinic, or X-ray controlled root-blocks can make a dramatic improvement, reducing pain whilst the disc lesion regresses.

## Cervical facet joint

### Findings

The problems present with an acute onset of neck pain, 'cricked neck', or pain of a more insidious onset, and the patient may have persistent discomfort. Examination shows an asymmetrical pattern of movement of the neck, with a hard end feel to passive neck range. Only with root entrapment at the lateral canal will the facet joints produce root symptoms, which are flared by movement, and then Adson's manoeuvre will be positive (see Glossary). Disc lesions may also be present and will complicate the findings.

### Cause

Either mechanical dysfunction between the vertebral segments or degenerative arthritis of the facet joints.

### Investigations

X-ray with 'oblique views' will display the lateral canal and any encroaching osteophytes, but MRI and/or CT scan are better investigations if a disc or other problems are also suspected. However, these investigations are probably not required clinically unless the patient is failing to make progress with treatment.

## Treatment

### Acute or root signs

(a) Ease inflammation and pain with a root-block or perifacetal cortisone. Electrotherapeutic modalities and non-steroidal anti-inflammatory drugs (NSAIDs) may help.

(b) Rest in a cervical collar if required, then mobilization and manipulation when the acute inflammation has settled.

### Chronic

(a) Postural correction – neck extension will narrow the lateral canal and load the face joints; therefore the head must be held straight on the neck. When the dorsal spine is slumped in flexion the neck is angulated into extension to allow the eyes to focus straight ahead. Looking at computer screens through bifocal spectacles, which 'near focus' at the lowest margin of the lens, increases this neck extension, so special glasses focused for the computer distance are advisable. Patients should correct their sitting posture by reforming their lumbar lordosis, reducing their dorsal kyphosis, and holding their head straighter on the neck. Holding a telephone between the ear and shoulder almost manipulates the normal neck and produces facetal problems. Headsets or earpieces are recommended.

(b) Manipulation of the neck – many chronic neck pains are eased by mobilizing the neck and treating any accompanying muscle spasm.

(c) Perifacetal injection or X-ray controlled facet injections.

(d) Rarely, surgical foramenotomy to the lateral canal will be required, if the root involvement fails to settle or the root damage is progressing.

---

### Caveat

Congenital abnormalities (e.g. hemivertebrae) often present in the child and adolescent, as may osteoid osteoma or secondary tumours (secondaries). Spinal lesions, such as syringomyelia, are often pain-free but have neurological signs which can be multiradicular.

## Sports

(a) In ball games the head is held still to focus the eyes on the ball whilst the body continues to move. The neck provides this coordinating link between eyes and body which is so vital that neck pain invariably interferes with performance. During the acute phase, sport is best avoided.

(b) The limited range of movement with chronic facetal osteoarthritis will provoke a change in technique, especially such as that required during the golf swing when a less full swing will have to be adopted, and in overhead sports.

(c) Tennis serving will have to be flatter, and badminton may prove impossible.

(d) Most difficult are contact sports, where there is a risk of more permanent damage, and the safe advice is to avoid the sport until better.

(e) Breathing during freestyle swimming with a flexed and then rotated neck can produce facetal problems. Indeed breaststroke with the head held out of the water can flare the lateral canal symptoms, producing pins and needles.

## Comment

Overall, one must be safe and the best advice is to avoid contact sport until better. CT scans help to assess long-term problems of facet joints much better than X-ray or MRI. Manipulation of the correct cases is the treatment of choice. Facetal injection of cortisone can be very effective.

## Stingers and burners [8,10]

The burner or stinger phenomenon is a transient neurological event characterized by pain and paraesthesia in the upper limb.

## Findings

Tingling, burning, or numbing sensations in a circumferential rather than a dermatome distribution.

Type 1   Bilateral arm pain and temporary quadriparesis = cervical stenosis.

Type 2   Pain lasting for at least 15 minutes, with dense paraesthesia (dead arm) = traction on the brachial plexus has occurred.

Type 3   Discrete transient root pain and traumatic motor weakness is shown by transient loss of function, with searing, lancinating pain

coursing down the arm. Paralysis is temporary, lasting 10–15 minutes. Often C6 numbness in the lateral three fingers can persist. Weakness of shoulder abduction and wrist extensors can be detected and brachial nerve tensioning tests are positive = nerve root irritation.

## Cause

Type 1   Axial loading of the neck.

Type 2   Lateral neck flexion away from, and shoulder depression on the side of, the pain.

Type 3   Hyperextension and rotation. Most commonly caused by a combination of extension and lateral flexion, compressing the lateral canal on the ipsilateral side, whilst causing traction of the roots on the contralateral side [8,10].

## Investigations

CT, MRI and electromyogram (EMG). The Torg ratio may be calculated to assess the possibility of further injury (see Glossary).

## Treatment

(a) Postural control, and neck strengthening.

(b) Electrotherapeutic modalities for inflammation and pain.

(c) Facetal or root block injections of cortisone.

(d) Surgery for the disc or facetal laminotomy.

## Sports

For American football, modify the shoulder pads so they are combined with a neck roll. Advise patients with a cervical stenosis (after analysis of spinal canal size) that they may be better changing sport [10].

## Comment

Although rugby and wrestling occasionally have this injury, it seems much more prone to occur in American football, possibly because of the head-on tackle, even though 'spiking' is banned.

## Ligamentous neck pain

### Findings

A full range of neck movements or symmetrical limited range of neck movements, which may be painful in full flexion and extension. There is tenderness to palpation over C7/T1 and/or the nuchal crest.

The patient invariably has functional or a true dorsal kyphosis and sits over a desk for long periods. There may be protraction of the head.

## Cause

Overload of the neck ligaments – usually at C7/T1, occasionally at the nuchal crest, from constant neck flexion, the 'head-hanger's' neck, or as part of the whiplash complex (see Whiplash injuries).

## Investigations

None are clinically required, apart from eliminating other causes.

## Treatment

(a) Correct the posture, first and foremost retraining a lumbar lordosis and reducing the dorsal kyphosis. Whilst sitting, back posture can be improved by raising the desk and lowering the chair. Sitting on a wedge seat, kneel-on style chair, or just dropping a knee towards the floor, will increase a lumbar lordosis, straighten the dorsal kyphosis and allow the neck to be held in a neutral position.

(b) Retraction exercises of the neck.

(c) Electrotherapeutic modalities to calm inflammation and ease pain.

(d) Muscle balance training.

(e) Sclerosant injections of the ligaments (see Glossary).

## Sports

Activity helps these people, as the muscles take over the major support of the head from the ligaments.

## Comment

Correction of posture should cure 95% of these patients.

# Myofascial pain

## Findings

There are likely to be signs and symptoms of the underlying cause (see below). The neck range may be full or symmetrically limited and/or painful, with a soft painful end feel as muscle spasm is induced, preventing a full range of movement. There are tender trigger points, usually over the trapezius and rhomboids. These can produce radiating pain to the arms and localized muscle spasm may be palpated.

## Cause

The muscle is held in constant tension, even when at rest. This may be post-traumatic or have become a habit to protect an underlying problem, such as a painful facet joint, disc or shoulder. It may, however, reflect psychological tension. The muscle spindle controls gamma efferent tone but whether the spindle itself is the trigger point is debatable.

## Investigations

Explore psychological causes if indicated. Physical investigations will only help diagnose the underlying causes and there do not seem to be markers that diagnose this problem.

## Treatment

(a) Explain muscle spasm, and how and why agonist and antagonist muscles can work even at rest. Explain that a limb may not move because no muscle is working, but equally may not move because the hard work of one muscle is being cancelled out by that of another. Therefore, when the muscles work against each other they produce constant tension, such that the muscle may even appear to be fatigued doing nothing.

(b) Physiotherapy to rebalance muscle tension [11].

(c) Treat any underlying mechanical cause.

(d) Electrotherapeutic modalities to calm inflammation; NSAIDs.

(e) Spray and stretch [12].

(f) Dry needling [13], acupressure or ultrasound to the trigger spot. Wet needling with an injection of steroid or local anaesthetic to the trigger points.

(g) Hydrotherapy to encourage muscle exercises.

## Sports

Most patients will not do any activity; however, exercise should be encouraged on a 'little and often' basis, with the explanation that muscles will ache when first trained but that this is a good thing (see Chapter 20).

NSAIDs may help at this time. Use hydrotherapy to encourage muscle work but reduce muscle load.

## Comment

Probably this area is less well understood and the underlying mental fear or psychological problems must be handled at the same time. A primary injury, such as to a shoulder, can be followed by a secondary problem, e.g. hunching and contracting the trapezius to protect from shoulder pain. This secondary cause can create further pain that may indeed be the presenting symptom. The principle of a primary and a secondary problem must be appreciated. Treat the primary cause and follow rapidly with treatment to the secondary cause, which is the habituated muscle spasm.

# Cervical rib

## Findings

The history can be confusing. It will contain elements of pain and, particularly, sensory neurological symptoms of pins and needles and numbness that can radiate to the hand. As symptoms become worse, motor symptoms of weakness appear, particularly at C8/T1, with weakness in the intrinsic muscles of the hand. However, weak forearm flexors may also be evident from the C7 involvement. These signs and symptoms are often intermittent or variable within the same patient, depending upon the amount of constriction the cervical rib is causing on the cervical plexus. They may be uni- or bilateral. The rib can sometimes be palpated. Roos' abduction and external rotation test is positive (see Glossary). Ipsilateral neck rotation followed by ipsilateral neck flexion may be limited with a hard end feel, bony block, which indicates a positive test. Adson's test may be positive (see Glossary) [14].

## Cause

A ligamentous band or bony projection deepens the thoracic outlet so that the exiting C8/T1 contribution to the cervical plexus is stretched up and over this band.

## Investigations

X-ray may show the bony rib at C7 and MRI can, though not always, display the ligamentous band. EMG may be helpful.

## Treatment

Postural control to elevate the pectoral girdle should relieve the traction on the nerve. Occasionally, surgery is required to release the ligamentous band.

## Sports

Unfortunately, almost all sports that involve arm movement will cause problems, and many work situations can also produce problems, particularly if poor posture is involved.

## Comment

This can be a difficult problem to diagnose accurately, and certainly to treat. Fortunately it is not a common condition.

# References

1 Barker S, Kesson M, Ashmore J, Turner G, Conway J, Stevens D. Guidance for pre-manipulative testing of the cervical spine for vertebrobasilar insufficiency. J Orthop Med 2000;22(1):24–27

2 National Health and Medical Research Council. Head and neck injuries in football. Canberra: Australian Government Publishing Service; 1995

3 Ryan AJ. Protecting the sportsman's brain (concussion in sport). Br J Sports Med 1991;25:81–86

4 Pickin M. A discussion of whip lash injury to the cervical spine. J Orthop Med 1995;17(1):15–23

5 Khan S, Cook J, Gargan M, Bannister G. A symptomatic classification of whiplash injury and the implications for treatment. J Orthop Med 1999;21(1):22–25

6 Gargan MF, Bannister GC. The long term prognosis of soft tissue injuries to the neck. J Bone Joint Surg 1990;72B:901–903

7 Gargan MF, Bannister GC. The comparative effects of whiplash injuries. J Orthop Med 1997;19(1):15–17

8 Watkins R (ed.) The spine in sports. St Louis: Mosby; 1996

9 Cyriax JH, Cyriax J (eds). Cyriax's illustrated manual of orthopaedic medicine, 2nd edn. Oxford: Butterworth-Heinemann; 1993

10 Castro FP Jr, Ricciardi J, Brunet ME, Busch MT, Whitecloud TS III. Stingers, the Torg ratio, and the cervical spine. Am J Sports Med 1997;25:603–608

11 Mottram S, Comerford M. Exercise therapy: spine. In: Hutson M, Ellis R (eds) Textbook of musculoskeletal medicine. Oxford: Oxford University Press; 2006. Ch. 4.3.12

12 Travell J, Simons DG. Myofascial pain and dysfunction. The trigger point manual. Baltimore: Williams and Wilkins; 1983

13 Chan Gunn C. Soft tissue pain-treatment with stimulation-produced analgesia. In: Hutson M, Ellis R (eds) Textbook of musculoskeletal medicine. Oxford: Oxford University Press; 2006. Ch 4.3.9

14 Tanner J. Pectoral girdle. In: Hutson M, Ellis R (eds) Textbook of musculoskeletal medicine. Oxford: Oxford University Press; 2006. Ch 3

## Further reading

Bruckner P, Khan K. Clinical sports medicine, 3rd edn. New York: McGraw-Hill; 2006

Hutson M, Ellis R (eds). Textbook of musculoskeletal medicine. Oxford: Oxford University Press; 2006

Reid D. Sports injury assessment and rehabilitation. Edinburgh: Churchill Livingstone; 1992

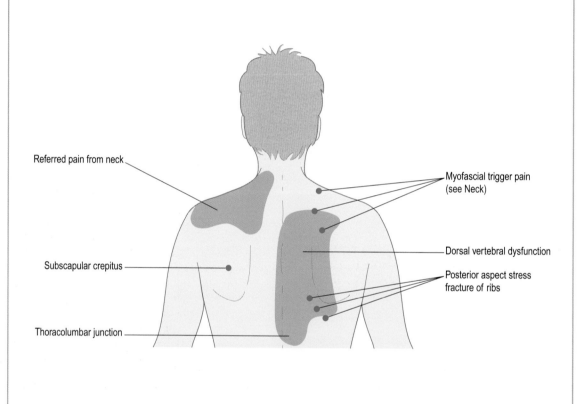

Referred pain from neck

Myofascial trigger pain
(see Neck)

Dorsal vertebral dysfunction

Subscapular crepitus

Posterior aspect stress
fracture of ribs

Thoracolumbar junction

# Chapter Four

4

# Dorsal spine

## Pain referred from the neck

The thoracic spine provides lateral flexion and rotation, but limited flexion. Overload or trauma within these positions may cause dorsal spinal dysfunction. It is unusual for a disc displacement to occur in this area, though not impossible.

### Caveat

All examinations of the dorsal spine must start with an examination of the movements of the cervical spine, and the cervical spine should be considered as the most likely cause if these tests produce discomfort or pain in the dorsal spine (see Chapter 2).

## Dorsal vertebral dysfunction

### Findings

The onset may be acute or chronic. Pain may be felt centrally, but it is usually to one side of the spine and may radiate to the anterior chest wall. Lateral or anterior chest pain without spinal pain may occur. The lower dorsal vertebrae may refer symptoms, T9 towards the abdomen and umbilicus and the thoracolumbar junction to the groin, via the ilio-inguinal nerve. Symptoms are often worse when lying down and better when sitting or standing, so the patient may sleep in a chair rather than in bed. Twisting to one side hurts. Breathing, coughing and sneezing may hurt. The pain is worse with movement. The higher vertebrae may refer pain to the arm or shoulder. (During clinical practice one notices referred pain towards the arm from the dorsal spine, even down at the T8 level. This may appear during palpation or injection of the facet joint and one should not reject these histories, but realize that referred pain from this area is still poorly understood.) Neck flexion may produce dorsal pain, but whether this represents classical referred pain, thoracic dural irritation, thoracic facet joint flexion or thoracic ligamentous stress is not clear. Rotation of the dorsal spine is worse to one side than the other. Dorsal spinal rotation should be tested while the patient is sitting on the couch, thus limiting pelvic rotation and enabling mainly dorsal rotation to be tested. Standing and stretching forward to touch the floor outside the opposite foot with the contralateral hand may be painful, and there may be local tenderness to palpation over the spine, facet joints or costovertebral joints. A similar test may be performed with the patient sitting and rotating to one side. The contralateral arm is pulled down and across the body; when the tender structures are felt to tighten, breathing out and stretching may exacerbate the pain. However this stretch can be used therapeutically after a local injection [1].

## Cause

The most common cause is from the facet joints, and possibly from the costovertebral joints, but dorsal discs do occur and degenerative disc disease is found quite frequently. This might well be the effect of chronic low-grade trauma from extension and twisting manoeuvres. Ligamentous pain, particularly from the interspinous ligaments, is common. The major areas that suffer interspinous ligament strain appear to be from T3/4 to T7/8 [1]. Many problems are due to too great a dorsal kyphosis, which may be postural or secondary to underlying bony deformity.

## Investigation

It is important to have considered, and if necessary excluded, the potentially serious differentials, especially cardiac and intrathoracic conditions and bone tumours. Most commonly, X-ray findings show a bony kyphotic spine, sometimes with long-standing wedging, and anterior osteophytes of no clinical significance, apart from reflecting dorsal discal degeneration. Schmorl's nodes reflect discal herniation into the body of the vertebrae and are probably of no clinical significance. Anterior wedge collapse reflects old Scheuermann's (see Fig. 2.2), osteoporosis, tuberculosis or secondary tumours, with a crush fracture. Tumours, cysts, syringomyelia and demyelinating causes are well displayed with MRI.

## Treatment

(a) As the most common cause is mechanical dysfunction, the symptoms respond to manipulation. This may have to be repeated frequently until the pain suddenly clears.

(b) Injection of cortisone to the facet joints.

(c) Mobilization and/or injection of the costovertebral joints under screening.

(d) Sclerosant injections (see Glossary) of supraspinous ligaments and facet joints [1,2].

(e) Posture (see Chapter 2).

(f) Extension exercises to the dorsal spine, and avoiding flexion and rotation.

(g) Self-manipulation by lying supine with the painful segment on a fist, handkerchief or tennis ball, and by using purpose-built dorsal spinal racks.

(h) A pillow placed in front of the chest whilst sidelying may limit the dorsal rotation that occurs when asleep and thus the stresses across the facet joints.

(i) Rarely, surgery to a disc.

## Sports

Dorsal facetal or costovertebral problems can occur outside sport and interfere with performance. However, sports with flexion and rotation, such as rowing, squash and golf, in addition to contact sports, can produce facetal dysfunction. High dorsal pain (T2/3) in a golfer is often caused by standing too close to the ball at the address position.

Gymnasts are reported to have a high instance of degenerative change in their discs at the thoracolumbar junction, but, when reviewing the literature, most information is presented as case reports [3].

## Comment

Manipulation helps most dorsal problems, which appear to be mainly facetal. The patient's relatives can be taught how to perform a straight lift and extension mobilization of the dorsal spine. Facetal hydrocortisone and sclerosants/prolotherapy will often settle the chronic cases. Dorsal cord lesions may have few signs or symptoms in the dorsal spine but may cause apparent lumbar problems, and undiagnosed leg pain requires investigation of the higher levels of the spinal cord, including the dorsal spine.

# Scheuermann's epiphysitis
## (see Chapter 2, Part 1: Cartilage end plate)

This occurs in teenagers and presents with a painful dorsal spine, which may have no mechanical signs (see Glossary.) Less commonly, Scheuermann's may present in the upper lumbar spine.

## Cause

A disturbance in the growth plates of the vertebrae, and herniation of the disc into the vertebral body. Scheuermann's is more common in the dorsal spine than in the lumbar spine.

## Treatment

Analgesics and NSAIDs may be given but education in core stability techniques, for both general day-to-day activities and sport, is essential. The symptoms are often quite refractive to treatment until the spine has fully developed (see Fig. 2.2). Correct, stabilized posture and relative rest help but a spinal brace may be required to maintain correct posture during growth.

## Sport

Sports are limited by pain, and training should concentrate on skills that do not flare the problem. Emphasis should be made to the patient and coach that these skills are trained and performed with core-stabilizing techniques. Contact sports should probably be avoided. It has not been established whether sports are a cause or effect of Scheuermann's.

## Comment

This is often quite refractive to treatment until the spine is fully developed.

## Costovertebral joint

The upper ribs move in a bucket handle plane whilst the lower ribs move in a pump handle plane, and mobilization techniques should utilize this variance. Whether the examination techniques can accurately differentiate this diagnosis from facetal pain is of some doubt (see dorsal vertebral dysfunction). Mobilization of the dorsal spine is effective in rowers and butterfly swimmers [4], and rowers should have a full kinetic chain evaluation from legs, pelvis and lumbar spine when they present with dorsal spinal pain [5].

## Myofascial pain

Myofascial pain has a local trigger point which may be eased with continued acupressure from the fingers, dry or wet needling [6], and spray and stretch techniques [7] (see Glossary: Myofascial pain).

## Fractured rib – traumatic or stress

A positive rib spring test raises the possibility of a rib fracture (Fig. 4.1) (see Chapter 6).

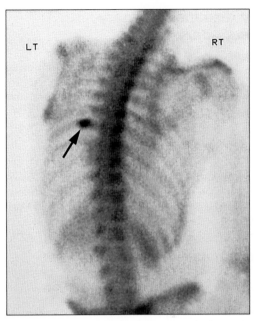

**Figure 4.1** • A bone scan shows an unusual posterior stress fracture of the ribs in a golfer. The more common site of presentation is at the mid- to anterior axillary line (see Fig. 6.1).

## Subscapular crepitus

Elicitation of this sign, by compression and rotation of the scapula on the chest wall, indicates rubbing between the scapula and thoracic wall (see Chapter 17).

## Costosternal joint/Tietze disease

Dorsal referred pain may radiate to the sternum, but localized tenderness or swelling over the costosternal joints is suggestive that this is the cause of the pain. Tietze disease is usually from rheumatoid or other inflammatory diseases. It is not always easy to determine whether the back or the chest is the source of the problem when the patient is lying down for the examination, as pressure on the sternum may cause the couch to irritate the spine, and pressure on the dorsal spine may irritate the costosternal joints, as the patient lies prone. To prevent this effect, the tests are best performed with the patient sitting (see Chapter 6: Costochondral cartilage pain/Tieze disease).

# Bony disease – primary or secondary

Constant pain, not worse with movement and often with atypical findings, suggests bony disease. A fracture may be worse with minimal movement. If in doubt, investigate further (see Fig. 2.7).

# Intrathoracic problems

If pain occurs with breathing, swallowing and on exertion rather than with movement, then consider intrathoracic problems such as pleural, myocardial, reflux oesophageal or mediastinal as a cause.

# References

1  Broadhurst NA, Wilk VJ. Vertebral mid line pain; pain arising from the interspinous spaces. J Orthop Med 1996;18(1):2–4

2  Cyriax JH, Cyriax PJ. The thoracic spine: sclerosants. In: Cyriax's illustrated manual of orthopaedic medicine. Oxford: Butterworth-Heinemann; 1993. pp. 195–196

4  Thomas PL. Thoracic back pain in rowers and butterfly swimmers: costovertebral subluxation. Br J Sports Med 1998;22(2):81

5  Davis BA, Flintoff JT. Diagnosis and management of thoracic and rib pain in rowers. Curr Sports Med Reports 2003;2:281–287

6  Chan Gunn C. Soft tissue pain-treatment with stimulation-produced analgesia. In: Hutson M, Ellis R (eds) Textbook of musculoskeletal medicine. Oxford: Oxford University Press; 2006. Ch 4.3.9

7  Travell J, Simons DG. Myofascial pain and dysfunction. The trigger point manual. Baltimore: Williams and Wilkins; 1983

# Further reading

Bruckner P, Khan K. Clinical sports medicine, 3rd edn. New York: McGraw-Hill; 2006

Cyriax JH, Cyriax PJ. Cyriax's illustrated manual of orthopaedic medicine. Oxford: Butterworth-Heinemann; 1993

Hutson MA (ed.). Sports injuries: recognition and management, 2nd edn. Oxford: Oxford Medical Publications; 1996

Hutson M, Ellis R (eds) Textbook of musculoskeletal medicine. Oxford: Oxford University Press; 2006

Keson M, Atkins E. The thoracic spine in sport. J Orthop Med 1999;21(3):80–85

Reid D. Sports injury assessment and rehabilitation. Edinburgh: Churchill Livingstone; 1992

Watkins RG (ed.). The spine in sports. St Louis: Mosby; 1996

# Chapter Five

# Lumbar spine

## Part 1 **Flexion-orientated lesions**

## Prolapsed or herniated disc

### Findings

The typical history involves a period of slouching, straining, lifting or pushing, with the back in a flexed position, followed by the slow onset of pain, coming on over a few hours, or sometimes overnight. Standing, flexion and side flexion are painful, and there may be a catch or deviation of the spine, when returning from flexion to neutral. Some backs may be deviated sideways. Straight leg raise, Lasègue's and slump test may be positive (see Glossary).

Motor signs in the leg indicate a nerve palsy from nerve root damage (see Chapter 2: Lumbar spine nerve root signs, p. 15) [1].

### Cause

The nucleus pulposus is squeezed in a posterior direction by flexion of the spine (see Fig. 2.6). When this happens gradually it is known as 'disc creep'. Typically, flexion will cause the disc to move posteriorly towards the spinal canal where it will cause pain from the nerves in the annulus and posterior longitudinal ligament or it will impinge on the dura itself, causing intense pain. If the prolapse extends further then it will compress the nerve root causing sciatica, which consists of, or has elements of, radiation of pain to the appropriate dermatome, 'pins and needles', numbness, fasciculations and muscle weakness (root palsy) (Fig. 5.1).

## Investigations

Clinically, these are not required if the signs are sufficient to make an accurate diagnosis. If there is no progress with therapy then MRI or CT scans will establish whether a sequestrum is present (Fig. 5.2), the level of the disc involved, and exclude other intraspinal pathology. If these investigations are not diagnostic then a surgical disc probe may be required. Under narcoleptic anaesthesia the discs, facet joints or sacro-iliac joints under consideration are injected to discover which reproduces the patient's concomitant pain.

## Treatment

(a) Rest in the acute phase may be required, though mobility should be encouraged as soon as possible.

(b) Posture to maintain extension.

(c) McKenzie extension exercises (see Glossary).

(d) Traction [2]. Traction has gone out of vogue, but one can try manual traction whilst examining the patient and, if this improves the symptoms, then traction will be of benefit. This can be manual, mechanical or postural. Postural traction may be increased by suspension couches, which hold the patient by the feet and then invert them to differing degrees. The patient can then use these couches at home when the disc creep is troublesome, which is often at the end of the day.

(e) Epidural [3].

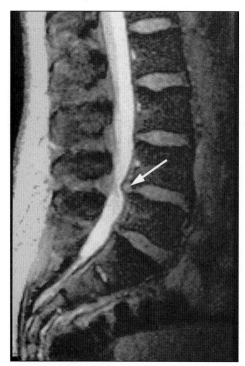

**Figure 5.1** • T1-weighted MRI showing a prolapsed lumbar disc impinging on the dura.

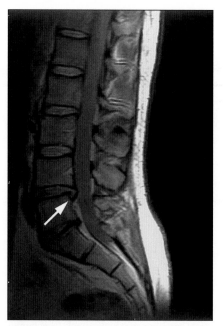

**Figure 5.2** • T1-weighted MRI shows a lumbar disc prolapse that has extended along the posterior aspect of the vertebral body as a sequestrum, which is unlikely to reduce with conservative measures and will probably require surgery.

**(f)** Adverse neural tensioning techniques (at the stage when the disc is still prolapsed, adverse neural tension exercises will increase the pain).

**(g)** Surgery – discectomy.

### Caveat

**Many so-called lumbar rolls, built into seats, are placed too low and push the pelvis forwards, thus increasing flexion of the spine. McKenzie's flexion exercises and flexion manipulations may make this type of disc worse (see Glossary).**

## Sports

Avoid all sports during a painful flare of a disc herniation, but see Annular disc or 'disc creep', Sports, below, for hints on how to avoid aggravating the injury when improvement has started.

# Annular disc or 'disc creep'

## Findings

The creeping disc, which some may call the annular disc, will often be the cause of lumbar pain and is brought on by sitting. Typically, the patient gets up from a seat with backache, is slightly stuck in flexion but manages, with extension exercises, to straighten up his or her back and reduce the pain, often entirely, and then walks away with no problems. Examination may reveal no diagnostic signs apart from a minor backache on flexion. Often the posture has a flat, straight spine and the patient sits slumped into a lumbar kyphosis (see Fig. 5.1).

## Cause

Movement of the nucleus pulposus posteriorly will stretch the annulus (see Prolapsed or herniated disc). However, note that the creeping disc usually does not impinge on the dura or nerve root.

## Investigations

None are clinically required, but see Prolapsed or herniated disc, above, if the lesion progresses.

## Treatment

Postural control to avoid spinal flexion, core stability training and extension exercises (see Chapter 2, Part 2: Posture).

## Sports

**(a)** After a hard game the ligaments are warm and more pliable, so the player should sit in the changing room with the lumbar spine in extension rather than slump exhausted with a flat or kyphotic lumbar spine. Increasing extension by sitting with one foot drawn under the bench, or with the knee pointing to the ground, should help.

**(b)** Cycling – if the back is troublesome then a posture that produces more lumbar lordosis must be utilized and this can be achieved by lengthening the bike frame, raising the handle bars and using tribars or a handle bar extension to lengthen the 'seat to hand' distance.

**(c)** Weightlifting – lifting weights will naturally increase intra-abdominal pressure, which must be contained by core stability techniques and a neutral back, with some lumbar lordosis (see Chapter 2, Part 1: Function of the vertebral column). As soon as the trunk and back are 'thrown in' to help produce the required strength, then lumbar stability has been lost and the exercise must stop. The specific muscles being trained are fatiguing and other muscles are being used to help out, invariably flexing the spine and straining the disc.

**(d)** Sailing – it is easy to sit slumped in a dinghy or boat, but postural lordosis should be maintained; here, a knee dropped towards the floor will be very helpful. Lumbar extension matched by core stability must be employed whilst lifting the anchor, winding the winch and pulling on the sheets.

**(e)** Windsurfing – many beginners, being unaware of the technique required to resist the force of the sail, are pulled into flexion, and this is exacerbated when trying to pull the sail up from the water. Experienced windsurfers, who use a harness and are capable of a 'deep water start', usually do have the correct technique, which involves flexing the knees and hips and stabilizing the extended spine.

**(f)** Golf – the golfer should stand with the upper body more upright, the arms held closer to the body and hips and knees flexed, as if sitting on a shooting stick. Whilst teeing up or picking the ball out of the hole, lumbar extension can be maintained by bending over one knee and resting the elbow on this knee for support, with the contralateral leg extended behind. Pulling the trolley with the palm of the hand facing downwards causes the back to twist, so the hand should be held palm up and close to the buttocks; thus allowing a normal neutral back posture to be maintained.

(g) Hockey – tackling and stopping techniques on Astroturf require the hand holding the stick to be held close to the ground, and dribbling to be in a crouched position. Players should be taught how to perform these techniques with flexed knees and hips, and emphasizing lumbar lordosis or lumbar neutral.

(h) Rowing – over-reaching produces a flexed lumbar spine, and, if the 'catch' is taken up in this position, then the disc will be stressed. A core-stabilized, lordotic posture will reduce the likelihood of back problems. Free weight training with the 'upright row' risks overloading the flexed back.

## Annular tear

### Findings

There is a history of lumbar pain, of varying intensity, which may have followed either a slow or acute-onset back injury. Though the pain is exacerbated by some movements, it has a somewhat undiagnostic variability in its pattern. Whilst signs of dural irritation may be present, sometimes the only sign is a 'swing round' effect of the spine during standing flexion or return from flexion. The problems seem resistant to treatment, rather dribbling on over time, or being exacerbated by certain activities.

### Cause

There is a tear in the annulus. Many discs can be seen on MRI scans to be herniated, although they are not causing the patient any pain; therefore it is thought that to produce discal pain there needs to be both a mechanical and a chemical element. Possibly, this annular tear is deformed by mechanical movement, but also keeps on producing chemical irritants [4] and so seems to persist over time.

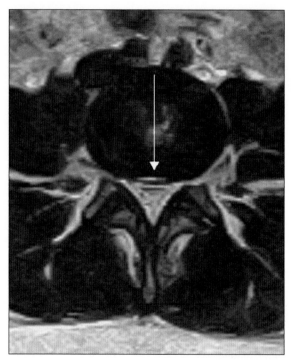

**Figure 5.3** • The annular tear can be seen on T2 or STIR-weighted images.

### Investigation

Only MRI shows up this lesion, on T2 and short tau inversion recovery (STIR) sequences – it appears as a bright signal at the very posterior edge of the disc (Fig. 5.3).

### Treatment

This disc does not respond to manipulation, and not usually to traction. Its response to an epidural is to have some relief, but no cure. Core stability training is essential to protect the annular tear from continuous overloading and, hopefully, allow it time to heal. However, this is a disc that may require intradiscal injection or ablation, with laser or radio-frequency treatment. Surgical ablation or a prosthetic disc replacement may sometimes be the only answer if problems are intolerable.

## Dural and nerve root adhesions

### Findings

The neurovascular bundle, and in particular the nerve roots, must be able to move, to adapt to the change in length produced by flexing or extending the limb. Adhesions from previous discal herniation or surgery will prevent the free movement of the nerve or dural tissue. This pull on the nerve produces pain, and the pain is exacerbated by bending or sitting, especially with straight legs, such as when lying in a bath or in bed. The pain will often wake the patient from sleep. Because the nerve is trapped, 'pins and needles', altered sensation, hyperaesthesia and continual pain may be presenting symptoms. If the dura is prevented from moving by the adhesions, then neck flexion, or even raising the arms, may produce back symptoms. Some history of trauma, or disc pathology, preceding the current problems will therefore also exist, and signs and symptoms from the primary cause may co-exist (see above, Prolapsed or herniated disc).

## Cause

Scar tissue is formed following inflammation within the spine, most commonly following a disc lesion, surgery or infection. A vital principle to be understood is that the dura, spinal cord and nerves must be able to move freely to accommodate the changes in body and limb position. This is most easily understood by appreciating that the shortest distance between two points is a straight line. So, when standing with an absolutely straight back, the distance from the top of the brain to the tip of the filum terminale will be shorter than when bending the head forward towards the knees. The neurovascular tissues, and in this case the dura, must be able to alter position to accommodate these changes. Equally, the sciatic nerve is stretched more by hip flexion combined with a straight knee and a dorsiflexed foot than when both the hip and knee are flexed and the foot plantarflexed. The restriction of dural or nerve movement, and the traction applied to them in overstretched positions, forms the basic principle behind dural stress tests, such as the straight leg raise and the Lasègue's, slump, and femoral stretch tests (see Glossary).

## Investigations

MRI scan, plus gadolinium, to differentiate fibrous scar tissue from the disc (Figs 5.4 and 5.5).

## Treatment

(a) Adverse neural tensioning (see Glossary).
(b) Epidural injections [3,5]
(c) Epiduroscopy [5]

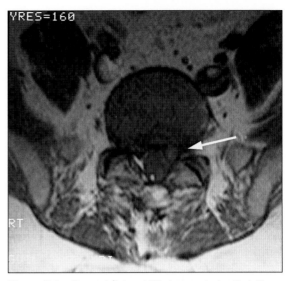

**Figure 5.4** • Pre-gadolinium MRI shows a lesion that fills the spinal canal (*arrow*).

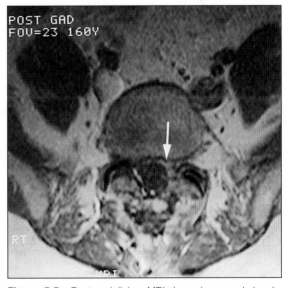

**Figure 5.5** • Post-gadolinium MRI shows increased signal within this lesion, suggesting fibrous scar tissue rather than a disc problem.

## Sports

Players may have to gradually play and exercise, within pain tolerance, whilst the nerve and dura free up enough to handle the range of movements demanded by their sport. It is particularly important to avoid positions of flexion or those equivalent to straight leg raising during this time, which may be many months. This could be considered as 'non-formal' or self-administered adverse neural tensioning (see Glossary).

## Comment

So often, the patients who almost grab you by the throat to emphasize the fact that they do have genuine pain will, in spite of a paucity of findings, have night pain and a slump test that is positive. Listen to these patients, for, even if these findings are not present, an epidural will dramatically improve their pain as much as in those that do have dural tensioning signs. However, the mechanical adhesions may not resolve. Adverse neural tensioning may be tried to free up and stretch out the nerve from the scar, but in my experience it flares patients to a degree that they find intolerable. Although I can see the logic of this treatment, I prefer time and the movements of daily living or sport to free up the scar tissue. I sometimes question whether the scar tissue does free up, or whether the peripheral neurovascular bundle, when stretched, lengthens at a ratio comparable with the 1 mm a day found in the Ilizarov leg-lengthening surgery. There does appear to be two elements to discal pain, one mechanical and the other chemical, and both are required to produce pain. Thus MRI scans, a year after a disc herniation, will display the still herniated disc, but if the patient has no dural adhesions there will be no pain.

## Lumbar ligaments

### Findings

#### Posterior lumbar ligaments

A ligamentous history is one of pain at rest, improving with activities but returning if the activities are prolonged. Thus, pure ligamentous back pain is worse first thing in the morning and when sitting or standing for a long time. However, it causes no trouble during games or with activities. It has been christened the 'cocktail party' or 'theatre goer's' back. These people get pain when standing around or sitting for a long time, and they have to have a 'little fidget', which eases the back. Once they start walking or moving, the pain settles. However, ligamentous pain does not always present in its pure form, but as an accompaniment to the mechanical problems of the facets and disc. Ligamentous pain may not be confined to the back but can also refer pain down the leg, often to the back of the knee.

## Inter- and supraspinous ligaments

There is no recognizable history that is pathognomonic of inter- and supraspinous ligament injuries. Palpation of the supraspinous ligament may be very tender, and this pressure at L5/S1 may refer pain down the leg. Indeed, whilst local injection around this ligament may also produce pain that is referred to the back of the leg, it may even cure leg pain in some patients.

## Cause

Stress from flexion, rotation, sheering, and compression and distraction to the pelvic ring on its posterior aspect, which may be more vulnerable around menstruation, or secondary to mechanical, disc, facetal or sacroiliac joint problems.

## Investigations

None are clinically diagnostic for posterior lumbar ligaments, although interspinous tears have been displayed with an injection of contrast medium and the appropriate scan.

## Treatment

(a) Electrotherapeutic modalities to calm pain and settle inflammation, such as ultrasound, interferential and shortwave diathermy; NSAIDs.

(b) Sclerosant/prolotherapy injections [6–9] (see Glossary).

## Sports

(a) Compression of interspinous ligaments or impingement of the spinous processes occurs in gymnastics or acrobatics, with severe local hyperextension, as in 'hanging baskets', walkovers, and gymnastic vaults. However, note that many of these athletes have multi-level spondylolistheses.

(b) Women who get perimenstrual backache experience a pain similar to that from the ligaments. The back seems less stable during menses, so that underlying mechanical instabilities may flare, and, though there is no reason not to compete, perhaps training should be lighter around the menstrual period.

## Comment

Although acute flares of ligament pain are helped by NSAIDs and physiotherapy, sclerosant/prolotherapy injections can give long-term relief and, indeed, may be the only treatment to relieve some ligamentous backaches. I have cured, with sclerosant injections to the posterior lumbar ligaments, a patient who presented after laminectomy surgery to his back with pain behind his knees. Equally, ligamentous backache that prompted full investigations of the kidneys (which proved negative) was also cured by sclerosant injections.

# Part 2 **Extension-orientated lesions**

This group is less homogeneous than the flexion-orientated lesions and the history must be listened to closely, as the variation in the minor elements gives a clue to the lesion (Fig. 5.6).

## Facet (zygapophyseal) joint

See Fig. 2.4.

### Findings

Lesions may be acute and tend to present as lumbar pain, without referral. However, experimental irritant injections into facet joints have produced referred pain in similar dermatomal patterns as root lesions. Groin pain is often referred from a facetal origin. As a disc degenerates, so the facet joints are brought into closer approximation and degenerative changes occur in the facets themselves, giving a more continuous pain that may radiate but invariably has a mechanical history of movement-induced pain. They may accompany disc pain, or continue after disc pain has settled, but they themselves do not produce numbness, or 'pins and needles', although their effect on the adjacent nerve root may. Extension and side flexion is painful, as may be full flexion. Dural stress tests are negative. Facet joint rocking and rolling hurts, as may local pressure over the relevant joint. Sacroiliac stress tests which are non-specific may also hurt (see Chapter 2; and Glossary: Facet and sacroiliac stress tests).

### Cause

(a) Impingement of one zygapophysis on its adjacent pair, caused by too much extension, which, posturally, is usually accompanied by lack of trunk and abdominal muscle tone and a slouched, lordotic, standing posture.

(b) Often, acute movements that disturb the alignment of the facet joints cause 'catching' pains.

(c) Pain may be secondary to an underlying disc lesion – the disc causing malalignment of the adjacent vertebrae, thus disturbing the facetal alignment, or the intervertebral discs becoming degenerate and thinner, bringing the facet joints into closer approximation.

(d) Osteoarthritis (OA) of the facet joints.

(e) Facetal cysts (Figs 5.7–5.9)

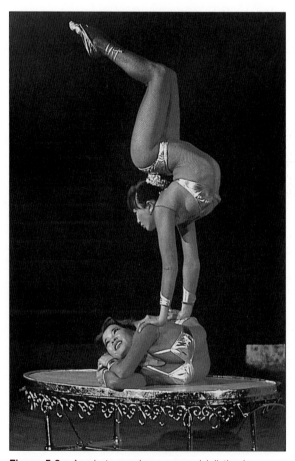

**Figure 5.6** • Acrobats may have a spondylolisthesis present at several levels of the lumbar spine.

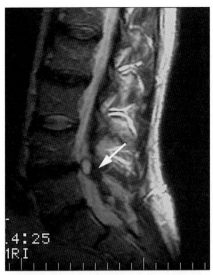

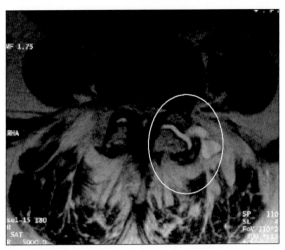

**Figure 5.7** • An intraspinal canal synovial cyst from the facet joint. An intrafacetal injection of cortisone relieved the problem.

**Figure 5.9** • A degenerate facet joint is more likely to suffer from an effusion and a cystic extension, as seen here.

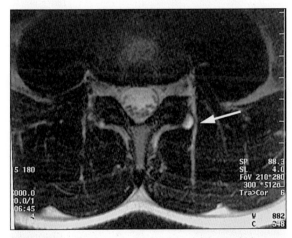

**Figure 5.8** • An extraspinal facetal synovial cyst that produced extension-orientated pain in a teenage tennis player.

## Investigations

X-ray will show established hypertrophic osteoarthritis; CT scans give a clearer picture than MRI of the facet joint and localized bony sclerosis enabling OA to be diagnosed earlier. However, MRI can display the presence of intraspinal, or extra-articular facetal, synovial cysts (see Figs 5.7 and 5.8).

Spinal probing (see Glossary) and endoscopy [5].

## Treatment

(a) Manipulation – facet joint dysfunction responds well to flexion, rotation manipulations. Self-manipulation and McKenzie flexion exercises will help. Massage relieves accompanying muscle spasm, which is often present.

(b) Electrotherapeutic modalities – these calm inflammation (e.g. interferential and shortwave diathermy).

(c) Posture – the patient should not try to increase lordosis, as for a disc, but should be allowed to slump into flexion. Softer beds are often more comfortable. If the patient stands with one foot raised on a box or the foot rail in a pub, this flexes the pelvis and reduces the compression between the adjacent facet joints, relieving the pain. 'Kneel-on chairs' and extension exercises make extension problems worse. A shooting stick or a bar stool may make standing tolerable for facetal problems by allowing a half-sitting position to be adopted.

(d) Cortisone – either perifacetal or intra-articular injections under screening give relief, but perifacetal sclerosants may be required for long-term relief.

(e) Cryo- or chemical rhizotomy, of the sinuvertebral nerve – this denervates the facets (see Chapter 2: Innervation).

(f) Surgical fusion.

> ### Caveat
>
> In adolescents the signs and symptoms are similar to facetal problems, but the diagnosis is likely to be an early stress fracture of the pars interarticularis.

## Sports

Though facetal problems can occur in all sports, they are particularly troublesome in extension-orientated sports (see Spondylolysis and stable spondylolisthesis). Older sportspeople are more prone to facetal OA and have to learn to avoid extension manoeuvres in sport.

## Comment

The general advice for backs is that one should sit up straight, but facetal problems are worse in extension, so many of the elderly who have facetal OA should be allowed to slump or perch on a chair and have soft beds. They are improved by flexion mobilizations. Manipulation may produce dramatic improvement and may also help realign adjacent vertebrae to allow the prolapsing nucleus pulposus to return centrally. Perifacetal sclerosants do seem to be successful and may even produce a chemical rhizotomy.

## Lateral canal entrapment and spinal stenosis

### Findings

The history is of back pain and, almost invariably, root pain down the leg, which is made worse by extension or walking around. The patient relieves the situation by sitting down, half sitting on the edge of a desk or shooting stick, and leaning forward or squatting. The nerve root may be irritated in the lateral canal by the facet joints, especially when enlarged with arthritis, and also by a lateral disc, when the history will have elements of disc pathology and some flexion discomfort. Whilst testing extension, the position should be held for a few seconds, as this time delay may be required before referred root pain is produced. Flexion, dural stress tests, straight leg raise, Lasègue's and slump tests may be positive if a prolapsed disc or nerve root adhesions are present (see Glossary).

## Cause

Entrapment of the nerve root in the lateral canal by a lateral disc, or more usually by a degenerate disc, and hypertrophic OA of the facet joints narrowing the lateral canal. Rarely, a facetal synovial cyst may be the cause (see Fig. 5.7). Spondylolisthesis will also narrow the canal.

## Investigations

Clinically are not required unless failing to progress, then MRI or CT scan (Fig. 5.10).

## Treatment

(a) Flexion manipulations or mobilizations. Traction in Fowler's position and/or home traction, such as a 'back swing', but a pillow under the knees to maintain lumbar flexion may be required.

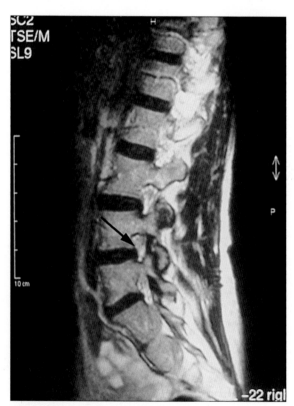

**Figure 5.10 •** Sagittal T1-weighted MRI clearly shows the lateral canal, with the nerve root and surrounding disc and facet joints (*arrow*). Discal prolapse or lateral protrusion, and facet joint hypertrophy, will narrow the lateral canal and compress the exiting nerve root.

(b) Permit the patient to have a postural, flexion slump (see Facet joint).

(c) Cortisone to the facets may settle inflammatory swelling around the nerve root.

(d) A paravertebral block placed in the lateral canal.

(e) Insertion of an interspinous separator such as the X stop.

(f) Laminectomy or laminotomy.

## Sports

Avoid extensions in sport – badminton and the tennis serve can exacerbate the pain. Facetal problems in a swimmer are reduced in backstroke but made worse by diving into the pool and by swimming the other strokes, which produce extension of the spine. The tennis serve should have increased knee bend to reduce back extension. Golfers need to avoid forcing extension on the follow through. This problem is most common in the older person (see Spondylolysis, below).

## Comment

Most 'back books' advocate good posture, which entails a lumbar lordosis, but this group with extension-orientated pain is helped enormously when they are given permission to slump or slouch. Techniques of self-manipulation, pulling the knees to the chest and rocking sideways can be really helpful in preventing recurrences.

# Spondylolysis and stable spondylolisthesis

Also known as stress fracture of the spine, bowler's back, and gymnast's back.

## Findings

Both the acute and chronic conditions, when inflamed, have persistent and usually unilateral, lumbar pain that is worse with movement. They frequently present in the adolescent. Certain sports are particularly associated with this problem. Lumbar extension is painful and ipsilateral side flexion may be painful. Straight leg raise, Lasègue's and slump tests are all negative. There are no abnormal neurological signs. The one-legged extension test and the Fitch catch are often but not invariably painful [10]. Facet joint rocking and rolling is often painful. There is local tenderness to palpation, which may be uni- or bilateral (see Glossary).

## Cause

This may occur idiopathically in 5- to 6-year-olds, without producing symptoms, and comes to the fore only when the back is stressed with extension manoeuvres. In extension, the facet above is thought to act like a chisel striking onto the pars interarticularis below. However, stress lesions of the pars interarticularis can be induced by sporting activities, especially repetitive rotation, extension, manoeuvres. Extension-orientated pain in an adolescent must always raise the possibility of this differential diagnosis. The lesion is possibly more common with a spina bifida occulta and a long isthmus of the pars interarticularis.

### Caveat

**The fracture may heal at one level but refracture at the next level above (a 'climbing' stress fracture).**

## Investigations

(a) Oblique X-ray shows a 'Scottie dog collar' which can appear sclerosed or lytic (Fig. 5.11).

(b) Planar bone scan may not display the lesion in the very early stages but a single photon emission computed tomography (SPECT) scan (Fig. 5.12) will be more diagnostic and should be requested at the same time [11]. X-rays may show a lesion that is then shown to be non-active on the bone scan, which indicates that this particular lesion has probably healed with fibrous union. The bone scan may then display a further hot lesion on the other side, which is the new active lesion. This was considered the gold standard investigation, but the MRI has become more accurate and has no harmful radiation, which makes it the first choice examination. However Masci and colleagues [10] still consider the SPECT scan to be the gold standard.

(c) CT scan with a reverse angle gantry is required to display the lesion, and with a cold, non-active lesion it will be the most accurate investigation (Fig. 5.13).

(d) MRI scan will reveal the medullary oedema in the pars on the T2- and STIR-related sequences (Fig. 5.14).

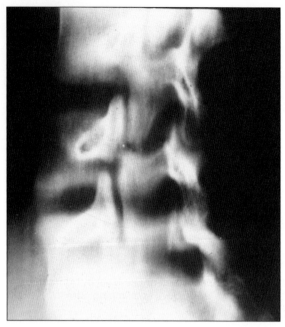

**Figure 5.11** • An oblique X-ray gives the 'Scottie dog' appearance. An apparent collar is produced by a pars interarticularis lesion.

> ### Caveat
>
> A positive lesion on X-ray may not be the cause of pain, and a hot bone scan will show whether this is an active lesion and may even show an active lesion that is not visible on X-ray. Generally, but not invariably, the bone scan-positive lesion is capable of healing and can be monitored on CT scanning. Medullary oedema can be seen on MRI but the cortical bone is not so easily visualized.

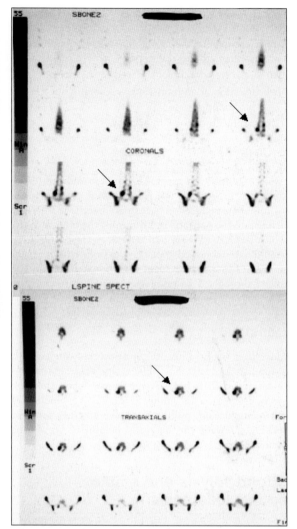

**Figure 5.12** • A planar bone scan may not show up a stress lesion, but a SPECT scan clearly displays the hot spot from the spondylolysis on coronal and transaxial scans.

An algorithm suggested to examine the pars is as follows [12]:

MRI Pars views

| Normal | Abnormal | |
|--------|----------|--|
| Stop | Age the lesion by SPECT and +/− CT | |
| | old and cold | new and hot |
| | stable or unstable | rest 3 months |
| | core stability, sclerosants, surgery | review |

## Treatment

(a) Three months' rest from the causative activity is usually sufficient. The lesion probably heals by bony union in cases where the bone scan is hot, and is considered to have healed by fibrous union if the bone scan is cold. CT scan is probably the best modality, besides pain, for monitoring healing.

(b) Cross-train for fitness using non-impact methods, such as cycling and rowing, and avoid

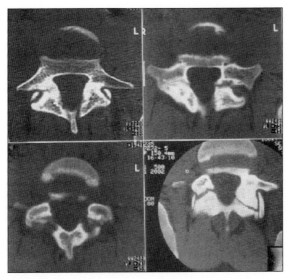

**Figure 5.13** • Various sites of stress fracture, from the pedicle to the pars, are shown by CT scans with a reverse angle gantry in different individuals (Dr Philip Bell).

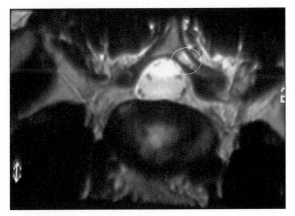

**Figure 5.14** • An MRI scan shows oedema in the pars interarticularis on the left.

swimming except for backstroke. Avoid running, especially downhill, if it produces discomfort.

(c) A stable spondylolisthesis may respond to manipulation as there is often a facetal element to the pain.

(d) Alter any causative technique (see below).

## Sports

(a) Gymnastics – extensions must be avoided during healing. However, note that, besides the generally accepted extension work, whipping giant circles on the rings to increase downward acceleration may force extension and be causative in male gymnasts.

(b) Cricket – fast bowlers who have a mixed bowling style are more prone to this injury. Bowlers should either be side on or front on, check with a coach. Youngsters should limit the number of fast balls they bowl, e.g. as recommended by the Australian Cricket Board [13]:

*Under 12 matchplay*: a limit of two spells of four overs, with approximately a 1 hour break.

Practice: 2 × 30 minutes practice sessions per week: 5 minutes short run, reduced pace; 20 minutes match speed/coach controlled; 5 minutes specific technique development.

*Under 16 matchplay*: A limit of two spells of six overs, with approximately a 1 hour break.

Practice: 2 × 40 minutes practice sessions per week: 5 minutes short run, reduced pace; 25 minutes match speed/coach controlled; 10 minutes specific technique development.

*Under 19 matchplay*: A limit of three spells of six overs, with approximately a 1 hour break.

Practice: 3 × 40 minutes practice sessions per week: 5 minutes short run, reduced pace.

(c) Swimming – avoid butterfly until healed. Other strokes are usually pain-free, but severe back extension with the pull phase in breaststroke may cause a flare. Diving into a pool may promote extension and therefore pain.

(d) Football – there is a fairly high incidence (10–12%) of this condition amongst the English Football Association selected youth at the National Training Centre. The cause is not yet understood but may be linked with jumping into extension to head a ball.

(e) Tennis – the problem can be caused by serving with too much back extension. The player may have to develop more knee bend during the serve to compensate.

## Comment

The physician must be aware of this problem and recognize that certain sports are prone to cause the problem. Whether screening of children for spina bifida occulta (of which there is thought to be an increased incidence) is cost-effective remains to be seen. Rest from causative activities is essential, but it is difficult to know precisely when youngsters should be returned to their sport. Resting for 3 months while medullary oedema is present or the bone scan is hot, which is thought to reflect healing, may be sufficient. The disappearance of the MRI T2 increased signal and the healing of the lesion visualized on CT helps monitor progress, but continuing pain, which may exist when MRI and CT appear normal, especially in sports like gymnastics, can be difficult to manage. Of note is that very active children may grow faster during an enforced period of rest. In a gymnast this increase in height alters rotational speed and thus performance. Parental and coach pressure to return the elite child to activities is extreme.

## L5/S1 disc

There may be a history of a disc problem, perhaps with dural tensioning signs, that is worse in extension (see L5/S1 disc prolapse in Part 3).

## L2/3 L3/4 disc and adhesions

### Findings

The patient often presents stuck in flexion, bent over, and is happier sitting and lying with the knees bent. The spinal canal is capacious at this level so a herniated disc has to be large to cause problems. The bent over position releases the stretch on the L2/3, L3/4 nerves because it allows a flexed hip, which shortens the functional length of the femoral nerve. Thus the opposite, the femoral nerve stretch test, is positive. There is often referred pain in the L2/3/4 area on the front of the thigh. However, it is *flexion* that produces the prolapse and, after the acute stage, extension exercises will help (see Chapter 2: The disc).

### Cause

Herniation of these discs is not so common as at L4/5 and L5/S1 but it is flexion manoeuvres that produce this problem. Often the patient stands with a straight, flattened spine, which seems to divert stresses on the lumbar spine to the higher segments. As there is more room in the spinal canal at this level, the smaller prolapses cause fewer problems.

### Investigations

(a) None are required if therapeutic progress is being maintained.
(b) MRI.

### Treatment

(a) Epidural.
(b) Root-block.
(c) These disc lesions heal in their own time, with analgesia, massage and electrotherapy to treat the symptoms.
(d) Posture to increase lumbar lordosis and reduce the high lumbar flattening is required once the disc has settled. Abdominal muscle tensioning and pelvic tilt may have to be reduced.

### Sports

See Part 1: Annular disc or 'disc creep'.

## Spinous process impingement

### Findings

There is a history of either a one-off forced and violent spinal extension or a mechanical history of repeated extension movements. There is local tenderness to palpation over the relevant spinous process. Worse on extensions, the pain is located centrally but can refer down the leg.

### Cause

An uncommon impingement of one spinous process onto another during excessive extension.

### Investigations

Apart from trauma where the spinous process may be fractured, not relevant.

### Treatment

Consists of modalities to calm inflammation, such as ultrasound, laser and local cortisone.

### Sports

This occurs in acrobatics, particularly the 'hanging basket', and in gymnastics walkovers, especially if the gymnast has a tendency to drop into extension at the low lumbar level L4/5–L5/S1 as opposed to extending upwards and then backwards, spreading the extension through all the lumbar vertebral segments. A whip into extension, as in circles on rings, or whip somersaults can produce this effect.

## Comment

I have rarely seen this problem, and only in the sports above. Individuals respond to cortisone, but must have the technique that produces the acute lordosis at one area corrected if possible. I have also seen congenitally absent spinous processes that permitted more facetal impingement.

## Part 3 **Mixed orientation**

### PART CONTENTS

Some painful back histories will have a combination of signs and symptoms that vary between extension and flexion because the lesion is unstable or changes its pattern as it progresses.

# L5/S1 disc prolapse

## Findings

### Normal pattern disc prolapse

(a) Flexion of the spine is painful and there may be an arc of pain, which causes the flexing spine to deviate sideways as it passes through this arc ('swing round'). This arc may occur on returning from flexion and the pain often causes patients to place their hands on their knees or hips to push up through it. This can occur with discs at other levels.

(b) Side flexion is more painful to one side than the other.

(c) Straight leg raise, Lasègue's and slump tests may be positive (see Glossary).

(d) Root signs will involve L5, extensor hallucis, extensor digitorum longus, extensor digitorum brevis, peroneals and/or S1, calf or hamstring weakness. Absent or reduced ankle jerk (see Chapter 2: Lumbar spine nerve root signs, p. 15).

(e) Extension manoeuvres ease the pain.

### Collar stud disc

This has the same pain pattern as a normal L5/S1 disc, but extension is painful as well, and may refer pain to the leg during this movement (see Fig. 2.8).

## Cause

This disc and the L4/5 disc are most at risk and a percentage of these disc prolapses are accompanied by a retroposition of L5 on S1, which creates a collar stud deformity of the herniating disc. This disc therefore can also present signs and symptoms mainly in extension; however, as the lesion regresses and the collar stud deformity is less marked, the symptoms become more flexion orientated. This disc must be treated as a separate entity when considering management as it is common and its pain patterns vary throughout treatment.

## Investigations

Lateral X-ray shows a small retroposition of L5 on S1 and a hollow in the inferior surface of L5 caused by the disc, whilst MRI scan shows the disc with a collar stud effect (see Fig. 2.8).

## Treatment

Initially, this disc problem is flared by both extension and flexion exercises, and, if severe, rest or epidurals may be required to calm the inflammation. In the early stages flexion is easier, and traction in Fowler's position and manipulation may help. Postural correction requires a more neutral position, not too much flattening nor too much lordosis. Later, as the disc herniation regresses, extension exercises may be tolerated.

## Sports

See Part 1: Annular disc or 'disc creep'.

## Comment

This is probably the most difficult disc to treat, and there have certainly been cases where early extension exercises have seriously exacerbated the problem (see Glossary, McKenzie flexion exercises). Mixed lesions can be made worse by both flexion and extension, but later one or the other McKenzie exercises may be of help. Postural correction and core stability exercises will have to be performed in the neutral position, not too far forward nor too far back.

# Unstable spondylolisthesis

See Spondylolysis and stable spondylolisthesis.

## Findings

An unstable spondylolisthesis may present with pain from the ligaments and facet joints. However, if the degree of slip progresses to involve the dura or, commonly, the lateral canal, then nerve root signs and symptoms will follow. In which case, dural stress tests and adverse neural tensioning will be positive, even in flexion, and, if severe, dural or root signs of the appropriate root level may be elicited. There may be a palpable step in the lumbar spine. Sacroiliac joint stress tests can be positive as this manoeuvre stresses the unstable vertebral segment (see Glossary).

## Cause

Slip of one vertebra on another due to bilateral pars interarticularis fractures at one level. Defined as grade 1 up to 25% slip, grade 2 up to 50% slip and grade 3 beyond 50% slip. It may present as an acute lesion or develop insidiously.

## Investigations

(a) Lateral X-ray will display and help grade the spondylolisthesis (Fig. 5.15).

(b) CT scans require a reverse-angle gantry to display the pars, but this view is not so good for showing any associated disc lesion.

(c) MRI scan, if there are dural signs, will display the extent of any disc involvement and the associated spondylolisthesis.

## Treatment

Most athletes will present with a grade 1; very few reach grade 2, or grade 3, which requires surgical fusion:

(a) If there are no dural signs then gentle manipulation will gap the facetal encroachment.

(b) Traction moves the proximal segment backwards [14], whilst Fowler's position (see Glossary: Traction), with the pelvis flexed on the lumbar spine, will also gap the facet joints.

(c) Sclerosant/prolotherapy injections to stabilize the unstable segment [7–9].

(d) A lumbar corset seems to provide support and comfort, though this must not be at the expense of ignoring core stability exercises.

(e) Home traction couches are cost-effective and can be used daily to relieve the pain at the end of a day.

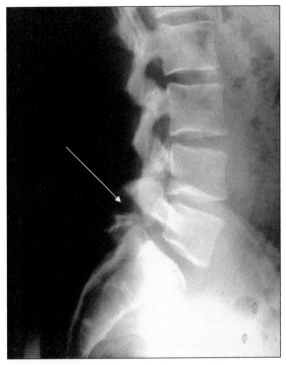

**Figure 5.15** • A lateral X-ray showing a grade 1 spondylolisthesis of L5 on S1.

(f) Surgery for grade 3 and for the unstable grade 1 or 2. There is possibly a greater indication for professional sportspeople to have surgery if the sport increases loads on their back.

## Sports

See under Spondylolysis and stable spondylolisthesis.

## Comment

Spondylolistheses may be pain-free but the problem arises from the instability of the segment. Many sportspeople do not want surgical stabilization and their problem can be controlled by home traction and sclerosant injections, plus avoidance of excessive extension exercises or axial weight-bearing. However, in certain sports or with large training loads, the patient may require surgical stabilization of the back before these exercises can be tolerated. Note that the pars interarticularis stress fractures may 'climb': as one level heals or is fused, so the stress is taken up to the level above and the stress injury appears in the higher segment.

## Lateral canal obstruction with disc

The older sportsperson is more likely to have facetal osteoarthritis and a narrowing of the lateral canal (see Fig. 5.10), so when nerve root symptoms that are worse with extension are found in the younger person, it suggests the lateral canal is obstructed by a lateral herniated disc (see Lateral canal entrapment and spinal stenosis).

## Sacroiliac joint

The sacroiliac joint (SIJ) is accepted as having a nutational (nodding) movement in the L-shaped joint of about 5 degrees and a downward movement of about 2 mm [15]. CT and MRI scans show osteophytes and areas of sclerosis or lysis, consistent with stress across the joint, that is not associated with systemic problems or ankylosing spondylitis (Fig. 5.16).

### Findings

A history of trauma and/or pain associated with the following:

(a) Running downhill. The foot checks the landing but the body weight continues its descent, producing a sacral down thrust and forward nutation relative to the ilium.

(b) Riding a horse. This can force abduction of the hip joints to the limit, at which stage any

further external rotatory pressures will be transferred to the pelvis, and thus the SIJ. If the patient has fallen from the horse, but the foot remains in the stirrup, then a traction jerk can be applied to the sacroiliac joint.

(c) Sacroiliac pain may be acute and debilitating after trauma, and this severity of response suggests ankylosing spondylitis.

(d) There may be an accompanying disc, facet joint or ligamentous history.

(e) Pelvic spring may be painful; however, if the patient supports the L5 segment by lying on a hand, and this relieves this sign, then the sign is probably negative for the SIJ and rather suggests segmental dysfunction. Other pelvic stress tests may be positive (see Glossary).

(f) Hip flexion may be painful because, after the hip has reached its limit of range, the passive flexion force applied by the examiner will continue the flexion moment into the spine and pelvis.

(g) The joint may be tender to local palpation and compression over the joint. Though pain may be referred down the leg from the SIJ, there is no history of 'pins and needles' or numbness, and dural stress tests are negative (see Glossary).

(h) Extension and full flexion may be painful.

### Cause

(a) Sacroiliac stress from a vertical compression force transferring foot impaction up to the spine. This may occur during a 'rear-end shunt' in a car, when the driver's foot is on the brake or clutch and the force is transferred up through the foot and leg to the SIJ.

(b) A shear force in the vertical plane, such as a foot caught in a stirrup, wrenching the leg away from the pelvis.

(c) Distraction occurs when the leg is forced or accelerated into adduction, such as during martial arts kicking.

(d) Compression occurs when the hip is stretched into external rotation, such as stretches in aerobics, in the lithotomy position, martial arts and some aerobic routines (Fig. 5.17).

(e) Increased relaxation of ligaments around menstruation or the third trimester of pregnancy allows greater movement in the joint and makes the SIJ more vulnerable to stresses.

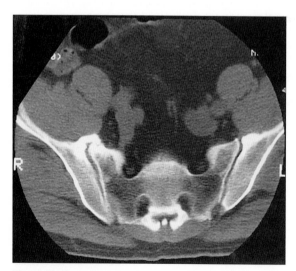

**Figure 5.16 •** A CT scan with a large right and developing left anterior osteophyte.

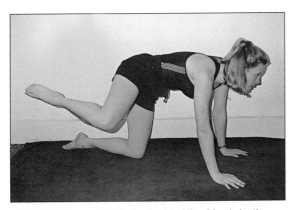

**Figure 5.17** • An aerobic routine involving hip abduction can stress the sacroiliac joint.

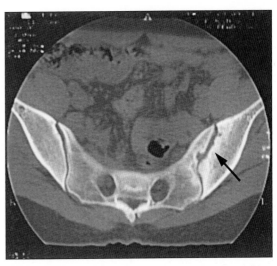

**Figure 5.19** • A CT scan showing ankylosing spondylitis. This 30-year-old HLA-B27-positive woman had normal X-rays and MRI. X-rays show ilial sclerosis, and total fusion of the sacroiliac joints may occur.

## Investigations

(a) X-ray and take bloods for HLA-B27, C reactive protein (CRP) and erythrocyte sedimentation rate (ESR) for ankylosing spondylitis (Fig. 5.19).

(b) Bone scan if a stress fracture or bony pain is suspected (see Fig. 5.18), and request that the MRI or CT scan is also taken through the SIJs and not just the spine (see Figs 5.16 and 5.19).

## Treatment

(a) Manipulation of the SIJ.

(b) Wear a sacroiliac belt following distraction injuries.

(c) Sacroiliac injections – cortisone.

(d) Sclerosant injections to the iliolumbar and sacroiliac ligaments.

(e) Anti-inflammatory drugs.

## Sports

In particular, SIJ pain is worse with:

(a) Martial arts – kicking.

(b) Running – worse on running downhill and on bend running. Running should be avoided until pelvic stress tests are negative.

(c) Pole vault – in the take-off leg when the drive and extension compresses the SIJ.

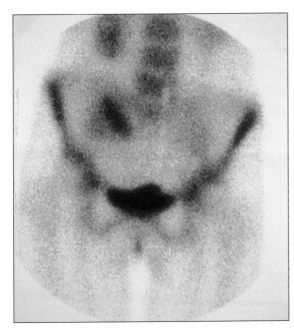

**Figure 5.18** • A bone scan shows a stress fracture across the sacral bone in an elite long-distance runner. (Dr Malcolm Bottomley)

(f) Stress fractures have been reported mainly in oligo/amenorrhoeic runners [16], but have been seen in other athletes who may be found to have a lower bone density (Fig. 5.18).

**(d)** Horse riding – external rotation: longer or shorter stirrups may reduce the amount of external rotation required. Internal rotation, which distracts the SIJ, may cause pain, in which case riding with very short stirrups may make this worse – ride longer until better. Shear forces can occur from the foot being caught in a stirrup during a fall.

**(e)** Aerobics – hip abduction movements, especially whilst kneeling, must be avoided (see Fig. 5.17). Do low-impact, not high-impact, training.

**(f)** Swimming – breaststroke may flare the SIJ; use a wedge kick or, if not a serious swimmer, just waft the legs.

## Comment

Dysfunction of this joint is both over- and under-diagnosed [17]. The pelvis forms a ring and, as disturbance of a ring structure affects more than one location, so one injury may produce, or be associated with, another injury. Thus, these SIJ problems are often associated with facet, disc or ligamentous lesions. The standard views used to investigate a back invariably do not include the SIJ so coronal obliques will be required for MRI or CT scanning. MRI may show early, painless stress lesions, and even grade 4 lesions, which suggest a stress of the sacrum, but the patient may have no presenting symptoms (see Fig. 8.17). Sacroiliac joint belts are of limited help. Manipulation may help the SIJ (although it may well be the accompanying facet that is being manipulated). Hydrocortisone has short-term relief but sclerosant injections provide long-term help, and have proved of great value [6–9].

## References

1 Cyriax JH, Cyriax PJ. Lumbar nerve roots. In: Cyriax's illustrated manual of orthopaedic medicine. Oxford: Butterworth-Heinemann; 1993. pp. 236–239

2 Cyriax JH, Cyriax PJ. Lumbar spine traction. In: Cyriax's illustrated manual of orthopaedic medicine. Oxford: Butterworth-Heinemann; 1993. pp. 221–225

3 Cyriax JH, Cyriax PJ. Lumbar spine epidural local anaesthesia. In: Cyriax's illustrated manual of orthopaedic medicine. Oxford: Butterworth-Heinemann; 1993. pp. 226–230

4 Milette PC, Fontaine S, Lepanto L, Cardinal E, Breton G. Differentiating lumbar disc protrusions, disc bulges and discs with normal contour but abnormal signal intensity. Spine 1999;24:44–53

5 Knight M. Endoscopically determined pain sources in the lumbar spine. In: Hutson M, Ellis R (eds) Textbook of musculoskeletal medicine. Oxford: Oxford University Press; 2006. Ch 3.2

6 Klein RG, Eek BC, DeLong B, Mooney V. A randomised, double blind trial of dextrose-glycerine-phenol injections for chronic low back pain. J Spinal Disorders 1993;6:22–33

7 Yelland M, Glasziou PP, Bogduk N, Schluter PJ, McKernon M. Prolotherapy, saline injections and exercise for chronic low back pain; a randomized trial. Spine 2003;29(1):9–16

8 Ongley MJ, Klein RG, Dorman TA, Eek BC, Hubert LJ. A new approach to the treatment of chronic back pain Lancet 1985;2:143–146

9 Dorman T. Prolotherapy. In: Hutson M, Ellis R (eds) Textbook of musculoskeletal medicine. Oxford: Oxford University Press; 2006. Ch. 4.3.12

10 Masci L, Pike J, Malara L, Phillips B, Bennell K, Brukner P. Use of the one-legged hyperextension test and magnetic resonance imaging in the diagnosis of active spondolysis. Br J Sports Med 2006;40:940–946

11 Read MTF. Single photon emission computed tomography (SPECT) scanning for adolescent back pain. A sine qua non? Br J Sports Med 1994;28:56–57

12 Dr Philip Bell. BUPA Wellness clinic, London

13 Foster D, John D, Elliott B, Ackland T, Fitch K. Back injuries to fast bowlers in cricket: a prospective study. Br J Sports Med 1989;23:150–154

14 Freiberg O. Lumbar instability in the young population; biomechanics, occurrence, new diagnostic and therapeutic methods. Paarvo Nurmi Congress Book from Advanced European Course on Sports Medicine: 50th Anniversary of the Finnish Society of Sports Medicine; 1989, pp. 208–210

15 Palastanga N, Field D, Soames R. Joints of the pelvis: sacroiliac joint. In: Anatomy and human movement, structure and function. Oxford: Heinemann Medical; 1989

16 Bottomley MB. Sacral stress fracture in a runner. Br J Sports Med 1990;24:243–244

17 McGill SM. A biomechanical perspective of sacro-iliac pain. Clin Biomech 1987;2:145–151

## Further reading

Bruckner P, Khan K. Clinical sports medicine, 3rd edn. New York: McGraw-Hill; 2006

Cyriax JH, Cyriax PJ. Cyriax's illustrated manual of orthopaedic medicine. Oxford: Butterworth-Heinemann; 1993

Hutson MA (ed.). Sports injuries: recognition and management, 2nd edn. Oxford: Oxford Medical Publications; 1996

Hutson M, Ellis R (eds). Textbook of musculoskeletal medicine. Oxford: Oxford University Press; 2006

Palastanga N, Field D, Soames R. Anatomy and human movement, structure and function. Oxford: Heinemann Medical Books; 1989

Reid D. Sports injury assessment and rehabilitation. Edinburgh: Churchill Livingstone; 1992

Watkins RG (ed.). The spine in sports. St Louis: Mosby; 1996

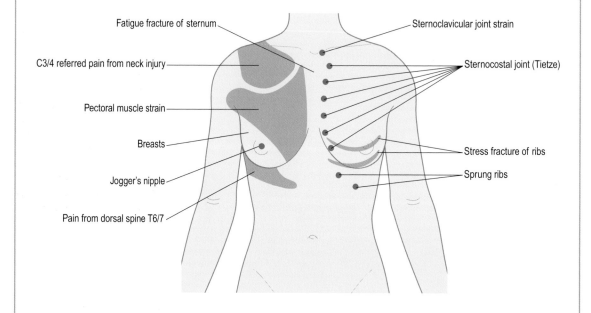

Fatigue fracture of sternum

C3/4 referred pain from neck injury

Pectoral muscle strain

Breasts

Jogger's nipple

Pain from dorsal spine T6/7

Sternoclavicular joint strain

Sternocostal joint (Tietze)

Stress fracture of ribs

Sprung ribs

# Chapter Six

# Anterior chest pain

## Systemic causes

Every history taken from someone with chest pain should take care to eliminate any cardiovascular problem, particularly concentrating on exercise-induced pain and disproportionate shortness of breath. People do not faint during exercise unless there is a problem with the heart, hypoglycaemia, hyperthermia or hyponatraemia.

Young people, under 30 years, are unlikely to suffer from coronary heart disease but their cardiac problems are likely to be arrhythmias, valvular dysfunction and hypertrophic cardiomyopathy, which may affect exercise. Long, tall streaks that play basketball and volleyball may have Marfan syndrome and be prone to aortic medionecrotic dissection. Chest infection, asthma and exercise-induced asthma should always be considered, as should pulmonary embolus for those on the pill or after long flights. Undiagnosed pulmonary bullae may rupture under the increased loads of training, and a pneumothorax may ensue. Reflux oesophagitis, which is reasonably common in cyclists, may be helped by pre-exercise antacids. Peppermint to bring up (or charcoal to absorb) gases can reduce gastric distension, and fizzy drinks should be avoided.

## Referred pain from the dorsal spine

Passive dorsal rotation with flexion and local palpation of the dorsal spine may produce pain that indicates this is referred pain (see Chapter 4).

## Referred pain from the neck

Test neck rotation, flexion and extension, side flexion, plus rotation in flexion for pain referred over the front of the chest in the C4 distribution (see Chapter 3).

## Fractured ribs – traumatic

The presentation includes a history of trauma and, in particular, a sharp catching pain on inspiration or movement that is localizable over a rib. No history of trauma is indicative of serious pathology complicated by a fracture. Complications include haemoptysis, tension pneumothorax, surgical emphysema and, more commonly, flail ribs, for which the patient should be given oxygen and referred to a trauma department. Management of these severe complications is dealt with in advanced trauma life saving and not in this book. The uncomplicated, rib-spring-positive, rib fracture will settle without treatment over 4–6 weeks, during which time non-contact sport may be played to pain tolerance.

# Costochondral cartilage pain/ Tietze disease

## Findings

Anterior chest pain that may be bilateral and is located over one joint or several joints. The history may be confusing because chest expansion to full inspiration and chest compression on full expiration may produce pain, as can coughing and slouching. There is local tenderness to palpation over the costochondral joint. Costochondritis and Tietze disease are not entirely synonymous: Tietze disease is systemic and has a swollen inflamed joint, the cause of which is still not fully understood.

## Cause

Tietze disease is a systemic inflammation that involves the costosternal joints [1], but in sport the problem is usually post traumatic, though not necessarily post impaction.

### Caveat

This rather confusing history of pain on expansion and also on compression of the chest, and therefore being flared with exercise, does raise the differential diagnosis of angina. It may also be very difficult to distinguish from referred dorsal pain, as rotation of the spine can hurt the costochondral lesion as well. Local palpatory pressure must be applied with the patient sitting, as pressure on the costochondral joint may also apply pressure on the dorsal spine when the patient is lying down, and vice versa.

## Investigations

None are clinically required to establish the diagnosis, but investigations to exclude intrathoracic or cardiac problems may be instituted on a 'better safe than sorry' basis. If the joint is swollen or not settling, look for systemic inflammatory disease as a cause.

## Treatment

Avoid compression of the chest and shoulder exercises that require pectoral muscle work. Modalities to settle inflammation, such as local ultrasound, laser, and particularly intra-articular cortisone, are beneficial. NSAIDs may help Tietze disease.

## Sports

No sport is obviously causative, but when the problem is present upper limb sports may have to be avoided until better.

## Comment

Costochondral pain is frequently confused with angina, but if the exercise ECG is normal then local palpable tenderness is diagnostic. The history can be confusing with both opposites; that is, both chest compression and expansion being painful. Ultrasound usually works over time but intra-articular cortisone can work rapidly.

# Sternoclavicular joint

## Findings

There is localized pain following trauma or with shoulder movements. There may be visible anterior subluxation of the clavicle on the sternum, or the sternoclavicular joint appears swollen. All shoulder girdle movements may be painful and the joint is locally tender to palpation. The pain may be referred up the front of the neck to the angle of the jaw.

## Cause

(a) Trauma.
(b) Shoulder girdle problems.
(c) Systemic inflammatory disease.

## Investigations

X-ray for fracture and disease changes. Full blood count, including CRP, ESR, anti-nuclear factor and rheumatoid factors. MRI will show inflammation of the joint [3].

## Caveat

Posterior subluxation of the clavicle is rare but can involve the great vessels from the aorta. Beware that soft tissue swelling does not lead to a misdiagnosis of anterior subluxation. Reduction may work but the subluxation may require surgical release [2].

## Treatment

Modalities to settle inflammation, such as ultrasound, therapeutic laser, cortisone injection into the sternoclavicular joint and NSAIDs, may be of value with inflammatory disease, and also following trauma. The natural history of anterior subluxation is good [2].

## Sports

The lesion often occurs following trauma; however, if a racket player stands front-on to forehand or overhead shots and does not rotate the dorsal spine, but forces retraction of the shoulder girdle, then the whole pectoral girdle, including the acromioclavicular and sternoclavicular joints, may become painful (see Figs 17.5 and 17.6).

## Comment

These really do very well with cortisone and, once calmed, often cause no more trouble, even on returning to racket sports. The above fault (see Fig. 17.5) is often demonstrated by the aggressive player with poor technique, who tries to hit hard from the front-on position, and must be corrected – this in itself may be curative.

## Fractured clavicle

Most fractured clavicles may be allowed to heal, even with some degree of displacement, and a guideline to return to sporting activity given to me by an orthopaedic consultant who specialized in motor cycling was: seven press ups – ride a horse; ten press ups – race a bike.

Stress fractures have been presented in a female gymnast [4] and unreported in a cricketer (see Fig. 17.7), but a pathological cause, such as through a cyst, should also be considered.

# Stress fracture of the ribs

## Findings

Usually, these occur around the anterior to mid-axillary line of ribs 4 to 7, with associated pain during the relevant sport. Breathing and coughing may produce a sharp pain and rib spring is positive. There is no referred tenderness from the dorsal spine, though a posterior angle stress fracture of the ribs can occur (see Fig. 4.1).

## Cause

Presumed to be from the irregular pull of the rib attachments of serratus anterior and external oblique muscles, plus rotational strains across the ribs [5,6].

## Investigations

X-ray is often negative, even in the late stages. A bone scan is the easiest to read for this problem, and is the best investigation if the diagnosis is unclear, but if the player is associated with certain sports that are classically connected with rib stress fractures then this should alert the clinician (see Sports, below, and Fig. 6.1).

## Treatment

Rest for 4–6 weeks from causative activity, and alter the poor technique.

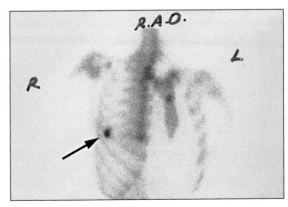

**Figure 6.1** • A bone scan shows a stress fracture of the ribs in a rower.

## Sports

(a) Rowing – it is possible that someone who is used to rowing one side of the boat, and who then switches to the other side, pulls too soon with the 'inside hand'. This is the hand that, when rowing the other side, travelled the furthest but now travels less far and has a different pull rhythm, which does not coincide with the arc of rotation of the oar. The serratus anterior or the external oblique would meet much harder resistance to this pull. A truncated arm pull-through and a decreased lay back position, plus a decreased lever arm, may yield a decreased risk of stress fracture [5].

(b) Golf – normally the body rotates through the shot. However, some golfers may slide their leading hip out sideways whilst striking the ball. In so doing, the left side is blocked out to stop the left side breaking away too soon and this can prevent a hook (either deliberately or accidentally); however, the pull from the arms is still powerful. This will stop the normal completion of the arm movement and cause a jerk-like pull over the muscle insertions into the ribs [6].

(c) Paddlers/canoeists – possibly pulling too hard with the ipsilateral arm, as opposed to pushing with the contralateral arm, is a cause of the injury.

(d) The condition has been reported in swimming [7].

## Comment

Chest pain and rib-spring positive, in the sports mentioned above, should warrant a bone scan if the clinician is unsure of the diagnosis.

## Sprung rib

### Findings

Surprisingly sharp, localized pain, found usually over the ninth costal cartilage, but also in all the floating ribs, that is worse on full inspiration and expiration. Simply flexing at the waist and performing abdominal exercises hurts, and the pain may interfere with sport to a disproportional extent.

### Cause

Usually, the ninth costal cartilage becomes unstable and flicks over the eighth rib. The cause is almost always traumatic.

### Investigations

None are clinically required; however, some of the differentials are serious and investigations to rule out other causes of abdominal or chest pain are justified.

### Treatment

The sprung rib is difficult to treat successfully. Modalities to settle inflammation, such as ultrasound, laser and local cortisone injection, can ease the pain, but they often require rest from abdominal and pectoral girdle activities for much longer than expected.

### Sports

The injury usually occurs in contact sports and, because breathing hurts, even aerobic cross-training may prove troublesome.

### Comment

Although physiotherapy and injections help, this injury can still require a long time to settle, and returning too soon to physical activity seems to flare the problem.

## Pectoralis tear

### Findings

This presents as an acute episode, when the resistance to the arm pulling into internal rotation is too great. Massive bruising and, later, a palpable gap in the pectoralis muscle around the anterior axillary line may be present. There is weakness and pain on resisted adduction of the arm across the body.

### Cause

Tear of, usually, the pectoralis major, when a violent, powerful adduction and internal rotation of the arm is resisted, such as when a player breaks away from a judo or rugby hold.

## Investigations

None are clinically required, but an ultrasound scan of muscle, which will assess the size of the tear, may be appropriate. Note the congenital absence of the sternal head with Poland syndrome [8,9].

## Treatment

(a) Try strapping the arm, or holding it in a sling across the chest, to shorten and approximate the pectoralis. The muscle does tend to reattach to the thorax but a gap may always be palpable and function weaker. After 3 weeks, the patient may start isometrics and gradually increase isotonic and isokinetic adduction. Build to 'bench press' and 'pectoralis (pec) decks', but work initially with narrow grip and gradually widen it.

(b) Surgery may be the appropriate treatment [10] and can produce a greater recovery of peak torque and work [11].

## Sports

Judo and wrestling are the most common causes. Here, the powerful adduction forces required for a hold or throw are resisted by the opponent to a degree sufficient to tear the muscle. Rugby and American football can produce similar problems.

## Comment

I have seen only a few, and my surgical colleagues thought they could not approximate the muscle tear as the tissue was too friable. Later, local attachment had occurred with a palpable gap and separation, but a return to almost normal function. However, Wolfe et al [10] and Hanna et al [11] feel surgery is the first line treatment, to achieve a postoperative return of strength and function.

## **Fatigue fracture of the sternum**

### Findings

This (single reported case) presented as an acute injury with sit-ups and acute chest pain, worse on coughing and movement. There was local tenderness to palpation [12].

### Cause

This is an unusual stress fracture that occurred as a complication of sit-ups in a body builder, but possibly

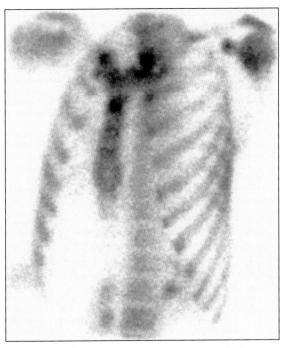

**Figure 6.2** • A bone scan shows stress across both sternoclavicular joints and the manubrium sterni. (Dr Philip Bell)

associated with pectoral muscle activity. Usually a sternal fracture is traumatic.

### Investigations

X-ray and bone scan for the fracture (Fig. 6.2) and CT or MRI scan to exclude underlying neoplasia. Blood tests to exclude leukaemias are advisable.

### Sports

Weight training.

### Comment

This is a very rare case and I have not seen a case myself. I do not know whether anabolic steroids were a factor or not.

## **References**

1 EMIS. Tietze syndrome; 2005. Available from: www.patient.co.uk/showdoc/40001294

2 Rockwood CA. Resection arthroplasty of the sternoclavicular joint. J Bone Joint Surg 1997;79(3):387

3 Higginbotham TO, Kuhn JE. Atraumatic disorders of the sternoclavicular joint. J Am Acad Orthop Surg 2005;13(2):136–145

4 Fallon KE, Fricker PA. Stress fracture of the clavicle in a young female gymnast. Br J Sports Med 2001;35;448–449

5 Karlson KA. Rib stress fractures in elite rowers. A case series and proposed mechanism. Am J Sports Med 1998;26:516–519

6 Read MTF. Case report – stress fracture of the rib in a golfer. Br J Sports Med 1994;28:206–207

7 Taimela S, Kujala UM, Orava S. Two consecutive rib stress fractures in a female competitive swimmer. Clin J Sports Med 1995;5:254–257

8 Poland A. Deficiency of the pectoralis muscle. Guy's Hosp Rep 1841;6:191

9 McGillivray BC, Lowry RB. Poland syndrome in British Colombia; incidence and reproductive experience of affected persons. Am J Med Genet 1977;1:65–74

10 Wolfe SW, Wickievicz TL, Cavanaugh JT. Ruptures of the pectoralis major muscle. An anatomic and clinical analysis. Am J Sports Med 1992;20:587–593

11 Hanna CM, Glenny AB, Stanley SN, Caughey MA. Pectoralis major tears: comparison of surgical and conservative treatment. Br J Sports Med 2001;35:202–206

12 Robertson K, Kristensen O, Vejen L. Manubrium sterni stress fracture: an unusual complication of non contact sport. Br J Sports Med 1996;30:176–177

## Further reading

Bruckner P, Khan K. Clinical sports medicine, 3rd edn. New York: McGraw-Hill; 2006

Hutson M, Ellis R (eds). Textbook of musculoskeletal medicine. Oxford: Oxford University Press; 2006

Reid D. Sports injury assessment and rehabilitation. Edinburgh: Churchill Livingstone; 1992

# Chapter **Seven**

# 7

# Abdomen

## Referred pain from the dorsal spine

Referred pain occurs with passive rotation of the dorsal spine, which, if it is the cause of the problem, should have segmental localized palpable tenderness in the spine (see Chapter 4).

## Sprung rib

Localized tenderness over the 9th to 12th costal cartilage (see same topic in Chapter 6).

## 'Stitch'

### Findings

Pain located in the subcostal area and which occurs early on during continuous aerobic exercise.

### Cause

Not known, but possibly due to splanchnic vascular contraction diverting visceral blood to the muscular system and causing an ischaemic type of pain. A proper warm-up to allow a more gradual redistribution of blood to the muscles seems to prevent the onset.

## Spigelian hernia

### Findings

There may be quite severe abdominal pain on exercise and very localized tenderness, with a small palpable pit in the abdominal muscles just lateral to the rectus abdominus. The pit is about the size of a little finger tip and is locally tender to palpation. 'Sit ups' can flare the pain.

## Cause

A small anterior abdominal wall defect that reaches the spigelian fascia.

## Investigations

None are of clinical importance in that MRI and real-time ultrasound invariably do not display the lesion. However, ultrasound may show some muscular inco-ordination. Ultrasound will also display the underlying abdominal organs to exclude them from the diagnosis.

## Treatment

Surgical repair of the defect seems to be effective.

## Sports

None are specifically relevant.

## Comment

I have seen only six cases, and all the patients had seen many doctors. The very local, tender pit was pathogno-monic and all other signs and investigations were unhelpful. All six cases were cured by surgery.

# Rectus abdominis

## Findings

Localized tenderness in the rectus abdominis, worse with sit-ups or resisted abdominals.

## Cause

Strain of the rectus abdominis, which usually occurs at one of the aponeuroses or close to the lateral wall of the rectus sheath.

## Investigations

Ultrasound scan may show unilateral hypertrophy (Fig. 7.1), a tear or muscular dysfunction; MRI may show localized muscle inflammation.

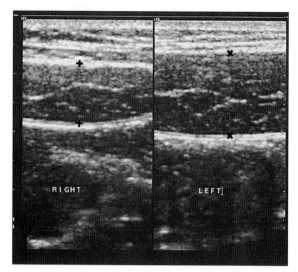

**Figure 7.1** • Ultrasound scan of a tennis player showing unilateral enlargement of the rectus abdominis (*between the two crosses*).

## Treatment

(a) Electrotherapeutic modalities to settle the inflammation.

(b) Stop sit-ups, and correct any sporting technical faults.

## Sports

(a) In general it is related to too many sit-ups during training. However, be alert to the possible abuse of anabolic steroids.

(b) Tennis – the serve may produce a unilateral, enlarged rectus abdominis, possibly because the left hip is pushed forward at the throw up, when the weight is transferred to the left side. The left hip cannot clear out of the way during the hitting phase and the rectus abdominis must 'pull the body through' the serve. Simply pulling harder with the abdominal muscles, to achieve a top spin serve, may increase the muscle loading and cause the strain, whilst the wind may disturb the accuracy of the throw up and influence muscle activity. MRI-positive, ultrasound-negative tennis players may survive a match or two, but they are best advised to retire and heal properly before returning to tennis [1].

## Comment

Not common but, if it occurs during a tennis tournament, it is frequently in its unilateral form (see Fig. 7.1), which can be quite debilitating and require local anaesthesia. I wonder if too many people work too hard on their sit ups for their rectus abdominis 'six packs'. These help flexion of the abdomen but do not stabilize the pelvis or the spine, which requires transversus abdominis work. Many sports do not require extra strong abdominal flexors.

## Epigastric discomfort

The differentials will include referral of pain from the dorsal vertebrae, cardiac ischaemia and, in the elderly, an aortic aneurysm. The epigastric causes of pain often reflect the increased acidity from tension, but in sports like cycling can indicate reflux oesophagitis or subdiaphragmatic compression from the stomach. An antacid, peppermint to 'bring up wind' or a charcoal biscuit to absorb gas will reduce this discomfort. Fizzy drinks, which are freely available at tournaments, can contribute to these problems.

## Conjoined tendon

Disruption of the conjoined tendons of the abdominal muscles causes pain in the groin and lower abdomen. There is quite marked tenderness to palpation through the inguinal canal of the external ring, which is dilated (see Chapter 8: Conjoined tendon injury).

## Pubic tubercle

Tenderness is found over the tubercle rather than the symphysis pubis, which suggests conjoined tendon disruption (see Chapter 8: Conjoined tendon injury).

## Inflammation of the pubic symphysis

There is a low abdominal ache with exercise, especially associated with groin or perineal pain, and tenderness to palpation is found over the pubic bones and symphysis (see Chapter 8: Traumatic osteitis pubis symphysis).

## Abdominal pains

Apart from the usual medical problems, where the cause is not from sport but whose presence may interfere with sport, check for melaena, which can be associated with long-distance running. No reason has been found for the melaena, though a 'slap' of the caecum has been postulated [2] and, in one case, supernumerary ligaments binding the gall bladder [3]. Runners' diarrhoea, which may be a more minor symptom from the same causative mechanism, is very common in long-distance runners.

## Renal pain

Haematuria and myoglobinuria can be associated with long periods of exercise or high-intensity exercise and in themselves are not indicative of renal disease (see Chapter 21).

## References

1   Personal communication. Conversation with Dr Philip Bell, Wimbledon tennis tournament doctor; 2006

2   Porter AM. Marathon runners and the caecal slap syndrome Br J Sports Med 1982;16(3):178

3   Dimeo FC, Peters J, Guderian H. Abdominal pain in long distance runners; case report and analysis of the literature Br J Sports Med 2004;38(5):e24

### Further reading

Bruckner P, Khan K. Clinical sports medicine, 3rd edn. New York: McGraw-Hill; 2006

Hutson M, Ellis R (eds). Textbook of musculoskeletal medicine. Oxford: Oxford University Press; 2006

Reid D. Sports injury assessment and rehabilitation. Edinburgh: Churchill Livingstone; 1992

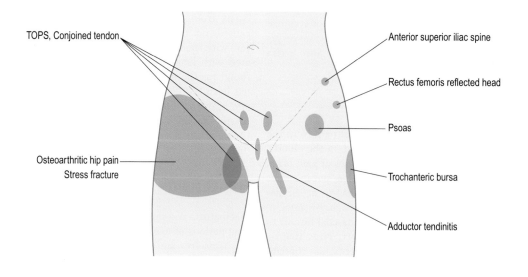

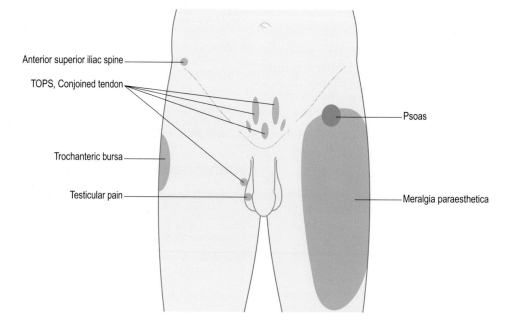

# Chapter Eight

8

# Groin

## CHAPTER CONTENTS

## Referred pain

The clinician must always check for referred pain from the spine, particularly the thoracolumbar junction from where the ilio-inguinal nerve supplies the groin (see Chapter 4: Dorsal vertebral dysfunction). Also examine the fourth and fifth lumbar segments for facetal problems as they also can refer pain to the groin (see Chapter 5, Part 2: Facet (zygapophyseal) joint). These lumbar segmental problems can be accompanied by sacroiliac joint (SIJ) and ligamentous problems, which by themselves can refer pain to the groin. For a starter, this makes accurate diagnosis of groin and pelvic pain difficult and, on top of that, the diagnosis of pelvic pain is difficult because the pelvis is a ring. If a ring structure is disturbed in one place, so a compensatory stress is placed elsewhere on the ring. Thus, a disturbance of the SIJ may physically disturb the pubic symphysis. Both structures will require treatment, but treatment of the primary cause, in this case the SIJ, is the only way to achieve a long-term cure (see Chapter 5, Part 3: Sacroiliac joint).

## Osteoarthritis of the hips

### Findings

Osteoarthritis (OA) commonly presents with pain in the hip or groin but it is also possible for there to be generalized thigh or knee pain but no hip pain. A low buttock ache may also be present and therefore it can be difficult to distinguish whether it is the back or the hip that is causing the pain. If initial back movements, tested whilst standing, bring on the pain, then sit the patient on the couch and repeat the tests; these should then be pain-free as the hip is no longer being moved. Equally, the extreme range of normal hip movements can load the pelvis and the back and cause back pain referred to the hip. Arthritic joint movements should hurt at the end of joint range, which may be restricted, either mechanically or by pain. The Trendelenburg gait and tests may be positive (see Glossary). The hip should be tested with the patient sitting, lying supine and prone. The signs may be different as the joint alignment is altered in each case but, overall, passive external and internal rotation of the hip, passive abduction and adduction, and flexion and extension are painful and/or limited.

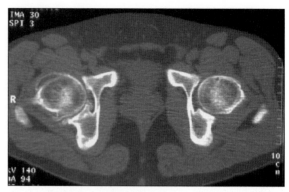

**Figure 8.1** • MRI displays gross areas of osteophytic overgrowth around the right hip joint.

## Cause

Degeneration of the articular cartilage, with cysts and sclerosis in the femoral head and/or acetabulum (see Glossary: Osteoarthritis). It is possible that sportspeople are more prone to OA, although a genetic link is also likely. The problem seems worse with impact sports, such as running and jumping. However, in therapeutic terms, total immobilization of a joint produces articular chondral degeneration of the adjacent surfaces as no synovial fluid can flow up the nutrient cannaliculi to nourish the cartilage. Hence, rehabilitation consists of non-impact exercises to move the joint and enable synovial fluid to be squeezed up the nutrient cannaliculi.

## Investigations

X-ray of the hips to look for osteophytes, a narrow joint space, cysts, sclerosis, and in a case of previous Perthes, the flattened femoral head (see Glossary: Perthes' disease; Fig. 22.15). MRI can show osteochondral damage before it is visible on an X-ray, but as the treatment is not altered by this investigation the extra cost incurred is probably not justified, unless one is trying to advise on future activity or assess a professional player's long-term employment prospects (Fig. 8.1).

## Treatment

(a) Electrotherapeutic modalities to calm the soft tissue inflammation, such as shortwave diathermy and interferential.
(b) Maintenance of muscle strength and fitness, by non-impact training (see Sports, below).

### Caveat

(a) An os acetabulare may limit hip range and this may affect martial arts performance by reducing the kicking range. Clinically, the pain is usually unidirectional (Fig. 8.2).
(b) Stress fracture of the femoral neck in the young, active, especially the oligo/amenorrhoeic runners.
(c) A patient with a fractured hip lies with the foot externally rotated.

(c) Injection of the hip joint with cortisone to calm any capsulitis.
(d) Sodium hyaluronate injection (see Glossary).
(e) Surgical replacement.

## Sports

(a) An arthritic joint must be moved within the pain-free range but the extreme ranges of movement should be avoided. Stop stretching and stop sports and exercises that force the joint to its outer, painful range.
(b) Non-impact training can be performed on a bike, the saddle may need raising if flexion of the hip is limited, and a rowing machine. Row within the pain-free range – by not 'coming too far forward' or 'laying back' too far. Whilst swimming, breaststroke should be avoided. If this is the only stroke available then a wedge kick, rather than a full frog kick, should be utilized to avoid pain.

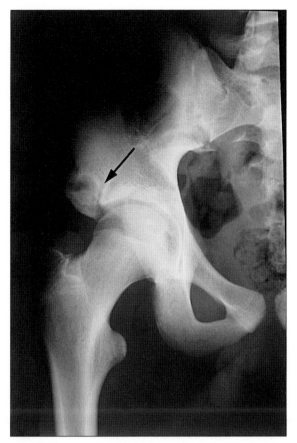

**Figure 8.2** • X-ray shows os acetabulare (*arrow*), which limited the range of some hip movements. This caused pain from impingement and a limited kicking range in a karate player.

(c) Quadriceps strength can be maintained with closed plus open chain exercises (see Glossary: Closed chain exercises). However, patients with osteoarthritis find open chain exercises less painful (see Chapter 20: Open chain and closed chain exercises).

(d) Golf, left arthritic hip – advise the patient to open the stance, use more arm swing and play a fade shot. Right hip osteoarthritis restricts the swing so that a hand and arm shot is required.

(e) Tennis – restrict play to doubles.

## Comment

I feel that there are two elements in the pain history, one capsular and synovial, the other bony. The soft tissue pain has a more continuous history, often being present at rest, whereas bony pain is associated more with movement, and especially weight-bearing. Physiotherapy, and a switch to non-impact sports, will help most people. Injection of the hip with cortisone helps the soft tissue problem and can be reserved for those with a lot of pain but little to see on X-ray. The injection can be repeated before special occasions, such as travel, holidays, etc. Patients seem to understand the need to take smaller steps, and swing both legs together when getting in or out of a car, if it is illustrated by an analogy such as being in a field surrounded by barbed wire, where one can run around inside the field with no trouble, but, if one tries to run outside the field, one runs into the barbed wire, which produces the pain.

## Labral tear of the hip

### Findings

The patient presents with anterior hip pain, which occurs in an individual, but repeatable, fashion. Certain movements of the hip are painful whilst others remain pain-free. Examination and repetition of these movements elicits the pain. There is no capsular pattern. Resisted muscle testing is not definitive.

### Investigations

X-ray and a bone scan of the hip are normal. MRI may show a capsular tear but sometimes the diagnosis is not possible until arthroscopy of the hip is performed.

### Treatment

Arthroscopic debridement of the tear, or live with the problem.

### Sports

No sports are particularly prone to this problem.

### Comment

This is one of the clinical examination conundrums, which invariably lead to further investigations. Not all patients are improved following their arthroscopy and debridement.

## Adductor muscle strain

### Findings

The onset may be acute or chronic. There is local tenderness over the adductor longus origin, or the musculotendinous junction, about 6 cm distal to the origin. If the adductor magnus is involved then tenderness may extend along the inferior pubic ramus to the ischial tuberosity. This lesion does not often present with lower abdominal pain (see Traumatic osteitis pubis symphysis (TOPS) and Conjoined tendon injury). Resisted isometric testing at the inner and outer range of the adductor muscles is painful. Resisted adductors are painful with the hip flexed.

## Cause

Chronic overuse of the adductor longus or magnus, which occurs with side steps, a side foot tackle, kicking, twisting, turning movements or a slide into abduction. If the force is high enough, or if the adductor contraction is blocked, the onset may be acute. An entheseal spur may form on the femur – the horse rider's spur.

### Caveat

(a) Exclude hip joint pathology.
(b) An adductor tendinitis may still be part of a TOPS or conjoined tendon complex, where resisted adductors are painful on testing. However, resisted adductor pain without local, palpable tenderness is not likely to be caused by the adductor muscle itself.

## Investigations

These are usually not required, but an adductor enthesopathy may display a positive bone scan and specific MRI views can display localized muscle inflammation and bony oedema. Occasionally myositis ossificans can occur, which is seen best on X-ray or ultrasound.

## Treatment

(a) Electrotherapeutic modalities to settle inflammation.
(b) Local hydrocortisone to settle inflammation.
(c) Massage techniques, such as deep or cross-friction, to reduce and realign scar tissue.
(d) Adductor stretches to limit scar tissue contraction.
(e) Isometrics to the adductors to help organize fibrocytes and maintain strength.
(f) Cross-train for fitness and start leg swinging movements, in and out of abduction.
(g) When fit to run, add the Achilles ladder through to sprints.
(h) Cross-over side steps and figure-of-eight movements. Start the kicking ladder.
(i) Rarely, surgical debridement or tenotomy.

See Chapter 20.

## Sports

(a) Acute injuries occur when side stepping, stretching for a tackle, or when a kick is blocked. Chronic injury often ensues but can come from recurrent twisting and stretching.
(b) In track and field, block starts and acceleration utilize the adductors, and if the psoas is weak – limiting the drive from hip flexion – then the adductors are required to work harder. Strengthening the psoas will thus help.

## Comment

This is a lesion that is often seen in its chronic phase. A steroid placed at the adductor longus origin, accompanied by immediate rehabilitation, often settles this lesion in 2 weeks. Then running and side steps rehabilitation can be added. Sometimes, the injection helps differentiate the adductor lesion from the conjoined tendon injury and TOPS, as the adductor lesion improves whilst the others are not affected.

## Conjoined tendon injury

See in conjunction with Traumatic osteitis pubis symphysis (TOPS).

## Findings

There is a history of groin pain and suprapubic or low abdominal pain. This may be severe enough to cause the patient to bend over double, and there may be an accompanying adductor lesion (see above). However, the conjoined tendon lesion, by itself, is not tender to palpation at the adductor origin, although resisted adduction does produce the symptoms. Besides breaststroke, even swimming backstroke or front crawl hurts. Turning over in bed may produce pain in the low abdomen.

Resisted abdominals hurt, as does palpation of the external ring through the invaginated scrotum. This is a rare lesion in women. If the external ring is not tender, and no diagnosis can be made, then, over a

2-week period, one may have to run the patient daily, through the Achilles ladder (high knees and sprints) to provoke the injury. Sometimes, after 2 weeks, the patient breaks through the pain and is cured, whilst with others the external ring becomes increasingly painful to palpation and the diagnosis is confirmed. Often the contralateral side may produce symptoms after the primary side has been treated.

## Cause

There is disruption or degeneration of the conjoined tendon of the abdominal muscles at their attachment to the pubic tubercle. A crypt hernia may be present. Because the pelvis may be considered as a ring, there may be two or more injury sites in conjunction, such as the sacroiliac joint and the pubic symphysis. The cause may be from performing excessive sit-ups, or from twisting and backing off movements, such as in basketball, or in midfield soccer players who, whilst defending, may have the ball played back and forth across them. Possibly a limited hip range will predispose to this condition because, if the body's rotation is limited at the hip, the stress is forced onto the next link in the chain, which is the pelvis. TOPS may be the end stage of a continuum of damage to the conjoined tendon and pubis.

## Investigations

(a) Though a bone scan will exclude any differential stress fracture, such as sacral or pubic, an MRI scan will display whether there is bone oedema and can display soft tissue damage.

(b) X-ray. Flamingo/stork/one-legged standing views are normal if the symphysis has not been disrupted and will also exclude osteoarthritis of the hip (see Glossary: Osteoarthritis, Stork view; Fig. 8.3).

(c) Abdominal herniograms may be positive but are of debatable clinical value. (See Traumatic osteitis pubis symphysis.)

## Treatment

(a) Inject the pubic tubercle with a local anaesthetic and hydrocortisone for short-term relief.

(b) Surgical plication of the conjoined tendon.

(c) Rest, which may take 12–18 months to bring about healing, but with controlled exercise may

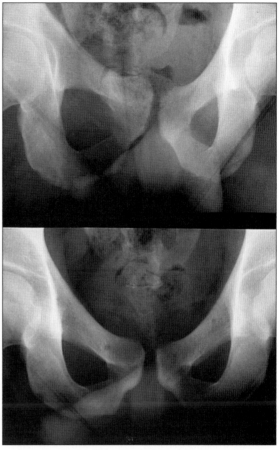

**Figure 8.3** • Flamingo or stork X-rays. If standing on one leg and then the other shows movement in the pubic symphysis greater than 2 mm, the pubic symphysis is considered to be unstable.

be the treatment of choice when surgery is not available.

(d) Controlled exercise. Cross-training on a bike (rowing or swimming may cause problems). Achilles ladder, then add cross-over, side step runs, plus figure-of-eight and kicking ladder (see Chapter 20). Reduce sit-ups and certainly avoid rotational sit-ups such as 'crunches'.

 Caveat

**There may be pubic tubercle or inguinal nerve sensitivity post operation, when an injection with a local anaesthetic and hydrocortisone will help.**

## Sports

This lesion has been reported as TOPS in many sports. However, there may be a continuum – the conjoined tendon being the precursor of TOPS. The overall impression is that twisting and turning movements with one foot fixed, such as stretching out for a ball, side stepping, or kicking is the major problem, for with good, small-step footwork, the conjoined tendon sufferer can often play squash (see Traumatic osteitis pubis symphysis).

## Comment

This is still a difficult diagnosis to make, and sometimes comes down to no other diagnosis being available, plus the patient fails to rehabilitate. There seems to be an increased diagnosis of this problem. Are there in fact more of these injuries, or are they being recognized more frequently? I do believe too many sit-ups are trained, especially with twists, for no improvement in performance. Some professionals are returned to their sports too soon after surgery, when they either break down again or get a contralateral injury. If this is a tear of the conjoined tendon then one must question the surgical placement of a mesh to control a hernia, as opposed to repair of the tendon. Excision of the inguinal nerve at the same time reduces pain rapidly, but is this treating the cause or blocking the symptomatology? Prophylaxis has to be the way forward.

## Traumatic osteitis pubis symphysis (TOPS)

### Findings

As for a conjoined tendon injury. The TOPS sufferer may describe the pain as radiating into the perineum or rectum.

### Cause

Degenerative changes are found in the pubis or pubic symphysis, which may be part of a disturbance of the pelvic ring. The pubic symphysis becomes unstable.

### Investigations

(a) X-ray. Stork/flamingo/one-legged standing views show an unstable pubic symphysis, with greater than 2 mm shift (see Fig. 8.3). X-ray of the later stages shows areas of lysis and sclerosis in the pubic symphysis.

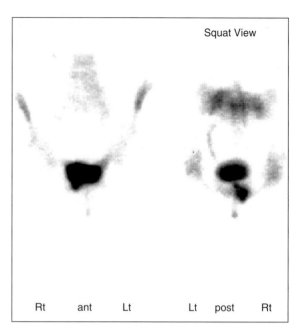

Squat View

Rt    ant    Lt          Lt    post    Rt

**Figure 8.4 •** Bone scans of the pubis should be taken in the squat position to separate the bladder signal from the bone signal.

(b) Bone scan. Squat views may be hot and asymmetrical (Fig. 8.4).

(c) Blood tests for HLA-B27, anti-nuclear factor and rheumatoid factor should be performed if the gracilis margin is fluffy or eroded (Fig. 8.5).

(d) Specific views on MRI may show bony oedema in the pubis and a fracture line (Figs 8.6 and 8.7), disruption of the symphysis capsule, both inferior and superior, and confirmed anteroposterior translation of the pubic symphysis (see Stress fracture of the pelvis: pubic ramus).

### Caveat

Fluffy erosion of the gracilis margin may be from either ankylosing spondylitis or rheumatoid arthritis (see Fig. 8.5), but ankylosis of the pubic symphysis is caused by ankylosing spondylitis (Fig. 8.8).

### Treatment

(a) Local anaesthetic and hydrocortisone into the pubic symphysis for temporary relief [1].

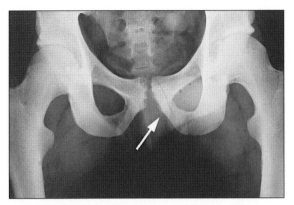

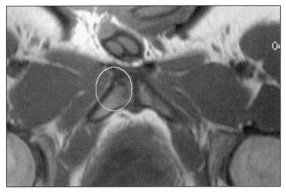

**Figure 8.5** • X-ray shows cysts and sclerosis, with erosion of the gracilis margin, in the pubic symphysis of a young footballer with ankylosing spondylitis (*arrow*). Groin pain and erosion of the gracilis margin may be the first presentation of ankylosing spondylitis.

**Figure 8.7** • A black line in the right pubic bone indicates a stress fracture.

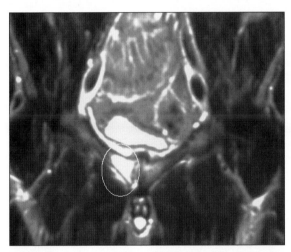

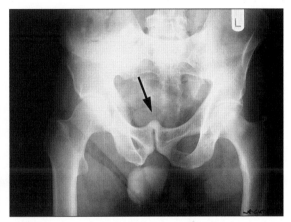

**Figure 8.8** • Ankylosis of the pubic symphysis and sacroiliac joints.

**Figure 8.6** • Bony oedema in the right pubis suggests that the stresses across the pubic symphysis are not all through the joint.

**(h)** Controlled rehabilitation and core stability (see Chapter 20).

## Sports

**(a)** Change of direction sports may cause the problem if the 'side to side' and rotational movements are not accompanied by good footwork. When the 'play' goes from side to side across the player, as in a midfield footballer, then the player has to stretch for the ball or to make a tackle. An extreme stretch will force external rotation of the hip to its end range. Because the hip can no longer contribute to abduction, the abduction force reaches the pelvis and the weakest point, the pubic symphysis, comes under load. Athletes with a limited hip range may be more liable to injury

**(b)** Rest and cross-train for 12–18 months.

**(c)** Try conjoined tendon repair, if less than 3 mm shift on stork views.

**(d)** Sclerosants to the sacroiliac joints to strengthen the pelvic ring [2].

**(e)** Pamidronate infusion or intramuscular injection may reduce the bone oedema and pain.

**(f)** Rarely, surgery to fuse the pubic symphysis if it remains unstable after the appropriate rest.

**(g)** Treat any systemic cause.

[3]. Players may have to channel the opposition in one direction to avoid the ball being played across them.

**(b)** When TOPS has occurred swimming is painful, and not just breaststroke but also backstroke and front crawl produce abdominal pain.

**(c)** Cross-training should be on a rowing ergo to maintain equal pressure on both sides of the pelvic ring, and then asymmetry of load, by cycling and running, can be added later.

**(d)** Sit-ups should be avoided.

**(e)** Running probably should not start for 12–18 months, and sprinting and high knee raises may be difficult until truly stable.

## Comment

TOPS may be the end point of an unstable pelvic ring, where the conjoined tendon strain is the early phase. Do we do too many sit-ups, and are they relevant, or is it twisting across the pubis that causes the problem? The erosion of the gracilis margin certainly must lead to investigation for ankylosing spondylitis in the young, and when this sign is present on X-ray it is often not recognized. TOPS can be considered as being equivalent to a fractured pelvis, which will take 18–24 months to heal, and so one should question whether the players are returned too soon to activities. In several cases of mine, like Chakraverty [2], sclerosants to the sacroiliac joints have helped stabilize the pubic symphysis. This may be utilizing the ring theory, where a ring cannot be disturbed in only one place, so at least two sites will be disturbed; therefore, if two sites are stabilized (the sacroiliac joints), the third (the pubic symphysis) will be helped.

## Rectus femoris origin

### Findings

Although the presentation may be of weakness when running or kicking, a careful history elicits an injury, an acute incident or low-grade pain with these activities, and this is particularly so in an adolescent when the episode may be acute. There is local tenderness over the anterior rim of the acetabulum or anterior superior iliac spine. Resisted, supine, straight leg raise is weak and can be painful, as may be resisted flexion of the hip. Quadriceps stretch is reduced and painful and the modified Thomas test is positive (see Glossary).

There may be variable passive hip signs, which are not diagnostic. In an adult, a slip, stumble or kicking may cause the injury, as well as gradual overload.

## Cause

An enthesopathy or, especially in the growth phase, avulsion apophysitis. This occurs at the acetabular reflexion or anterior inferior iliac spine (Figs 8.9 and 8.10; see Chapter 10: Torn rectus femoris muscle).

### Caveat

**(a)** This injury is prone to myositis ossificans. carry out X-ray or ultrasound on the patient who has a history of getting worse, with or without treatment, over the 5 days post injury (Fig. 8.11).

**(b)** Weakness – check L3/4 nerve root of the lumbar spine.

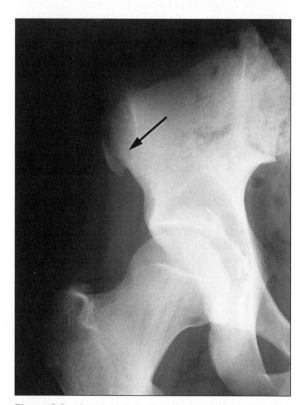

**Figure 8.9 •** Anterior inferior iliac spine avulsion is the most typical finding in an adolescent following a sprint race (*arrow*).

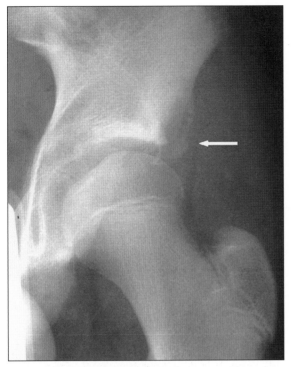

Figure 8.10 • Avulsion of the reflected head is not common, though tenderness of this area is a typical finding with rectus femoris injuries.

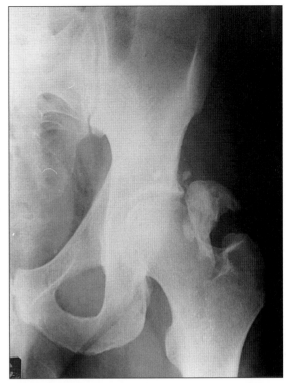

Figure 8.11 • Myositis ossificans in the rectus femoris origin.

## Investigations

An X-ray will display an avulsion or myositis ossificans (see Fig. 8.11). Diagnostic ultrasound will show the myositis, tear, and probably the avulsion and it is the investigation of choice if a 'hip pointer' haematoma is suspected.

## Treatment

(a) RICE (see Glossary). The patient may require crutches for the first few days.

(b) TENS or interferential can provide minimal contractions of the rectus femoris in the early treatment and rehabilitation of adolescents limited by pain.

(c) Stretch the quadriceps, especially with hip extension.

(d) Lying supine to extend the hip and then raise a straight leg, with no added weights, until the patient can manage 20–25 repetitions without pain, then add weights when free of pain.

(e) Quadriceps ladders.

(f) Kicking ladder (see Chapter 20: Knee ladder).

(g) If myositis ossificans is developing then only rest and stretch gently until the myositis is 'mature', plus prescribe an anti-inflammatory such as indomethacin.

(h) This injury often takes a while to heal and can be monitored by testing any weakness of straight leg raise rather than by assessing pain, which disappears from the later stages of healing.

## Sports

(a) This injury is associated with kicking but may also be seen in the first few 100 metre sprint races of the summer, especially in the adolescent.

(b) Baseball players may slide into base and traumatize the soft tissues, producing a haematoma over the iliac crest.

## Comment

This is more common than expected and the persistent hip pain is often caused by rectus femoris weakness. The adolescent often has an avulsion or enthesitis that takes several weeks to settle. Myositis is quite common in the adult. This injury was common in mini-rugby until tackling over the try line was abolished. The try scorer would often kneel down to score and the tackler would pull the try scorer's back and hip into extension, avulsing the rectus femoris origin.

## Psoas strain/bursitis

### Findings

Groin pain with, or following, hill running, high knee drills or running on muddy ground when the foot has to be pulled out of the ground. Sometimes running bent over, as in field hockey. Passive hip flexion beyond 90° produces groin pain and resisted hip flexion at 90° is painful. There is tenderness to palpation at about two fingers' breadth, lateral to the femoral artery at the groin. Psoas stretch is tight and painful (see Glossary: Thomas test, modified). Straight leg sit-up, or leg raise may cause pain. A weak psoas may cause anterior knee pain or adductor tendinitis as psoas weakness reduces active hip flexion, thus encouraging a low knee, valgus movement, and it can present with atypical movement patterns when trying to run (see Chapter 11).

### Cause

Inflammation of the psoas bursa. Weakness and strain of the psoas muscle with, occasionally, avulsion or enthesopathy of the lesser trochanter (Fig. 8.12)

### Investigations

Clinically not required. Ultrasound can show increased signal in a bursa and helps guide the injection, but an X-ray and bone scan are required to exclude avulsion of the lesser trochanter. MRI if not progressing.

### Treatment

(a) Electrotherapeutic modalities to settle inflammation of the bursa, such as ultrasound and interferential.
(b) Local injection of the bursa with cortisone.
(c) Massage, stretching of the hip and isometric hip flexion at 90° to control scar tissue.

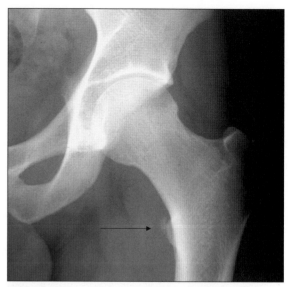

**Figure 8.12** • Avulsion of the psoas attachment at the lesser trochanter.

(d) Cross-training and rest from hip flexion, especially if there is an enthesitis or avulsion of the lesser trochanter.
(e) Isometric hip flexion at 90°, for strength.
(f) High knee drills of the affected leg whilst standing on the other.
(g) Achilles ladder. Concentrate on the high knee section (see Chapter 20).

### Sports

(a) This is often seen in runners, especially runners who carry their knees low and often into valgus, who then start speed drills or hill running, which requires a higher knee lift.
(b) Field hockey and cross-country skiing can produce the problem in the unfit – one by a crouched running style, the other by an overload when the leg is swung forwards.

### Comment

The psoas weakness, which reduces hip flexion and therefore speed and acceleration, may go unnoticed, but it should be looked for in many knee, leg and ankle problems. Rehabilitation of this muscle may be the key to settling the other problems. The lesser trochanteric enthesitis takes patience and time to settle.

# Stress fracture of the femoral neck

## Findings

There has often been a period when the patient has noticed a low-grade ache in the groin when running, but some present with an acute exacerbation of pain. The pain may radiate to the knee or even be referred to as sciatica. Sitting lumbar spine movements are pain-free but there are capsular signs in the hip, or bizarre undiagnostic signs and protection of hip movements. If in doubt, investigate for a stress fracture.

## Cause

Overload of the femoral neck through impact training or running. Two types are recognized: the superior surface (tensioning) type in Babcock's triangle, and the inferior surface (compression) type in Ward's triangle (see Glossary). However an intertrochanteric variety may also be encountered. The superior type is prone to complete fracture and subsequent avascular necrosis, even after surgical pinning. Beware mid- to long-distance, underweight, female runners with oligo/amenorrhoea (the female athlete's triad) as they are more prone to osteoporosis and atypical stress fractures.

## Investigations

Atypical hip pain and thigh pain in runners and army recruits [4] should be bone scanned. The advantage of the bone scan at this stage is that it will show up pubic, pelvic and femoral shaft lesions that may enter the diagnostic differentials. An X-ray as a first line might display the diagnosis, but is often negative. If the area to be MRI scanned is localizable to the hip area, this would be the investigation of choice as MRI will also display any hip joint pathomechanics. Consider a CT scan for further assessment of the extent of the stress fracture, particularly if there is a black line on MRI.

## Treatment

### Tensioning type (superior surface)

(Figures 8.13 and 8.14)

(a) Initial treatment is non-weight-bearing until the patient can stand without pain. At this stage they may weight-bear with crutches, then walk with a stick, and finally walk unsupported. A trial of non-impact cross-training, such as

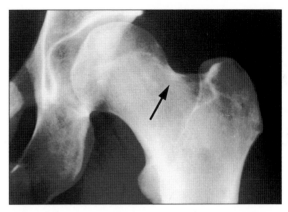

**Figure 8.13** • Fortunately the area of sclerosis in the superior surface of the femoral neck suggests healing of this stress fracture. CT scan would be required to exclude non-union (*arrow*).

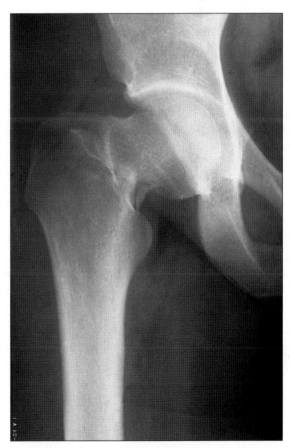

**Figure 8.14** • A disaster in a young athlete: this tension stress fracture has completed and will need surgical pinning. Avascular necrosis may still occur.

rowing, swimming or cycling, may be started when the patient has no pain at rest.

(b) When pain-free walking is obtained, gradually introduce running on soft ground with shock-absorbing shoes.

(c) Achilles ladder when running skills and technique might also be improved (see Chapter 20).

(d) Observe frequently, this is the problem stress lesion. If CT has shown an extension of the lesion beyond the cortex into the medulla, or there is failure to progress, then surgical pinning should be considered.

## Compression type

Treat similarly to the tensioning type, but this type usually heals without surgery (Fig. 8.15).

## Both types

Patients of both types require:

(a) training advice on how to increase distance and speed (see Chapter 20)

(b) cross-training for endurance training (runners) – only using running for tempo, pace training and speed work

(c) diet and weight checks, particularly for oligo/amenorrhoeic runners – and consider a hormonal assay and bone density scan.

## Comment

Because of the disaster caused by avascular necrosis, it is better to investigate with a scan and put the patient on crutches if there is the slightest doubt that a stress fracture might exist (Fig. 8.16). Subtrochanteric stress fractures are reported [5]. These intertrochanteric stress fractures seem to occur in the less skillful runners and power walkers where, perhaps, an altered muscular pattern is at work on the femur.

## Stress fractures of the pelvis: sacrum

See Chapter 5.

## Findings

Sacroiliac pain that is worse on impact. The back movements are pain-free, but sacroiliac and pelvic compression tests are positive.

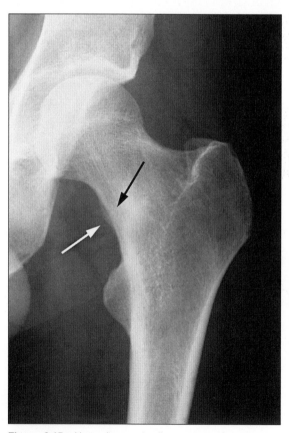

**Figure 8.15** • X-ray shows a healing compression stress fracture (*arrows*). This lesion, unlike the tension stress fracture, is unlikely to fracture completely.

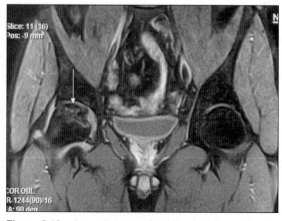

**Figure 8.16** • Avascular necrosis of the right femoral head.

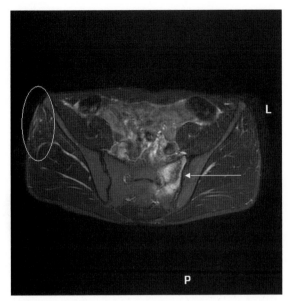

**Figure 8.17** • An MRI scan displays a tensor fasciae latae muscle lesion (*circle*) and a left-sided stress fracture of the sacrum (*arrow*). Though this appeared to be MRI grade 4, it was painless, symptomless, and not visible on CT. The MRI changes had settled in 6 months.

## Cause

This is an uncommon overuse fracture, possibly from unaccustomed repetition sprints on a Tartan surface, found in oligo/amenorrhoeic track and field athletes (see Chapter 5, Part 3: Sacroiliac joint) [5], though it has been reported in army recruits [6] and seen in runners with altered stride patterns due to other injuries (see comment below).

## Investigations

MRI (Fig. 8.17) or bone scan (see Fig. 5.18). Note that the sacroiliac joint can appear hot. A CT scan may be required for pain-free grade 4 MRI lesions that are found incidentally, as they can be invisible on CT , thus permitting exercise to continue to a limited extent.

## Treatment

Non-impact, cross-training for 8–12 weeks. Check diet and hormonal status of the oligo/amenorrhoeic patients and include bone densitometry in both male and female.

## Sports

(a) Long-distance female road runners, but has been seen in men, extending into the ilium [7].

(b) Elite recruits [6].

## Comment

An uncommon lesion. An elite athlete realized, 1 month before a major championship, that at these high levels races were won by sprinting at the end of a 5000 or 10 000 m race. She suddenly added large numbers of repetition sprints around the bend to her training, with disastrous results (see Fig. 5.18). Another patient strained his tibialis anterior at work but ran with an altered style, which produced a tensor fasciae latae strain, followed by a bursa over the iliac crest. An MRI scan at that time also showed a grade 4 stress fracture in the contralateral sacrum. This fracture was totally pain-free. It was not visualized on CT scan and was invisible on MRI 6 months later (see Fig. 8.17).

# Stress fractures of the pelvis: pubic ramus

## Findings

There is atypical pelvic pain, which may refer to the pubis and perineum or down the leg. It is worse with activity. Examination must exclude pain from lumbar referral, hip, adductors, and hamstrings.

## Cause

Though this fracture can be seen in a fall of the elderly, in sport it is an uncommon, overuse fracture, usually of the inferior pubic ramus but occasionally in the superior pubic ramus. It is found mainly in long-distance oligo/amenorrhoeic female runners. However, MRI scans for pubic symphyseal pain are also showing fracture lines in the pubis rather than the ramus. This is covered in this chapter under Traumatic ostetis pubis (see Figs 8.6 and 8.7).

## Investigations

X-ray may show callus because the athlete has trained through the pain, producing a chronic lesion (Fig. 8.18). However, when there is referral of pain and the exact source of pain is unknown then the bone scan is the best investigation. MRI scans display early oedema and the fracture line (see Figs 8.6 and 8.7).

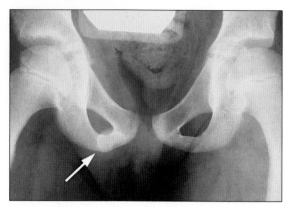

**Figure 8.18** • Callus in the inferior pubic ramus from a stress fracture (*arrow*).

## Treatment

Cross-training without impact for 6–8 weeks, then train via the hamstring ladder (see Chapter 20). Check the hormonal state and diet of the oligo/amenorrhoeic athlete (see Chapter 21: Bone density/osteoporosis).

## Sports

Female long-distance road runners.

## Comment

In sport, I have seen this lesion only in oligo/amenorrhoeic female, long-distance runners.

## Obturator nerve entrapment [8]

### Findings

There is exercise-induced medial thigh pain, commencing in the region of the adductor muscle origin and radiating distally along the medial thigh. The patient may have to be sent out to exercise just before the clinical examination. Hyperextension of the thigh may reproduce the symptoms.

### Cause

Entrapment of the obturator nerve by thick fascia overlying the short adductor muscles.

### Investigations

Electromyogram of the obturator nerve is invariably positive. Obturator nerve block will produce weakness in the appropriate muscle, and a cuticular patch anaesthesia in the mid-medial thigh.

### Treatment

Surgical release or alteration in activity.

### Sports

Seen mainly in Australian rules football, but soccer, running and netball have reported cases.

### Comment

This is not a common diagnosis, but in cases of non-responding groin pain, even with MRI scan showing some oedema over the pubic bone and adductor origin, this diagnosis must be considered. The referral down the thigh and the feeling of altered sensation and perhaps weakness are indicative. My running patient, treated conservatively, stopped his quadriceps stretching exercises, reduced his mileage and settled without further treatment.

## Neuroma

Many sportspeople have suffered trauma around the pelvis, and some superficial nerves may be caught in scar tissue. Checks should be made for local point tenderness, especially over the iliac crests, for the long cutaneous nerve to the thigh and in any inguinal hernial or conjoined tendon repair.

## Meralgia paraesthetica

Pain over the anterior aspect of the thigh, with local point tenderness sited somewhere from the iliac crest to the upper mid-thigh (see Chapter 10).

## Os acetabulare

Probably seen incidentally on X-ray (see Glossary; Fig. 8.2), but it can limit the range of hip movement where, in sports like gymnastics, hockey goalkeeping and marshal arts, it is a problem.

## Inguinal glands

Apart from the usual systemic, perianal and genital causes, athletes should be checked for tinea pedis and tinea cruris. Infected or chronic lacerations in the lower limb from opponents' studs are often causative.

## Inguinal hernia

Diagnosed by a bulge, swelling and palpable cough impulse over the external ring (see medical textbooks).

## Femoral hernia

This is not a common lesion and is, quite often, a difficult diagnosis to make. There is tenderness, and perhaps a swelling, in the femoral triangle, usually in a female (see medical textbooks).

## Torsion of the testis

Examination reveals a painful testis lying in the horizontal plane. If this cannot be reduced into a pain-free vertical plane then urgent surgery is required to save the testis.

## References

1   Holt MA, Keene JS, Graf BK, Helwig DC. Treatment of osteitis pubis in athletes. Results of cortico steroid injections. Am J Sports Med 1995;23:601–606

2   Chakraverty RC. A case of osteitis pubis secondary to unilateral sacroiliac joint instability treated with prolotherapy. J Orthop Med 2003;25(1):10–13

3   Williams JG. Limitation of hip joint movement as a factor in traumatic osteitis pubis. Br J Sports Med 1978;12:129–133

4   Stoneham MD, Morgan NV. Stress fractures of the hip in Royal Marine recruits under training: a retrospective analysis. Br J Sports Med 1991;25:145–148

5   Leinberry CF, McShane RB, Stewart WG, Hume EL. A displaced subtrochanteric stress fracture in a young amenorrheic athlete. Am J Sports Med 1992;20:485–487

6   Kiuru MJ, Niva M, Reponen A, Pihlajamäki HK. Bone stress injuries in asymptomatic elite recruits. Am J Sports Med 2005;33:272–276

7   Bell P. Discussion during joint consultation; 2004

8   Bradshaw C, McCrory P, Bell S, Brukner P. Obturator nerve entrapment. A cause of groin pain in athletes. Am J Sports Med 1997;25(3):402–408

## Further reading

Bruckner P, Khan K. Clinical sports medicine, 3rd edn. New York: McGraw-Hill; 2006

Hutson M, Ellis R (eds). Textbook of musculoskeletal medicine. Oxford: Oxford University Press; 2006

Reid D. Sports injury assessment and rehabilitation. Edinburgh: Churchill Livingstone; 1992

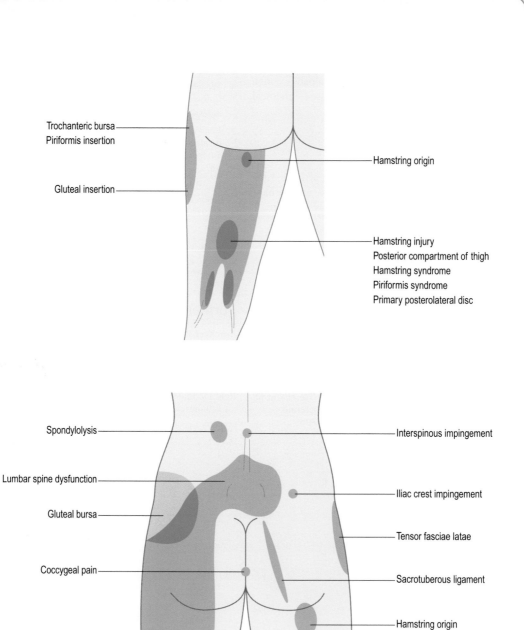

Trochanteric bursa
Piriformis insertion

Gluteal insertion

Hamstring origin

Hamstring injury
Posterior compartment of thigh
Hamstring syndrome
Piriformis syndrome
Primary posterolateral disc

Spondylolysis

Interspinous impingement

Lumbar spine dysfunction

Iliac crest impingement

Gluteal bursa

Tensor fasciae latae

Coccygeal pain

Sacrotuberous ligament

Hamstring origin

# Buttock and back of thigh

## Referred pain

Pain from a primary posterolateral disc, usually L5/S1, may exist in the back of the thigh without accompanying back pain, and examination of the spine must be the first part of the clinical examination. Both facet joints and the sacroiliac joint can also refer pain to the thigh and must be excluded as causative before examin-

ing for more local causes (see Chapters 2 and 5). Pelvic pain is difficult to diagnose. Some injuries seem to have discernable patterns whilst others require further investigation to establish a diagnosis. An MRI scan may show oedema in the hip stabilizers, for which we have no recognized diagnostic pattern. These hip stabilizers are the rotator cuff of the hip and may prove to be as important to management as the rotator cuff is to the shoulder.

### Caveat

**Abnormal painless muscle swelling around the pelvis and upper thigh may be sarcomatous.**

## Hamstring syndrome

### Findings

The patient gives a history of sciatica, with night pain, leg pain, 'pins and needles' and numbness that is worse with exercise. This is differentiated from spinal sciatica by testing the patient whilst sitting. When the back is tested with the patient standing, the back movements will also stress the leg muscles, which may be the source of pain. If the back is tested with the patient seated then the leg muscles do not contribute and pain is likely to be from the back. Peripheral nerve stress tests, straight leg raise and Lasègue's test are positive, but the slump test, Valsalva and Kernig's test are negative as the dura is not involved in the lesion (see Glossary: Dural stress tests). Straight leg raise may be worse with internal rotation of the hip, as this bows the sciatic nerve across the biceps femoris at its attachment to the ischeal tuberosity. Localized tenderness over the lateral ischeal tuberosity may be palpated and may produce leg pain.

## Cause

The sciatic nerve is bowed and irritated by the biceps femoris attachment to the ischeal tuberosity.

## Investigations

X-ray to exclude avulsion of the ischeal tuberosity but, if in doubt, bone scan or MRI for a tuberosity lesion, or MRI scan of the lumbar spine to exclude a disc lesion. The MRI probably does not display the bowing of the sciatic nerve around the biceps femoris. EMG is probably not much help.

## Treatment

Adverse neural tensioning with the leg internally rotated, together with perineural cortisone injection around the lateral ischeal tuberosity to reduce inflammation. Surgical release of the biceps femoris origin [1].

## Sports

None are of clinical relevance. Rehabilitate via the Hamstring ladder (see Chapter 20).

## Comment

Rare. I have seen only two cases and both did well with adverse neural tensioning and cortisone around the tuberosity, although, in several cases in Finland, surgery has been successful [1].

# Piriformis syndrome

## Findings

Similar to the hamstring syndrome (above) but no ischial tenderness is palpable. It may be worse with resisted, external rotation of the flexed hip, or passive, internal rotation of the flexed hip.

## Cause

The sciatic nerve is compressed between the gemelli or, as a variant, passes through, as opposed to beneath, the piriformis.

## Investigations

(a) X-ray to exclude bony causes from the hip, pelvis and ischial tuberosity.
(b) Bone scan, or MRI the pelvis to exclude stress fractures and ischial enthesitis.
(c) MRI to rule out other causes, especially disc lesions.

## Treatment

Adverse neural tensioning and, possibly, a cortisone injection of the piriformis origin at the sacrum may help. Surgery to free the nerve.

## Comment

Very rare, and difficult to diagnose. In fact there are a wide number of differing criteria postulated for the piriformis syndrome [2]. I find the criteria that I have given above help me most in my management. I do not think this is the same problem that occurs after a case of an established disc and sciatica. Here, I wonder if the lack of movement, sustained by the sciatic nerve, allows adhesions to tether it as it passes through the greater sciatic notch. An injection of steroid over the inferior border of the sacrum, close to the notch, may help this type of sciatic pain.

# Hamstring muscle injury

## Findings

There is a history of an acute, non-traumatic injury during activities, with or without bruising tracking down to the back of the knee. (The bruising may appear 3–4 days after the incident.) There is pain on stretching or resisted testing of the hamstring. The hamstring is best tested with the patient lying prone so the leg can be tested against resistance, with a flexed knee and a straight knee. Resisted knee flexion and straight leg hip extension are painful. The hamstring lesion may be able to resist the examiner without pain, so the chair test can be utilized during the consultation to increase the loading on the hamstring (see Glossary: Chair test). A chronic hamstring injury with no bruising is more difficult to assess, because straight leg raising will be painful and Lasègue's test is often ambiguous, suggesting the possibility of referred pain from the back. The slump test stretches the hamstring and invariably produces pain, but this pain is not relieved when the patient raises his or her head during the slump test. Local tenderness over the ischeal tuberosity suggests possible avulsion [3,4] or enthesitis, whereas local, palpable tenderness in the muscle is usually 6 cm off the origin or over the muscle lesion itself.

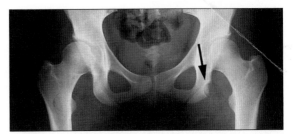

**Figure 9.1** • X-ray shows a discrete avulsion of the ischial tuberosity caused by stretching into front and back splits.

## Cause

A tear or sprain of the hamstring. The hamstring crosses two joints. Contraction of the hamstrings should extend the hip and flex the knee. Occasionally the hip is flexed whilst the knee is flexed and this paradoxical movement is known as Lombard's paradox. This paradoxical movement can be overloaded during the change of cadence from the acceleration to the cruise phase of sprinting (about 30–40 metres into the race), bending whilst running (reaching for a ball, dipping for the line), or checking hard for a side step. Although the quadriceps/ hamstring ratio is often quoted at 70% on isokinetic testing at 90° per second, the balance in fact alters at faster speeds, depending on the sport [5]. Most become less quadriceps dominant, and indeed runners may become hamstring dominant. Some isokinetic tests (unreported from my clinic) in the prone position (extended hip) displayed a weakness in the hamstring that was not displayed when the hamstring was tested sitting (flexed hip). Tests also suggest that either the weak or the strong leg might be damaged, the strong leg presumably overworking to make up for the weak leg. Thus rehabilitation may have to be designed to train the weak, non-damaged muscle as well. EMG studies show that the hamstring decelerates the extending knee ready for impact (co-activation of the hamstring and quadriceps), so that downhill running or a sudden dip in the ground can upset this coordination, producing a tear [6]. Thus a forced hurdles-style stretch can often provoke contraction of the hamstring, the very muscle one is stretching, and produces an avulsion of the hamstring origin at the ischium (Fig. 9.1). A violent fall into hip flexion can avulse the hamstring origin [4] (Fig. 9.2).

## Investigations

(a) X-ray, bone scan or MRI if avulsion of the ischium is suspected [4] (see Figs 9.1, 9.3 and 9.4).

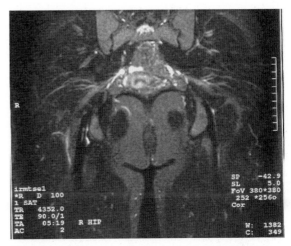

**Figure 9.2** • MRI shows a degenerative tear in the right hamstring tendon, and an ischial bursa from a fall backwards that forced a straight leg 'piked' flexion at the hips.

### Caveat

A primary posterolateral disc may present with no back pain, only leg pain. Straight leg raising, Lasègue's and slump tests may be positive, and resisted hamstrings should not hurt. A history of gradual onset of pain and no acute hamstring episode suggests a disc lesion. Any history of 'pins and needles' or numbness suggests a nerve lesion. An epidural is often required but long, strong traction [7], McKenzie extensions and extension posture may reduce the disc herniation faster (see Chapter 5).

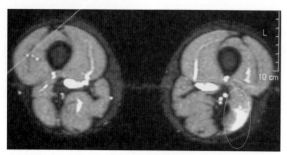

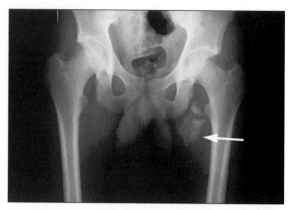

**Figure 9.3** • Though a clinical diagnosis and progress through rehabilitation governs the management of hamstring injuries, the oedema or a tear seen on MRI can help elite teams plan their selection strategies.

**Figure 9.5** • Myositis ossificans in the hamstring, which suggests that a small ischial avulsion has also occurred.

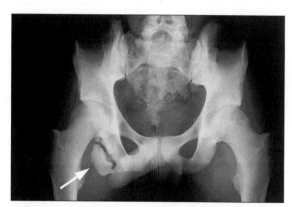

**Figure 9.4** • This avulsion of the ischial tuberosity is chronic, having remained attached by fibrous union and continued to grow. They frequently result in symptomatic non-union and should be fixed surgically [8].

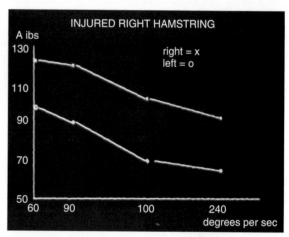

**Figure 9.6** • Isokinetic dynamometry shows that the undamaged leg is the weaker leg and that the damage has occurred in the stronger leg. Clinicians cannot assume that strengthening of the damaged leg is the correct management.

### Caveat

Very occasionally, an acute hamstring muscle tear may keep bleeding within the fascial compartment and produce an acute compartment syndrome. Increasing pain at rest must be taken seriously (see Posterior compartment of the thigh).

**(b)** Real-time ultrasound and MRI scan will display a haematoma, and the MRI can show oedema, intratendinous lesions (Fig. 9.5) and an ischial bursitis (see Fig. 9.2). Ultrasound may show scarring.

**(c)** Isokinetic dynamometry at varying speeds, both sitting and prone, can display a weakness which may not be in the damaged leg (Fig. 9.6) (see Cause above).

### Treatment

**(a)** RICE (see Glossary).

**(b)** Electrotherapeutic modalities to calm inflammation. Massage techniques, such as effluage and frictions, to remove fluid and any haematoma, plus cross-friction to encourage fibrocyte orientation.

**(c)** Aspiration of any haematoma, under ultrasound guidance, will hasten recovery.

**(d)** Stretching to prevent scar contraction.

(e) Hamstring ladders – bottom and top (see Chapter 20). Note that sometimes the injured leg may be the strong leg; therefore the weak, undamaged leg must be strengthened and trained.

(f) Cortisone to the ischial tuberosity if the ischial bursa is inflamed (see Fig. 9.2), or the scar tissue is adhesive, followed by hamstring stretching and the rehabilitation ladders.

(g) Epidural. There does appear to be some neural element causing persistent hamstring pain, in which case an epidural can be highly successful in curing this problem, especially if the slump test is just positive.

(h) Surgical debridement of the tuberosity or resuture of any avulsion [3].

(i) Early resuturing of avulsed hamstring origin ruptures [4,8].

(j) Sacroiliac joint manipulation is thought to occasionally alter the relative position of the pelvis, and thus the tension of the hamstring origin from the ischial tuberosity. This therapy may be treating only referred pain.

## Sports

This injury can occur in most sports, and rehabilitation should be completed before attempting match competition. A previous hamstring injury predisposes to a further injury so rehabilitation must be satisfactorily completed. Hamstring training should be maintained even when the athlete is back to full competition.

## Comment

This is a common injury. The primary posterolateral disc is often misdiagnosed as a hamstring lesion and I have seen ischial avulsion several times from the hurdles-type stretching exercises. The hurdle-style stretch should not be forced because this stimulates the co-activation of the hamstring as the knee straightens. I feel ballistic stretching should also be used to train up hamstring co-activation (see Chapter 20). An epidural can prove very effective with patients who do not seem to progress with their hamstring lesion and who have a possible 'slump positive'.

## Piriformis muscle

### Findings

Pain in the buttock and towards the greater trochanter at its posterior aspect, where it is tender to palpation.

There may also be referred pain towards the anterior hip, the lateral aspect of the thigh and the knee. However, sometimes the referral of pain is along the inside of the thigh to the knee. Weakness of external rotation of the hip; resisted external rotation of the hip may be painful.

### Cause

A tear or strain of the external rotators and hip stabilizers, usually at the insertion on the greater trochanter, although the whole muscle may be involved and may be part of the hip external rotator group that is causing the problem.

### Investigations

None are clinically relevant unless progress or the diagnosis is in doubt, in which case an MRI may show inflammation of the external rotators of the hip [9] (Fig. 9.7).

### Treatment

(a) Treatment to calm inflammation, such as ultrasound or laser, and cortisone injections to the insertion. Occasionally injecting the origin may help.

(b) Massage techniques to organize scar tissue, such as frictions to the insertion.

(c) Stretching of piriformis into internal rotation to prevent scar contraction. Place the affected leg in the 'figure-of-four' position (see Glossary) and then pull the leg and pelvis together, to flex the hip towards the chest.

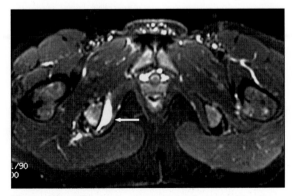

**Figure 9.7** • MRI shows a haematoma from an obturator internus tear. The frequency and clinical picture of injuries to the pelvic and hip stabilizers has not yet been quantified. (Dr Philip Bell)

**(d)** Isometrics to resist external rotation of the hip – for scar organization and strength.

**(e)** Balancing on one leg without allowing the trochanter to stick out, with the femur in varus. Holding a half squat on one leg, but ensuring the pelvis does not swing forwards on the ipsilateral side, which happens if the piriformis and external rotators are weak and therefore cannot maintain the external rotation of this hip (see Figs 20.11 and 20.12).

**(f)** Orthotics will help limit internal rotation of the hip during function, and thus reduce the work required by the piriformis.

## Sports

The running athlete must learn to run 'tall' by stabilizing the pelvis (see Glossary, Core stability) and not allowing the pelvis and hip to collapse into internal rotation during heel strike and lift off. 'Running tall' can be achieved only by strengthening and using the external rotators of the hip.

In golf, hitting into a closed left hip may cause a problem – open out the left foot.

## Comment

This muscle group is as important for hip stability as the rotator cuff is for the shoulder and must be rehabilitated as emphatically.

## Gluteal bursa

### Findings

Diffuse pain over the upper and outer quadrant of the gluteal muscles that is worse with active hip extensions, and therefore when running. Pain on resisted, prone, straight leg hip extension and perhaps passive hip flexion. There is local tenderness on deep palpation, in the upper and outer quadrant of the gluteal muscles.

### Cause

Overuse of the gluteal muscles during unaccustomed exercise. Usually from running, climbing and hill walking, but maybe from aerobics and martial arts.

### Investigations

None are clinically required.

## Treatment

**(a)** Electrotherapeutic modalities to settle the inflamed bursa, such as ultrasound and interferential.

**(b)** Local cortisone over the tender area, adjacent to the bone where the bursa lies.

## Sports

This injury probably occurs more in aerobic and fitness classes that concentrate on hip extension exercises. Some martial arts employ a hip extension when training for back kicks. Occasionally a stiff-legged style of running will flare the gluteal bursa.

## Comment

Not common. In most clinical cases an increase in exercise, which has concentrated on the gluteals, has been the cause. Any injection must be placed in the upper outer quadrant to avoid the sciatic nerve.

## Trochanteric bursa

### Findings

There is gradual onset of pain over the greater trochanter, which is worse when lying on that side or when the legs are crossed. The pain may refer down the outside of the leg to the lateral aspect of the knee. The lumbar spine is pain-free, and most hip movements are pain-free, but passive adduction and internal rotation, which stretch the bursa, may hurt. Resisted abduction may be painful, and there is local tenderness to palpation over the greater trochanter. If the iliotibial tract is tight then Ober's test may be positive (see Glossary).

### Cause

Inflammation of the bursa, lying between the iliotibial band and the greater trochanter, which is caused by increased functional femoral anteversion, producing a functionally tight iliotibial band. Sitting crossed legged, standing on one leg, running on a camber when the lower leg becomes inflamed, twisting dances and direct trauma may be causative. Check for overpronation at the feet as this can functionally increase internal rotation at the hip (see Glossary).

### Investigations

None are clinically relevant, unless there is failure to progress, when a diagnostic ultrasound scan may show

## Caveat

**Trauma over the greater trochanter may produce a haembursitis that requires aspiration.**

the bursa, especially a haembursitis, and, in the chronic case, MRI may have T2-weighted or STIR-related sequences that are positive (Fig. 9.8).

## Treatment

**(a)** RICE (see Glossary).

**(b)** Electrotherapeutic modalities to settle inflammation, such as ultrasound, laser and interferential.

**(c)** Cortisone injection of the bursa.

**(d)** Massage techniques, such as frictions, to relieve adhesions.

**(e)** Stretch the iliotibial tract to reduce friction across the greater trochanter.

**(f)** Avoid sitting with crossed legs and standing on one leg with the hip out sideways. Avoid carrying a child on the hip.

**(g)** Orthotics to reduce femoral anteversion.

**(h)** Strengthen the external rotators of the hip, including the piriformis and gluteals.

**(i)** Surgical Z-plasty to the iliotibial tract.

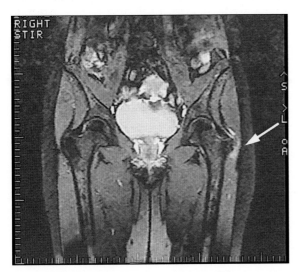

**Figure 9.8** • STIR sequence MRI displays a left trochanteric bursitis (*arrow*).

## Sports

Race walkers rarely get this problem, although the 'rolled through' running style that mimics the race walkers may be causative. The causes above may give a clue to the problem during exercise, but camber running should be avoided (see Glossary).

## Comment

Not common and probably over-diagnosed as a bursa, when the hip stabilizers are the underlying problem. The inflammation responds well to cortisone but not desperately well to physiotherapy. Avoidance of the cause, and alteration of the faulty mechanical skill, is important to prevent recurrence.

# Sacrotuberous ligament strain

## Findings

Deep buttock pain, exacerbated by the movement described in Cause, below. Tender on palpation over the superior surface of ischial tuberosity and along the ligament to the sacrum. This tenderness is best palpated with the patient lying prone. The knee of the side being examined rests on a chair alongside the couch so that the hip is flexed to 90°.

## Cause

Caused by a strain of the sacrotuberous ligament, which runs from the ischial tuberosity to the sacrum. The strain occurs when the body weight is on one leg that is flexed at the knee and hip, and at which stage the body is externally rotated and extended towards that leg, such as whilst digging a hole and throwing a spadeful of soil sideways and backwards.

## Investigations

None are clinically required, but this can be one of those unclear diagnoses and may warrant a bone scan or MRI to exclude other problems.

## Treatment

**(a)** Electrotherapeutic modalities to settle deep inflammation, such as interferential.

**(b)** Injection of the superior surface of the ischial tuberosity with cortisone.

**(c)** Passive hip flexions and massage to reorganize the ligament.

**(d)** Avoid the causative factors (see Cause and Sports).

## Sports

Squash – does not usually occur during a game but during a coaching session; and to the coach! The drill can involve the coach playing a repeated, backhand high clearance from close to the front wall. During a game the coach will push away from the shot, but during the drill he or she may remain static over the flexed hip, but add rotation and extension, to watch the trajectory of the shot and the movement of the player being taught. It is safe but sore to play with this problem.

Golf – occurs on the non-dominant side, when the golfer hits into a closed, locked hip.

## Comment

This is not a common injury, but when it occurs it produces a long-lasting, deep buttock pain. Steroid injection to the superior surface of the ischial tuberosity definitely helps.

## Tensor fasciae latae strain

### Findings

Mainly found in long-distance runners but also in some martial arts. Resisted abduction of the thigh is painful, and it is locally tender to palpation under the iliac crest at its origin. The clinician should check for oversupination, camber running, downhill running and, in martial arts, 'round the head' kicks. Piriformis and the other hip stabilizers may be weak.

### Cause

This is a rare injury, caused by a strain of the muscle origin under the iliac crest, owing to overuse, but can be a secondary injury to 'running round' a primary problem elsewhere.

### Investigations

None are clinically required, though MRI will display muscle oedema (Fig. 9.9) and sometimes a bursa over the iliac crest.

### Treatment

Electrotherapeutic modalities, such as ultrasound and laser, will settle inflammation, as will local cortisone.

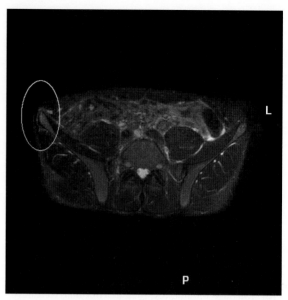

**Figure 9.9** • Tensor fasciae latae (TFL) strain under the lip of the ilium. Oedema can be seen in this MRI in the TFL and a bursa over the right iliac crest can be seen.

Reduce the amount and intensity of training and correct the skill faults (see Findings, above).

### Sports

**(a)** Mainly found in untrained long-distance runners when the other hip stabilizers are weak and a supinated foot strike is strong.

**(b)** Round the head and abduction kicks may cause problems in martial arts.

### Comment

A rare problem that does well with cortisone, but correction of hip stabilizer weakness is essential. The patient in Figure 9.9 damaged his anterior tibialis by holding a door up with his foot while he fixed the hinges. When he returned to running, he then produced a tensor fasciae latae injury that progressed to an iliac crest bursitis and a painless grade 4 stress lesion of his contralateral sacrum.

## Posterior compartment of the thigh

### Findings

**(a)** This is an uncommon injury of long-distance running, being worse when the speed is increased and when running on roads. The pain settles with rest and slowing down, although, if severe, it may last for 24 hours. Clinical examination after the event reveals little [10]. The differential is of a hamstring injury, which unlike this injury is found to be sore with repetition sprinting or with resisted hamstring testing.

**(b)** Continued bleeding after a hamstring tear, which will present with increasing pain, tenderness and swelling and will need urgent surgical release.

## Cause

**(a)** Chronic – possibly caused by increased vascularity of the hamstrings with exercise, and therefore swelling of the muscle, which is confined by the fascia. This compression reduces the blood flow, causing a relative ischaemia during activities.

**(b)** Acute – continual bleeding from a hamstring tear (see above, Hamstring muscle injury).

## Investigations

Required to rule out differentials as no tests are diagnostically positive:

**(a)** X-ray.
**(b)** Diagnostic ultrasound – especially if continued bleeding is the cause.
**(c)** MRI of the back and leg.
**(d)** EMG to exclude neuromuscular causes.
**(e)** Bone scan to exclude bony causes.

## Treatment

**(a)** Urgent surgery for the acute compartment syndrome.
**(b)** Stop running long distance and/or a surgical fascial split for the chronic cases [10].

## Sports

Long-distance running.

## Comment

Very uncommon. I have seen only two chronic cases, which both went to surgery with variable results. I have had only one acute case of ongoing bleeding – over 3 to 4 days – a medical student, son of a doctor!

## Coccygeal ligament

There is tenderness on palpation of the coccyx both externally and per rectum, and local tenderness alongside the coccyx over the sacrococcygeal ligaments. The pain responds well to local cortisone injection around the sacrococcygeal ligaments (see Chapter 2, Part 2: Coccygeal pain).

### Caveat

**Coccygectomy is usually unsuccessful, but, in some cases of hypermobility of the coccyx that can be proven by showing increased flexion of the coccyx on the X-ray taken when sitting (as opposed to standing), surgery may be tried as a last resort.**

## Iliac crest impingement and hip pointer

This is an extension problem in gymnasts and acrobats and is associated with walkovers. Local tenderness to palpation develops over the iliac crest and may be an impingement injury. The injury is improved by rest, cortisone injections and electrotherapeutic modalities to settle inflammation. The 'walkover' in gymnastics is often performed with acute extension at the lower lumbar segments, as opposed to spreading the extension over the whole lumbar spine.

The hip pointer occurs in baseball, particularly when the batsman is sliding into a base, legs first. There is friction, which traumatizes the soft tissues over the iliac crest and can produce a haematoma, requiring aspiration and physiotherapy to clear the debris. I have not as yet seen this in cricket where the fielder is sliding feet first after the ball so that the ball can be picked up and thrown quickly.

## References

1 Puranen J, Orava S. The hamstring syndrome. A new diagnosis of gluteal sciatic pain. Am J Sports Med 1988;16:517–521

2 Remvig L, Ellis RM, Patinjn J. Piriformis syndrome: definitions, reproducibility, and validity of diagnostic procedures and results of efficacy trials. J Orthop Med 2004;26(2):67–76

3 Kurosawa H, Nakasita K, Saski S, Takeda S. Complete avulsion of the hamstring tendons from the ischial tuberosity. A report of two cases sustained in judo. Br J Sports Med 1996;30:72–74

4 Oravo S, Kujala UM. Rupture of the ischial origin of the hamstring muscles. Am J Sports Med 1995;23:702–705

5 Read MT, Bellamy MJ. Comparison of hamstring/quadriceps isokinetic strength ratios and power in elite tennis, squash, and track athletes. Br J Sports Med 1990;24(3):178–182

6 Osternig LJ, Hamill J, Lander JE, Robertson R. Co-activation of sprinter and distance runner muscles in isokinetic exercise. Med Sci Sports Exerc 1986;18:431–435

7 Cyriax JH, Cyriax PJ. Indications for traction. In: Cyriax's illustrated manual of orthopaedic medicine, 2nd edn. Oxford: Butterworth Heinemann; 1993. p. 222

8 Servant CT, Jones CB. Displaced avulsion of the ischeal apophysis: a hamstring injury requiring internal fixation. Br J Sports Med 1998;32: 255–257

9 Klinkert P, Porte R, de Rooje T, de Vries AG. Quadratus tendinitis as a cause of groin pain. Br J Sports Med 1997;31:348–350

10 Peltokatho P, Harjula A. Posterior compartment syndrome of thigh in runners. Sports Medicine in Track and Field Athletics: Proc. 1st IAAF Medical Congress, Finland; 1983. pp. 57–59

## Further reading

Bruckner P, Khan K. Clinical sports medicine, 3rd edn. New York: McGraw-Hill; 2006

Hutson MA (ed.). Sports injuries: recognition and management, 2nd edn. Oxford: Oxford Medical Publications; 1996

Hutson M, Ellis R (eds). Textbook of musculoskeletal medicine. Oxford: Oxford University Press; 2006

Reid D. Sports injury assessment and rehabilitation. Edinburgh: Churchill Livingstone; 1992

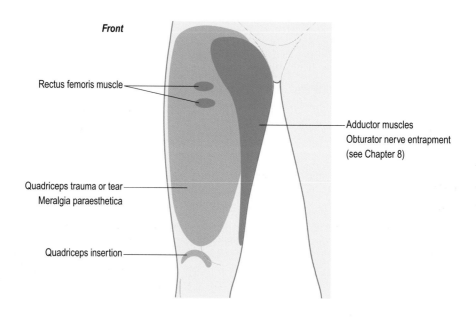

***Front***

Rectus femoris muscle

Adductor muscles
Obturator nerve entrapment
(see Chapter 8)

Quadriceps trauma or tear
Meralgia paraesthetica

Quadriceps insertion

# Chapter Ten

# Anterior thigh

## CHAPTER CONTENTS

## Referred pain: lumbar nerve root L3/4

### Findings

The presentation may or may not be with lumbar pain, but pain may refer onto the anterior thigh, shin and the top of the foot, which may have 'pins and needles', numbness and hyperaesthesia. There may be painful, fixed, lumbar flexion and back movements that provoke leg pain. Femoral stretch and prone lying knee flexion are positive (see Glossary: Dural stress tests). The knee jerk may be absent and the quadriceps weak, but this is not a pain-induced weakness. Hip rotation, tested in the sitting position so as not to involve the back, is pain-free. There is no history of trauma, swelling or bruising (see Chapter 5).

### Cause

L3/4 disc or lateral canal entrapment of the L3/4 root; L2/3 is referred more to the groin.

## Referred pain: hip

### Findings

When the back is tested with the patient sitting on the couch then little mechanical pressure is applied to the hip. When the hip is involved then lumbar movements are pain-free, but hip rotations, flexion, abduction and adduction are painful and refer pain through to the knee (see Chapter 8).

### Caveat

**Thigh and knee pain, without hip pain, is a common presentation of the slipped capital femoral epiphysis in adolescents.**

## Trauma to the quadriceps

### Findings

There is a history of an acute episode of direct trauma or blocked quadriceps muscle action. Swelling of the thigh may occur, and, if the bleeding is extrafascicular (peripheral muscle bundle tear), the bruising will track down, under gravity, towards the knee. This early bruising is indicative that the injury will heal fairly rapidly, whereas swelling with no bruising is indicative of a central tear (intrafascicular) or haematoma, which heal much more slowly. There is pain on testing resisted quadriceps, and the pain is worse on the stairs, with squats, straightening the knee and kicking. There is a limited quadriceps stretch and the modified Thomas test is reduced (see Glossary; Fig. 22.25).

## Cause

There has been direct trauma to quadriceps, especially whilst contracting the muscle. Blocking of a fast quadriceps movement, such as a kick blocked by a tackle, tears the muscle (Glossary, Blocked movement).

 **Caveat**

If, whilst sitting, passive knee flexion remains less than 90° after a few days, beware the onset of myositis ossificans, especially if the injury is near the femur. Gradual increasing pain over 5 days suggests myositis ossificans has developed, or is developing. Increasing swelling and pain over 12–24 hours means bleeding is continuing into the muscle (Fig. 10.1).

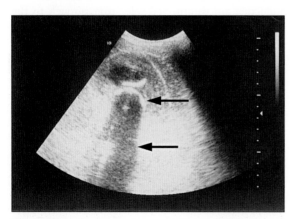

**Figure 10.1** • Real-time ultrasound displays a dark haematoma with bright reflection from the myositis ossificans near the bone. The bone shows as a white line with shadow beneath (*arrows*).

## Investigations

Diagnostic ultrasound scan for any haematoma and myositis ossificans, or X-ray for myositis ossificans.

## Treatment

(a) Pressure and RICE (see Glossary).

(b) In the early stages, aspirate any haematoma, under ultrasound control.

(c) Electrotherapeutic modalities to encourage healing and removal of tissue debris, such as ultrasound.

(d) Massage to remove tissue debris and realign healing fibroblasts.

(e) Electrotherapeutic modalities, such as interferential, to encourage early muscle contraction within the pain-free range.

(f) Stretch the quadriceps to prevent scar contraction.

(g) Isometric exercises followed by isotonic exercises (see Chapter 20).

(h) Quadriceps ladders (see Chapter 20).

(i) Myositis ossificans may develop in 15% of patients with severe injury [1] (see Glossary).

## Sports

Occurs in sports where a quadriceps movement may be interrupted or blocked extrinsically, or direct trauma can occur.

## Comment

Early management of this lesion has to be observed for the suspected onset of myositis ossificans. If this is thought likely then active treatment must be stopped, and rest instituted. NSAIDs (such as indomethacin) can be very beneficial when used early. Bisphosphonates may have a place.

## Torn rectus femoris muscle

### Findings

There is an acute or chronic history, with pain in the upper mid-quadriceps, which is worse on running, kicking, squats and stairs. Sometimes the history is not so much of pain, but a weakness or incoordination during the above movements. The lesion is locally tender with two gaps, invariably palpable, about 6 cm apart in the upper mid-thigh. Resisted knee extension with the hip flexed may be pain-free, but supine lying, resisted straight leg raise is weak or painful, and the modified Thomas test is tight (see Glossary: Thomas test; Fig. 22.25).

## Cause

Sometimes from a blocked quadriceps action (see Glossary: Blocked movement), but the lesion can develop insidiously, presumably from microtears. Kicking and sprinting are often causative, as this muscle exhibits Lombard's paradoxical movement (see Glossary: Lombard's paradox).

## Investigations

None are clinically required. Real-time ultrasound scan may be used to monitor the progress of the lesion. This lesion has often been clinically diagnosed as a sarcoma because of the irregular shape created by the double tear, but ultrasound will clarify the diagnosis. A leiomyosarcoma, which occurs in this area, is pain-free, larger, and has a more diffuse mass.

## Treatment

(a) The chronic phase is difficult to manage and the lesion slow to heal, but maintaining quadriceps stretching, the quadriceps ladders for training (see Chapter 20), and playing within tolerance helps. Sometimes rest from sport, but maintaining stretch and quadriceps rehabilitation, is required.

(b) The acute tear is treated with pressure, RICE and then as for a quadriceps tear (see above, Trauma to quadriceps).

## Sports

No specific sport is responsible for this injury, but a weak psoas is often found when this lesion is present.

## Comment

The chronic phase seems to niggle on without getting totally better, but then if the tear gets worse, and completes, the pain eases and the muscle heals to normal function, but with the indentations from the tears still palpable.

# Ruptured quadriceps

## Findings

Total separation of a muscle produces a painless muscle contraction on resisted muscle testing, but this is unusual in the quadriceps where a partial tear occurs, and resisted quadriceps is painful, even producing inhibition. There is bruising and swelling, which may also be around the knee in the acute phase, with a deformed quadriceps on contraction (Fig. 10.2) (see above, Trauma to quadriceps).

## Cause

Partial or complete rupture of the quadriceps, often close to the patella insertion.

## Investigations

(a) Although careful clinical examination should establish a diagnosis of the complete rupture, this lesion has been missed by clinicians [2]. If there is any doubt, ultrasound should be employed to establish the diagnosis. Minor quadriceps tears, grades 1 and 2, and quadriceps expansion lesions may require diagnostic ultrasound or MRI (Fig. 10.3) to display them.

(b) Ultrasound scan to locate any haematoma that is suitable for aspiration, or to monitor the lesion (see Chapter 11, Part 2C: Quadriceps expansion).

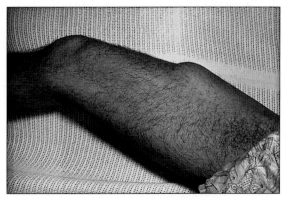

**Figure 10.2** • A previously ruptured quadriceps, now functioning perfectly normally in spite of the deformity.

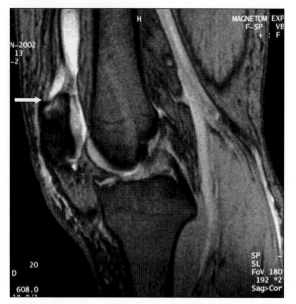

**Figure 10.3** • Partial rupture of the quadriceps tendon with underlying bone bruising in a motorcyclist whose knee slider caught the ground.

## Treatment

(a) RICE (see Glossary).

(b) Electrotherapeutic modalities to settle inflammation and remove tissue debris.

(c) Isometric exercises to organize scar tissue and build muscle strength.

(d) Stretching to prevent scar contraction.

(e) Closed chain exercises to maintain proprioceptive control and to strengthen the muscle.

(f) Quadriceps ladders, plus the knee (kicking) ladder, if required (see Chapter 20).

(g) Total ruptures heal well without surgery (see Fig. 10.2); possible surgical repair.

## Sports

The injury occurs in sports that can block quadriceps movement, or overload can occur with weightlifting – when steroid abuse must also be considered.

## Comment

Not that common, and certainly quadriceps function returns to normal without surgery in the total rupture. However, if the rupture is close to the insertion into the patella, or the athlete is elite, then surgical repair is of benefit.

## Meralgia paraesthetica

### Findings

Pain and numbness over the front to the lateral side of the thigh, but the focal point of tenderness may range from the anterior superior iliac spine to the upper one-third of the thigh.

### Cause

Compression of the lateral cutaneous nerve of the thigh, usually as it passes from deep to superficial through the subcutaneous fascia.

### Investigations

None are clinically required, and an EMG is rarely of value.

### Treatment

Relieve the cause of pressure, and if required inject cortisone around the tender focal compression area of the nerve. Surgery to release the nerve from the stenotic fascia is required if the problem fails to settle.

### Comment

A prime cause in sports players is compression of the nerve by the tight elastic around the top of the leg, from pants or shorts, and the tender spot may be palpated under the compression band left in the skin by the elastic. Alteration of the elastic compression cures most!

## Stress fracture of the femur

### Findings

A history of pain in the hip, thigh or knee that is worse with activity, which is invariably running or marching. Onset of non-traumatic pain in the hip or the thigh, worse with running or walking, that is not clinically diagnosable must be treated as a potential stress lesion. The patient should be given crutches if a potential diagnosis of a tension stress fracture of the hip is made. (see Chapter 8). Femoral shaft stress lesions usually have pain with hopping on the affected leg and with transaxial stress across the femur. The patient sits on the couch with the legs hanging over the side. The examiner places one arm under the thigh as the fulcrum and the other presses the knee towards the floor. When the fulcral arm is under, or near the stress lesion, the patient experiences pain. This is sometimes called the fulcrum test [3].

## Cause

Overload during running. Stress fractures in the femur occur at the subtrochanteric level and along the shaft of the femur, where it is an uncommon lesion.

## Investigations

(a) X-ray is the first-line investigation, but is often negative.

(b) MRI localized over the painful area, but as the lesion can occur anywhere along the length of the femoral shaft, and pain is referred somewhat variably, then a bone scan will display the whole length of the femur and the pelvis so that the possibility of referred bone injury from the hip or pelvis may also be detected (Fig. 10.4).

(c) Bone density (see Chapter 21).

(d) Female athletes triad (see Chapter 21: Bone density/osteoporosis).

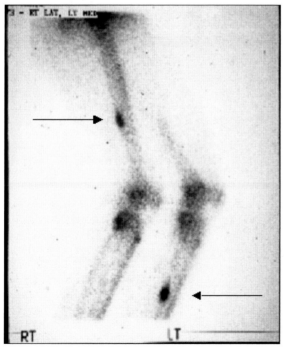

**Figure 10.4** • A bone scan shows a right femoral shaft stress fracture and a left tibial stress fracture. The biomechanics of this patient are likely to be abnormal. (Dr Philip Bell)

 **Caveat**

**If in doubt, rule a stress fracture out. Beware of pathological fractures.**

## Treatment

Non-weight-bearing on crutches, followed by a gradual introduction of weight-bearing and repeat testing, but, beware, the subtrochanteric [4] and tension femoral neck lesion can fracture (see Fig. 8.14).

## Sports

A possibility in all impact sports, but running and power walking are particularly noted for this injury. Beware the amenorrhoeic athlete.

## Comment

The femoral shaft stress fracture is not common. Why at times the stress occurs in the subtrochanteric region as opposed to the femoral neck is not understood, but I wonder if power walking and a hamstring-pull style of running might be causative.

## References

1 Reid D. Myositis ossificans. In: Reid D. Sports injury assessment and rehabilitation. Edinburgh: Churchill Livingstone; 1992. pp. 583–589

2 MacEachern AG, Plewes JL, Bilateral simultaneous spontaneous rupture of the quadriceps tendons. J Bone Joint Surg 1984;66:81

3 Johnson AW, Weiss CB, Wheeler DL. Stress fractures of the femoral shaft in athletes: a new treatment algorithm. Am J Sports Med 1994;22:249–256

4 Leinberry CF, Mcshane RB, Stewart WG, Hume EL. A displaced subtrochanteric stress fracture in a young amenorrheic athlete. Am J Sports Med 1992;20:485–487

## Further reading

Bruckner P, Khan K. Clinical sports medicine, 3rd edn. New York: McGraw-Hill; 2006

Reid D. Sports injury assessment and rehabilitation. Edinburgh: Churchill Livingstone; 1992

Hutson M, Ellis R (eds). Textbook of musculoskeletal medicine. Oxford: Oxford University Press; 2006

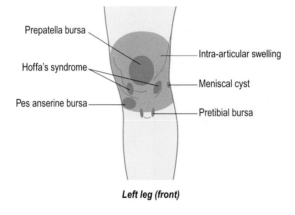

*Left leg (front)*

# Chapter **Eleven**

11

# Knee

## Part 1  **The swollen knee**

### PART CONTENTS

**A. Hot, swollen knee**

**B. Acute swelling within 4–6 hours
of trauma**

The clinician must consider the differential diagnoses of a hot, swollen knee, as some presentations may appear to have a knee that is cold to the touch (see Hot, swollen knee).

# Infection, gout and inflammatory arthritis

## Findings

All may present with a history of non-traumatic onset, although gout and infection may follow soon after some trauma. The history includes pain, warmth and swelling, sometimes with reddening. The knee is warm and usually painful to the touch, and painful on all movements, either active or passive. There is usually enough synovial swelling to make the bulge test, ballottement and patellar tap positive (see Glossary: Ballottement, Bulge test), but gout may only have soft tissue thickening.

## Investigations

Aspirate the joint and examine the aspirate by microscopy, culture and sensitivity. Polarized light is required for crystal arthropathy, gout or pseudogout. Autoimmune antibodies can be tested from the aspirate.

Blood test for rheumatoid factor, autoimmune profile and HLA-B27; though *Salmonella* and *Shigella* can produce an acute reactive arthritis, it is more common in the individual with a positive HLA B27. Lyme disease should be considered. Though non-specific urethritis (NSU) can occur at all ages, the young and the travelling sportsperson are more prone to this disease. Atraumatic monarthritis should have an aspirate and blood taken, which should be tested for chlamydia, gonorrhoea, and syphilis.

## Treatment

Systemic, reactive and infective arthritis are not covered in detail in this book. Refer to medical or rheumatological textbook for details of management (and see under headings in Part 1C).

# Acute swelling – general

The history includes an acute traumatic episode, with pain and swelling. Almost no one can continue to play on after the injury. The bulge test, ballottement, or patellar tap are positive for intra-articular swelling (see Glossary: Bulge test). In the presence of this rapid swelling, it is best to assume that a haemarthrosis has occurred, but the joint should be aspirated to confirm the diagnosis. The aspirate should be left standing for 5–10 minutes to allow fat globules, if present, to separate out. Fat globules within the aspirate are diagnostic of a fracture. If facilities are available then an MRI is most diagnostic.

# Anterior cruciate ligament tear

## Findings

The acute episode has a history of rapid swelling, within 4–6 hours of a twist, fall or impact on the knee.

The subacute or chronic problem has a history with a causative injury in the past that was accompanied by rapid swelling of the knee. However, patients do appear who give a past history of some trauma to the knee that did not grossly affect them at the time, but clinical examination shows them to have suffered an anterior cruciate ligament (ACL) tear. Pain is often not a presenting symptom and words such as 'jumps', 'gives way', 'unstable', or 'can't trust it' are used. The knee may be painful on active and passive movement. Ballottement, or patellar tap, is usually positive in the acute or subacute stage, whereas a positive bulge test is more common in the chronic case because this sign is present with less fluid. Anterior draw and Lachman test are positive. Arthrometry displaying increased translation is indicative, and some surgeons use a measure of this laxity as an indication for surgery. The pivot shift may be positive, but may only be obtained with the patient anaesthetized. The quadriceps and hamstrings are often weak (see Glossary for the various tests).

## Cause

Direct trauma and/or a twisting fall ruptures or partially ruptures the ACL. It may be part of O'Donoghue's triad [1] (see Glossary). Incorrect sporting technique or tricks, such as sitting on the back of skis then standing upright whilst moving, can be causative.

### Caveat

**O'Donoghue's triad may have had dislocation of the knee, so check for popliteal artery damage.**

## Investigations

(a) Diagnostic aspiration to display a haemarthrosis, which has no fat globules unless there is an accompanying fracture.
(b) MRI scan with sagittal obliques at about 15°.
(c) Examination under anaesthetic, and arthroscopy.

## Treatment

At this time management is still contentious. Despite early repair, late repair, or non-surgical management, ACL rupture leads to the early onset of degenerative changes [2]. The professional athlete will want an early return to sport and early surgery. Accompanying meniscal damage will hasten degenerative change and should

be dealt with, even without the ACL being repaired. Arthrometry guides some surgeons, who believe that laxity is the problem, whilst others believe that rotational and functional stability are the important indices. A conservative approach is to rehabilitate the knee over 6–12 weeks, and if functional control for daily living or the sport has not been achieved then reconstruct the ACL [2,3]. One indicator for this control is the ability to nullify the pivot shift. If, after 6–12 weeks of rehabilitation, the patient cannot control the pivot shift then, probably, he or she will not be able to control this instability in life or sport:

(a) Reduce the fluid by aspiration, electrical modalities and NSAIDs.
(b) Stabilize the joint with a brace or elastic support.
(c) Quadriceps and hamstring strength, particularly hamstring [4], should be trained by isometrics and electrical modalities, progressing to closed chain exercises. Open chain exercises may be as effective.
(d) Balance and proprioceptive exercises.
(e) Training with zig-zag hopping, and big 'hop and hold' landing.
(f) Hamstring ladders (see Chapter 20).
(g) Cross-train for aerobic fitness.

## Sports

(a) Knee braces cannot be worn during competition whilst playing rugby, football and other contact sports, but may be of help in non-contact sports.
(b) Ski bindings must be able to release upwards and sideways at the toes, as well as at the heel, so that the backwards fall may be protected [5]. Falling techniques may be taught to prevent cruciate ligament damage in skiers [6] (for which techniques such as sitting on the back of the skis and then standing up whilst on the move have been blamed).

## Comment

Many elite games players, even in rugby, play with absent ACLs [7], and one often finds clinically lax cruciate ligaments, with no functional disability, when examining the knee for something unrelated. Whilst the muscles around the knee are working, the knee is held under control. It is when the knee is relaxed – when checking a ball in soccer, or releasing the skis from the slope before turning to stop – that trouble may occur.

The functionally stable knee seems to be able to prevent the pivot shift from occurring (except under anaesthetic), and the clinical persistence of the pivot shift during rehabilitation may be a warning that this knee will not do well with conservative management.

## Tibial spine avulsion

### Findings

There is pain, an inability to support the weight on this leg and an acute swollen knee following a history of trauma. The bulge, ballottement or patellar tap are positive, and a knee aspirate, after standing for 5–10 minutes, shows a lipohaemarthrosis, with fat globules rising to the surface. The anterior draw and Lachman tests (see Glossary) are positive, but the patient may protect the knee from these tests because of pain. The patient is usually young.

### Cause

As for ACL tear, but in children and adolescents the attachment of the anterior cruciate at the tibial spinal enthesis is weaker than the ligament itself and avulses before the ligament tears.

### Investigations

(a) Diagnostic aspiration for a haemarthrosis, which contains fat globules.
(b) X-ray, with tunnel views, to show the tibial spine.
(c) CT or MRI.

### Treatment

Early surgical reattachment of the spine, followed by rehabilitation along the same lines as for the ACL tear (see this chapter).

### Sports

See Anterior cruciate ligament tear.

### Comment

This emphasizes the advantage of diagnostic knee aspiration. In certain circumstances X-ray and MRI facilities are not available, and indeed the timing of the swelling may be in doubt. Whereas an ACL can be managed conservatively, the anterior tibial spine should have early surgical reattachment. The reattached tibial

spine should heal entirely and leave no long-term problems.

## Tibial plateau fracture

### Findings

There is a history of acute swelling following trauma and the patient cannot weight bear. The bulge test, ballottement and/or patellar tap are positive (see Glossary: Bulge test). There is pain on active or passive movement of the joint.

### Investigations

After leaving the diagnostic aspirate to stand for 5–10 minutes, the haemarthrosis shows fat globules separating out: a lipohaemarthrosis. X-ray of the knee with tunnel views, CT and MRI scans will show the fracture.

### Treatment

Refer for orthopaedic surgical opinion and repair (Fig. 11.1).

## Peripheral meniscal tear

### Findings

An acute swollen knee after a twisting and/or falling injury. There may be a history of locking, clicking or giving way. McMurray's or Apley's tests (see Glossary) may be positive and there is tenderness on palpation of the joint line.

### Cause

Tear of the peripheral attachment of the meniscus, which has a blood supply and can therefore bleed.

### Investigations

(a) Diagnostic aspiration of a haemarthrosis that shows blood but no fat globules.
(b) MRI – may show the meniscal tear, or because the lesion is peripheral it may be difficult to interpret.
(c) Arthroscopy should be diagnostic.

### Treatment

Surgical repair is the treatment of choice, and then follow the knee ladders for rehabilitation (see Chapter 20).

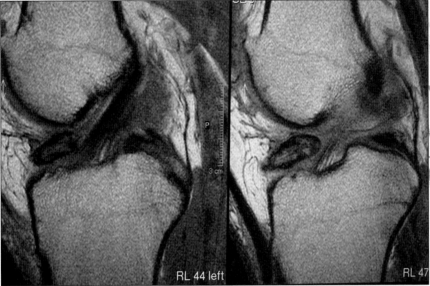

**Figure 11.1 •** A detached tibial plateau fracture that has healed as a loose body.

## Sports

Rehabilitation can involve non-impact cross-training until the knee is recovered sufficiently to train via the knee ladders (see Chapter 20).

## Comment

The best outcome follows early repair, within a few weeks. Thus an early MRI and, if in doubt, diagnostic arthroscopy is of value.

## Dislocated patella

### Findings

(a) The patella dislocates to the lateral side of the knee but may reduce spontaneously with pressure on the lateral side of the patella or require sedation to achieve reduction.

(b) The patient may present after the incident because of pain but with a history of immediate swelling. However, this may in fact be a description of the displaced patella or a haemarthrosis, and, because the knee capsule ruptures, the swelling may be generalized around the knee rather than confined to the joint. Bruising may occur later.

(c) Pain on quadriceps loading.

(d) Clarke's test remains positive for some time after the patella is reduced.

(e) A positive ballottement or bulge test may persist for some time.

(f) Apprehension test is positive for some time after.

(g) The patellar facets, usually medial, remain tender to palpation for some time after.

(h) The lateral femoral condylar articular surface remains tender to palpation for some time after.

(See Glossary for the various tests).

### Cause

(a) A traumatic, extrinsic impact dislocates the patella.

(b) Recurrent dislocation (see below).

### Caveat

**Many normal knees that suffer patellar dislocation will develop chondral or osteochondral damage on the deep surface of the patella or lateral femoral condyle [8]. In contrast, the abnormally lax patella may suffer recurrent dislocation without any damage being caused to the underlying bone; this is because the patella and femoral condyle do not grind across one another during the dislocation (Fig. 11.2).**

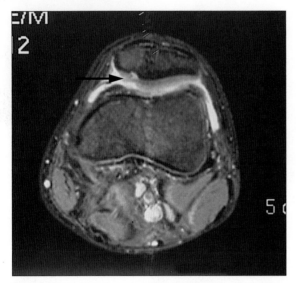

**Figure 11.2** • MRI scan shows an osteochondral defect in the medial facet, confirmed at arthroscopy following traumatic patella dislocation in the normal knee.

## Investigations

None are clinically required unless the patient fails to progress, then X-ray and MRI scan for osteochondral damage. Consider arthroscopy for osteochondral damage and a possible loose body. Record the ligament laxity score (see Glossary: Beighton–Horan score). Ultrasound will aid the diagnosis of the extent of capsular damage and subsequent healing.

## Treatment

(a) Reduction of the dislocation and aspiration of any haemarthrosis, if present.

(b) Possible open repair of the ruptured lateral capsule [9,10].

(c) Electrical and physiotherapeutic modalities to relieve pain, settle soft tissue swelling and maintain muscle strength.

(d) Low load, high repetition exercise. Increase the loads as improvement in pain tolerance permits.

(e) Correct any pronation at the foot, functional valgus at the knee and weakness of the external rotators of the hip as these will hinder healing by promoting lateral tracking of the patella.

(f) Control patella maltracking with a patella brace or McConnell strapping techniques, as the lateral capsule is usually either ruptured or lax.

(g) Cross-train by rowing, cycling, backstroke or freestyle swimming (not breaststroke).

(h) Closed chain leg exercises.

(i) Progress to the knee ladders.

(See Chapter 20 and Glossary).

## Sports

Osteochondral damage will take much longer to heal, and may prevent deep knee bends or much quadriceps power being applied to the knee until it has healed. Cross-training and low load, high repetition weights may have to be maintained for a considerable time.

## Comment

Acute dislocation in a normal knee is a severe injury and only 60% may return to their previous sporting activity with no or minor limitations [8] (see Part 2B: Subluxing patella).

## Posterior cruciate ligament tear

### Findings

(a) Acute – acute painful swelling following a history of trauma. The sag sign may be positive.

(b) Subacute and chronic – a history of trauma followed by an unstable knee (see Anterior cruciate ligament tear). The tibia subluxes in a posterior direction with the knee flexed at 90°, producing the sag sign. The posterior draw sign, which increases the sag sign, is positive (Fig. 11.3).

### Caveat

**The anterior draw test may appear positive as the knee moves forward from the posterior, subluxed position to the normal position. In the acute case, check the popliteal artery is intact.**

### Cause

Trauma to the knee and rupture of the posterior cruciate ligament, which may also be part of a major ligamentous disruption.

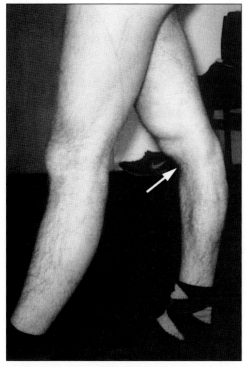

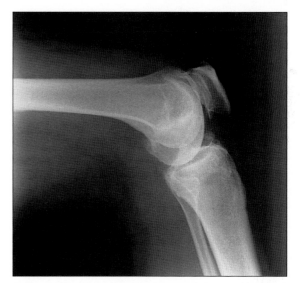

**Figure 11.4** • Osteoarthritis of the knee and patellofemoral joint.

## Osteoarthritis of the knee

### Findings

There is a history of previous damage, trauma, or non-traumatic gradual onset of pain. The knee contours appear larger. The bulge test, ballottement, or patellar tap may be positive if synovial fluid is present (see Glossary: Bulge test, Balottement). There is limited extension and flexion, with a painful, hard end feel on passive movement. There can be a secondary valgus or varus effect at the knee, owing to unicompartmental damage. There may be ligamentous pain from collateral ligament strains when the knee is stressed into varus or valgus (Fig. 11.4).

### Cause

Degeneration of the articular cartilage, more frequent after meniscectomy, cruciate ligament damage or intra-articular trauma. There may be eburnation (see Glossary), with cystic and sclerotic bony changes.

### Investigations

(a) X-ray – note uni-, bi-, or tri-compartmental degeneration may occur.
(b) MRI or CT scan for early osteoarthritis or a chondral flap, which may show up on these scans when the X-ray is virtually normal (Fig. 11.5).

**Figure 11.3** • The sag sign for posterior cruciate damage is positive in this knee, even when standing.

### Investigations

(a) Diagnostic aspiration of any haemarthrosis. There are no fat globules present unless accompanied by a fracture.
(b) MRI scan to show the posterior cruciate ligaments.
(c) Diagnostic arthroscopy.

### Treatment

(a) Usually is conservative. A similar management programme to the anterior cruciate ligament tear may be followed, but with a greater emphasis on quadriceps strength than on the strength of the hamstrings.
(b) Surgical repair.

### Sports

See anterior cruciate ligament tears.

### Comment

This isolated injury is far less common than anterior cruciate ligament tears, and requirements for surgery are much more debatable [11].

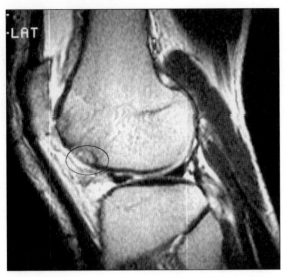

**Figure 11.5** • MRI showing an osteochondral defect in the femoral condyle.

## Treatment

(a) NSAIDs and electrical modalities to ease pain and swelling.

(b) Activity rather than rest [12].

(c) Quadriceps isometrics to maintain strength but not work the joint surfaces (see Glossary: Isometric/isostatic muscle contraction).

(d) Low load, high repetition weights, as isotonic or isokinetic exercises, particularly to the quadriceps (see Glossary: Isokinetic muscle contraction, Isotonic muscle contraction).

(e) Non-impact loading of the joint (rowing, cycling or swimming, not breaststroke) with low load, high repetitions.

(f) Possibly orthotics for the feet, and posterior tibialis rehabilitation, to prevent valgus stress at the knee.

(g) Knee brace, if the valgus or varus stress is causing ligamentous pain.

(h) Intra-articular injections of sodium hyaluronate [13].

(i) Injection of cortisone to settle the swelling and pain from the synovium.

(j) Arthroscopic washout.

(k) Arthroscopic debridement and drilling. Surgical correction of clinical genu varus and genu valgum.

(l) Replacement prosthesis.

## Sports

(a) Impact loading from running, jumping, etc., is not desirable. Rowing, cycling and swimming are the most suitable activities.

(b) Play doubles at tennis, rather than squash or badminton.

(c) Weight training should use low loads and high repetitions.

(d) Aquarobics/hydrotherapy reduces the stresses across the joints whilst maintaining mobility.

## Comment

A joint has to move so that synovial fluid is forced into the nutrient canaliculi of the chondral cartilage. A joint fixed in one position for too long will show localized degeneration at the areas of contact. Thus movement of the joint helps, but, because the shock-absorbing properties have been diminished by cartilage degradation, the impact should be reduced. Orthotics may help to reduce the valgus or varus effect at the knee. The vicious cycle of pain, inactivity and weak quadriceps must be broken by the relief of pain and rehabilitation exercises. The rowing machine, swimming and cycling are good non-impact exercisers for OA joints. Chair seats should be higher than the knees so that the sitting knee angle is increased, which will reduce the quadriceps loads required for standing up. Intra-articular injections of cortisone may dramatically relieve discomfort, and an arthroscopic washout can prove very effective. A 'wet' knee seems to survive better than a dry knee, where eburnation seems to occur faster. Sodium hyaluronate, which is equivalent to synovial fluid, helps but is it more effective in dry knees (see Glossary: Eburnation)?

## Meniscal tear

### Findings

(a) The history may be of slow-onset pain, but usually follows a more acute episode involving twisting in a flexed, weight-bearing, knee position.

(b) The knee may stick, lock, click and have pain on twisting and turning. Episodic catching, with long periods clear, suggests a parrot beak tear.

(c) Joint effusion may or may not be present.

(d) McMurray's test is usually positive, but a negative test does not exclude a tear. Apley's grinding test is positive but, again, a negative test does not exclude a tear.

(e) The joint line is tender to palpation.

(f) A unilateral block to extension in a non-osteoarthritic knee is a meniscal tear until proved otherwise.

(g) The duck waddle test is positive.

See Glossary, for details of the tests.

## Cause

Degeneration, and then fimbriation, of the meniscus, which often follows a traumatic twist of the knee, usually from a stumble, blocked twisting movement or other extraneous force that can tear the meniscus. The C-shaped menisci can move, but can become trapped and torn by rapid squatting, as in bunny hops, or an awkward squat with rotation, which the 'duck waddle' mimics (see Fig. 22.4). There are various types recognized: bucket handle, parrot beak, radial tear (associated with meniscal cysts), and a horizontal cleavage tear (Fig. 11.6).

## Investigations

Undiagnosed swelling, and pain on twisting movements, requires an MRI (Fig. 11.7). However, a complete, full history of swelling and locking, clinical signs of a passive extension block to the knee and normal cruciate ligaments should go straight to arthroscopy.

## Treatment

Small tears that do not lock the joint may well settle over time without treatment. A parrot beak or radial tear may settle with time, but partial meniscectomy is usually required for most meniscal tears and, especially for peripheral tears, meniscal resuturing is undertaken.

### Comment

The history often gives the diagnosis, but a block to extension is a most important sign. An unstable knee (posterior/anterior cruciate ligament disruption) may lead to meniscal damage. MRI grades of meniscal damage exist, where degeneration may be intra-substance and mistaken for a tear. A tear should be visible on T2 or STIR sequences as well as T1 and, if not, it is more likely to be degeneration of the meniscus. Clot implantation may be the way to preserve the meniscus [14].

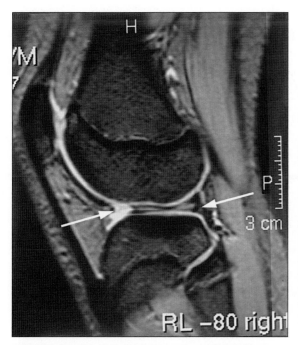

**Figure 11.6** • T2-weighted MRI showing a horizontal cleavage tear in a discoid meniscus (between the *arrows*).

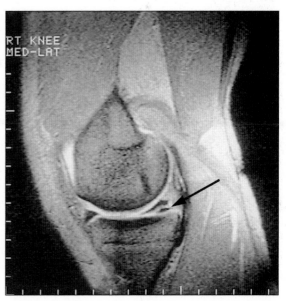

**Figure 11.7** • T2-weighted MRI with a posterior horn tear.

## Loose body

### Findings

There is a diagnostic history of episodic locking or catching with knee movements. Synovial swelling may be present. However, see Osteoarthritis of the knee, Meniscal tear, Osteochondritis dissecans and Cruciate ligament tear, which can all produce loose fragments.

### Cause

A fragment (or fragments) of meniscus, chondral cartilage or bone is detached and interferes with joint articulation. If the loose body remains in the intercondylar notch, it may cause no trouble.

### Investigations

X-ray with tunnel views, CT and MRI. All may still be negative in the presence of a cartilaginous loose body.

### Treatment

Arthroscopic removal, and management of the causative lesion.

### Sports

(See Osteochondral defect, below).

### Comment

The history of intermittent catching or locking is more diagnostic, as all investigations may be negative, even in the presence of a loose body.

## Osteochondral defect and osteochondritis dissecans

### Findings

This is mainly found in teenagers and it is often the final diagnosis in undiagnosed knee pain. There may be synovial swelling and a history of a loose body (see this chapter, Loose body). An osteochondral defect in an adult may have a history of degeneration, following wear and tear and/or trauma.

### Cause

Localized separation of a small area of articular cartilage and underlying bone. Osteochondritis dissecans is almost always found on the convex surface of a joint – the femoral condyles in the knee – and this may represent a compression stress fracture. However, an osteochondral defect may occur on all surfaces, as it may follow trauma or precede osteoarthritis.

### Investigations

X-ray, but progress to MRI or CT scan if not seen on X-ray but suspected clinically. MRI displays early osteochondral damage particularly well (see Fig. 11.5).

### Treatment

If the fragment is unseparated, avoid impaction exercises until healed, otherwise arthroscopic debridement and removal of the loose body.

### Sports

Osteochondritis dissecans is an adolescent injury that may be more frequent in sports played on artificial playing surfaces, such as field hockey, where the surfaces are harder, there is less slide of the foot and the knee is used in a deeper squat to make a tackle. Osteochondral lesions may be treated by non-impact, low load exercises, but surgery may allow the patient to return to impact sports sooner.

### Comment

It is often a missed diagnosis. In my opinion, active sporty adolescents who want to play their sport do not have psychological painful knees, and athletes whose pain prevents them playing a sport have a physical problem somewhere. Osteochondritis is often the hidden cause (see Chapter 21: Psychology). A joint's only protection from osteoarthritis is by maintaining articular cartilage, and it must be preferable to maintain this as long as possible, by giving time for it to heal – by incremental loading of the joint – rather than to undertake surgical debridement of the articular cartilage. If cartilage fragments are locking or catching the knee then arthroscopic lavage and articular cartilage trimming may help, but we must ask ourselves what debridement and cartilage drilling does, long term, that is more advantageous than giving time for articular cartilage to repair, especially in the young.

## Recurrent dislocation or subluxation of the patella

(See Anterior knee pain syndromes.)

## Unstable knee

The patient complains of feeling that the knee gives way or they cannot trust it (see Anterior and Posterior cruciate ligament tears, Meniscal tear, Subluxing patella and Loose body).

## Baker's cyst

The patient has a feeling of tightness behind the knee, especially on squatting (see Part 5: Posterior knee pain).

## Rheumatic conditions – basic management

The basic management for any atraumatic, non-mechanical joint disease is to aspirate the joint, and then, if the aspirate is cloudy, to send it for microscopy, including polarized light, culture, and sensitivity. Bloods for full blood count, CRP, ESR, autoimmune profile, and relevant antibodies to *Chlamydia*, *Shigella*, and *Salmonella* should be taken. Note any possible link to Lyme disease and be aware that gonorrhoea and syphilis are on the increase. Note any skin manifestation of psoriasis, which can present as a monarthritis and affect the knee. Seek a rheumatologist's opinion.

## Synovial chondromatosis

Diagnosed on X-ray; this requires surgical clearance of the loose bodies, if symptomatic (Fig. 11.8). See rheumatology books for further details.

## Pseudogout

Calcium pyrophosphate deposition (Fig. 11.9). Polarized light microscopy of the aspirated fluid confirms the cloudy deposit. Cortisone may produce dramatic relief with intra-articular deposition of the calcium. It may occur within the meniscus. See rheumatology books for further details.

## Reactive arthritis

Often in HLA-B27-positive individuals, following *Salmonella* or *Shigella*-type infection. Non-specific urethritis, especially *Chlamydia*, is quite a common cause of reactive arthritis (see Hot, swollen knee). See rheumatology books for further details.

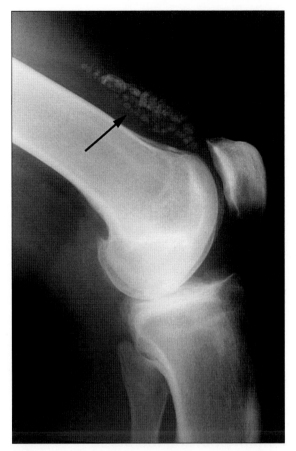

**Figure 11.8** • Synovial chondromatosis requiring surgical washout.

## Rheumatoid arthritis

The joints are more painful in the morning. There is a thickened synovium and maybe a joint effusion, with a capsular pattern to the pain. The joints may be warm and distorted. Children may present with a monarthrits, from juvenile chronic arthritis. It is an Rh seropositive arthritis. Patients probably can withstand and benefit from non-impact exercise in a rheumatalogical, non-active, phase. Take a rheumatological opinion. See rheumatology books for further details.

## Other seropositive or seronegative arthritides

Should be considered with a monarthritis or multiple joint pains, plus morning stiffness, pain of insidious onset, and no history of trauma. Check for psoriasis,

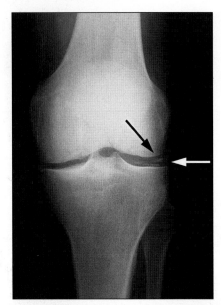

**Figure 11.9** • Calcium pyrophosphate, pseudogout, within the meniscal substance.

take bloods for autoimmune screening and seek a rheumatological opinion. See rheumatology books for further details.

## Pes anserine bursa/ semimembranosus bursa

Pain and swelling over the proximal medial tibia (see Part 3: Medial knee pain; Fig. 11.26).

## Hoffa's fat pad

Swelling limited to either side of the patellar tendon, which increases with the knee in extension and may be tender to touch (see Part 2: Anterior knee pain).

## Meniscal cyst

Firm, localized, palpable swelling over the lateral joint line of the knee, but it may present anteromedially or anterolaterally on the joint line (see Part 4: Lateral knee pain).

## Deep infrapatellar bursa or deep inferior pretibial bursa

Painful swelling around both sides of the tibial tubercle (see Part 2: Anterior knee pain).

## Prepatellar bursa (housemaid's knee)

Swelling localized superficially over the patella (see Part 2: Anterior knee pain).

## Effort-induced thrombosis (Paget–von Schroetter syndrome)

Pain and swelling at the back of the knee and the calf, worse with exercise (see Chapter 12 and Glossary).

# Part 2 Anterior knee pain

## PART CONTENTS

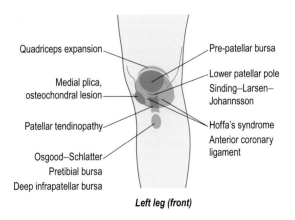

Quadriceps expansion

Medial plica, osteochondral lesion

Patellar tendinopathy

Osgood–Schlatter

Pretibial bursa

Deep infrapatellar bursa

Pre-patellar bursa

Lower patellar pole Sinding–Larsen–Johannsson

Hoffa's syndrome Anterior coronary ligament

*Left leg (front)*

## Referred pain – general

Referred pain from the third and fourth lumbar segment and from the hip (see Chapters 5 and 8) should be excluded before examining the knee.

## Maltracking of the patella

A maltracking patella generally tracks more laterally between the femoral condyles. The cause can be anatomically distant from the knee, from increased functional anteversion at the hip or overpronation at the foot, both of which increase functional valgus at the knee. Anatomical variations at the knee can also increase a valgus knee action. This valgus action tracks the patella laterally. The pain, however, is medial, around the patella.

### General findings for faults at the hip, knee and foot

(a)  There is diffuse, poorly localized, anterior knee pain.

(b)  All have functional valgus at the knees on the half squat test (Figs 11.10 and 11.11).

(c)  Patellar apprehension is often positive (see Glossary).

(d)  The medial patellar facets are tender to palpation.

(e)  Clarke's test is painful or inhibited (see Glossary).

(f)  The running style tends to be a low knee carry, with a windmilling effect of the lower leg such that, when the patient is seen soon after exercise, they may also present with tender capsular ligaments of the knee.

(g)  Pain whilst sitting with the knees bent. Some patients also sit on a chair or the floor with their knees close together but their feet out to the side, and the knees in valgus and external rotation.

(h)  The step down test displays the functional valgus movement at the knees (see Glossary).

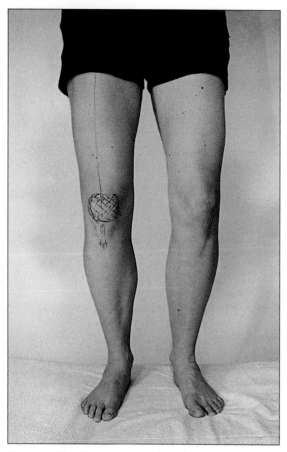

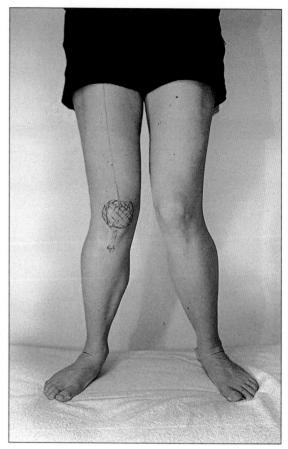

**Figure 11.10** • The Q angle is subtended by a line drawn from the femoral head to the middle of the patella and from this point to the insertion in the tibial tubercle. The Q angle is normally less than 15°. During this half squat test the knees have remained over the feet, maintaining normal patella tracking.

## Fault at the hip

The findings are as described in General findings, above, but, in addition, the patient has anatomical or functional anteversion of the femur. Those with anatomical anteversion of the hip stand with their feet together and straight legs, but the patellae squint inwards. Internal rotation of the hip is marked, but external rotation limited. The feet do not overpronate. The external rotators of the hip are weak. Patients with functional anteversion have poor core and pelvic stability and will drop the weight-bearing hip forwards and inwards, or the greater trochanter will protrude further laterally. These mechanisms encourage the knee to move into a functional valgus.

**Figure 11.11** • This half squat test produces a functional valgus at the knees, increasing the Q angle and producing functional pronation at the feet – a cause of maltracking.

## Fault at the knee

(a) Problems are as described in General findings, above, plus patients stand with their knees in valgus, because of either too much fat around the thighs or a laterally placed tibial tubercle or narrowing of the medial compartment from osteoarthritis of the knee.

(b) There is tenderness over the tibial (medial) collateral ligament on valgus stressing and palpation.

(c) The medial plica may be tender to palpation (Fig. 11.12).

(d) There may or may not be anatomical overpronated feet, but the patient will overpronate in function as the feet follow the effect of the knees (see Fig. 11.11).

(e) The posterior tibialis is weak on resisted testing.

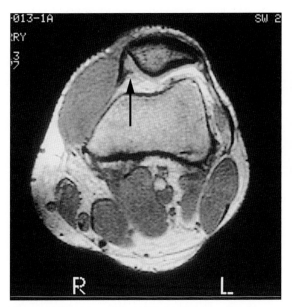

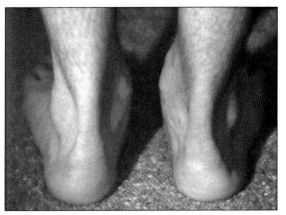

Figure 11.13 • Overpronated feet can cause ankle, knee, hip and back problems. True flat feet (pes planus) are not a problem and can occur in Olympic gold medal sprinters.

Figure 11.12 • T1-weighted MRI showing a medial plica (*arrow*).

(f) Weiberg's 2+ patella, patella alta, or patella baja, may be present.

(g) The bayonet sign may be present.

See Glossary for various tests.

## Fault at the feet

The findings are as described in General findings, plus:

Group 1   The basic anatomical stance is normal, but the feet are overpronated, with weak posterior tibialis on resisted testing (Fig. 11.13).

Group 2   There is limited talar dorsiflexion (congenitally flattened talus, or trauma to the talar dome) and therefore, in function, the foot pronates to create an apparent increase in functional range of ankle dorsiflexion. The pronation shifts the knee into valgus.

Group 3   Tarsal coalition may prevent the feet from adjusting to rough ground, so the knees must make this adjustment, with valgus or varus movements (see Fig. 14.3).

## Cause

The angle between the hip joint, quadriceps origin and the mid-point of the patella lying normally between the femoral condyles, and the mid-point of the patella and tibial tubercle, is increased beyond 15° (an increased Q angle) (see Figs. 11.10 and 11.11). The patella therefore lies towards the lateral femoral condyle, causing strain on the medial capsular structures plus decreased interchondral pressure between the medial patellar facet and the medial femoral condyle, so disuse fimbriation occurs over the medial patellar facets. Chondral cartilage requires pressure between adjacent articular surfaces to squeeze synovial fluid into the nutrient canaliculi.

## Investigations

### Fault at the hip

None are clinically required, except to exclude other problems, such as hip or bony lesions.

### Fault at the knee

(a) X-ray with skyline views to assess the Weiberg type, and lateral X-ray to establish whether patella baja or alta is present (see Glossary).

(b) CT or MRI, between 10 and 40° of knee flexion, can display the lateral, patella maltracking.

### Fault at the feet

Podiatric assessment is required to assess the cause for overpronation (see Fig. 11.13). Lateral X-ray of the ankle, to exclude a flattened talar dome, and check there are no tarsal coalitions for which CT may be required to evaluate further (see Fig. 14.3).

## Treatment

### General

Capsular and ligamentous pains can be eased with NSAIDs and electrical modalities. Lateral patellar tracking or rotation can be reduced or prevented by McConnell taping, or a patellar brace with a patellar restraining ring, and exercises to strengthen and coordinate the vastus medialis obliquus muscle [15]. A weak posterior tibialis should be rehabilitated and strengthened.

### Fault at the hip

Treat with strengthening and balancing exercises for the external rotators of the hip. The patient should walk and stand tall at the hip and pelvis, pulling the hips into external rotation by muscle tension. Concentrate on the knee staying over the first and second toes in one-legged half squats (see Figs 20.11 and 20.12) and whilst cycling or going up stairs. Weak external hip rotators allow the pelvis to swing into adduction and the knee to follow into valgus (see Chapter 20, general exercises for ankle, knee, hip and back). Orthotics may reduce functional pronation and thus reduce the work required from the hip rotators, but perhaps long-term development of strength in the external hip rotators is the priority.

### Fault at the knee

(a) Rehabilitation exercises are the same as those for Fault at the hip, above; however, if the thighs are too fat to allow the knees to touch, as is often seen in adolescents, they must lose weight.

(b) Corrective orthotics in the shoes, for overpronation, but note that a high arched foot can functionally swing too far into pronation and be unable to return to supination for lift off. Orthotics will reduce this range of movement and thus also its effect on the knee.

(c) Surface EMG, biofeedback training to the vastus medialis obliquus may help establish normal patella function.

(d) Running repeats the same movement angle across the knees, whereas 'change of direction' sports will vary this angle, and thus the tracking of the patella. Hence change of

direction sports suit the maltracking knee better than running.

(e) Calm any ligamentous strains (e.g. medial collateral) with electrotherapeutic modalities, NSAIDs or cortisone injection.

(f) Surgery, such as a lateral release, or tibial tubercle realignment, but only if conservative treatment fails.

### Caveat

**The medial subcutaneous fat pad at the knee can confuse diagnosis. It may be sore in the cold and on squeezing. It often changes colour with temperature, and ultrasound may help reduce the patient's discomfort from this problem.**

### Fault at the feet

See Figure 11.13

Corrective orthotics are required, as well as the corrective exercises for the cause from the hip and knee.

Group 1    Posterior tibialis strengthening. The psoas may need strengthening to encourage knee lift during running, allowing the swing phase to complete before foot strike.

Group 2    A heel raise may help, as in the standing position it moves the talus and foot towards plantar flexion. There is then a greater range of dorsiflexion available, before anterior impingement of the talus against the tibia occurs. Pronation of the foot to avoid this impingement is thus avoided. A shorter stride pattern should be advocated, and high knee drills prescribed to encourage lift off of the foot at the mid-stance phase, rather than pushing through to toe off, at which stage the limited dorsiflexion of the foot induces a functional pronation. Use of orthotics other than a heel raise may help, but if pronation is the way out of the limited dorsiflexion, they can make the situation worse.

Group 3    May have to accept the problem and increment loads more slowly, or consider taking up a non-running sport.

## Sports

(a) Change of direction sports cause fewer problems than running because the femur/patella positions alter, in contrast to being repeatedly maltracked, as in running.

(b) Swimming breaststroke and butterfly increase the valgus stress at the knee.

(c) Riding a horse may be helped by using longer stirrups to reduce knee valgus. A forefoot varus can be corrected by a wedge attached to the stirrup.

(d) Hill running can cause problems if knee lift is poor. The swing phase is not completed before foot strike, thus the foot lands in external rotation and pronation.

(e) Running on a camber may produce functional valgus on the higher side.

(f) The knee must be maintained in line over the foot during 'step ups'. Astride jumps taken too wide increase functional knee valgus.

(g) Bicycles must have play in the foot cleat so the knee is not locked into one position, and forefoot varus must be corrected at the pedal with a wedge on the shoe or the pedal. Vastus medialis obliquus function is encouraged by training with a raised saddle, and the knees should move in line with the feet, over the pedals.

(h) Some runners who land into the mid-stance phase instead of heel strike will run onto a soft pronating foot and the knee will suffer both overload and tracking problems. These people work very hard to run, going nowhere fast, rather like running on a jelly! (See Part2C: Problems of overload.)

## Comment

Patellar maltracking is the cause of the very common 'young adolescent girl's knee', and children after about 8 or 9 years of age may gain long-term correction and dramatically improve their athletic performance by using orthotics. However, orthotics are not the answer to all problems, as the three different types have different primary faults, which must also be corrected. Not all clinical trials have divided anterior knee pain into the possible differing mechanisms so that various clinical trials may not be cross-comparable and cannot be relied upon [16].

# Subluxing patella

## Findings

(a) This may present as the child who is always messing about, because they often stumble or may even fall, and when seen immediately after the incident there is nothing wrong.

(b) Signs of maltracking are present (see Maltracking of the patella).

(c) The patellar apprehension test is markedly positive.

(d) The medial patellar facets are tender to palpation.

(e) Weiberg's 2+ patella, patella alta, or patella baja may be present.

(f) The bayonet sign may be present.

(g) A high Beighton–Horan score is common.

(h) Clarke's sign may be positive.

(i) There is usually no underlying osteochondral lesion or synovial swelling.

See Glossary for diagnostic tests.

## Cause

(a) Patello-femoral incongruency such as patella alta, baja and Weiberg 2+.

(b) Increased Q angle, which is usually anatomical but may be functional (see Figs 11.10 and 11.11).

(c) Ligamentous laxity.

Subluxation of the patella laterally occurs more readily in the presence of ligamentous laxity and/or maltracking problems at the knee. Subconsciously the patient recognizes that, when the knee is bent and held into valgus, quadriceps contraction will move the patella laterally and thus dislocate the patella, so the quadriceps contraction is inhibited, causing a fall or stumble.

## Investigations

None are clinically required, but X-ray will establish patella variants and a laterally placed tibial tubercle. A previously normal knee may have underlying chondral damage, and MRI will be required to display the lesion.

## Treatment

Stabilize the lateral patellar tracking with the McConnell strapping regimen (see Glossary) [16]. This may prove too fiddly for active youngsters, or an allergy to plaster may occur, so a patella-stabilizing brace will be more effective. Correction of maltracking at all levels; that is at the hip, knee and feet. Lateral release or tibial tubercle transposition may be required as a last line, and surgery may not be very successful in the abnormal knee [17]. The previously normal knee that has been dislocated and is suffering recurrent subluxation may require medial reefing of the capsule as well as lateral release [18].

## Sports

People with this condition do struggle in almost all sports until the patella is braced (see Maltracking of the patella).

## Comment

One is pleasantly surprised how well these people do with a simple, relatively inexpensive, neoprene patella stabilizer, plus core and pelvic stability training combined with vastus medialis obliquus muscle work. Those who have a high ligamentous laxity score usually require orthotics for overpronated feet, and these feet require treatment, let alone to correct the effect on the knees.

## Medial plica syndrome

### Findings

Maltracking of the knee (see Maltracking of the patella). There is a palpable tender medial plica.

### Cause

The medial plica flicks over the articular corner of the medial femoral condyle and becomes thickened and painful.

### Investigations

None are clinically required unless the patient is not responding to conservative management of tracking problems. X-ray and MRI to exclude other problems. MRI can visualize the plica, but whether it is diagnostic of a pathological lesion is debatable (see Fig. 11.12).

### Treatment

(See Maltracking of the patella). Treat the inflammation of the plica with electrotherapeutic modalities or cortisone to the plica. Surgical division of the plica will be required if it does not respond to conservative measures.

## Sports

See Maltracking of the patella.

## Comment

This is probably treated surgically too frequently, before correction of tracking problems has been achieved, and in my opinion surgical plical resection and lateral release should only follow good adequate conservative management. I have seen a crescendo of repeat operations following early unsuccessful surgical intervention.

# General findings with overload problems

All have a history of pain on squatting, walking up or down stairs and on hills, jumping, checking fast to stop, and kicking, both with the striking and the supporting leg. Resisted quadriceps, active straight leg raise and/or bent knee extension are painful. The one-legged squat test or a step down test (see Glossary) may be the only positive finding if the lesion is mild.

## Cause

Damage to the quadriceps, patella or patella tendon mechanism caused by the application of too much quadriceps work – both too long and too strong.

## Treatment

(a) Overpronation produces a soft, mobile foot, which does not return to supination in time to firm up the forefoot for propulsion. This is like running off jelly, and therefore knee extension has to produce the impetus. These individuals have a short stride and tend to run into mid-stance, rather than heel or forefoot strike. They work really hard to produce a heavy, laboured, running style, driven by the quadriceps, which become overloaded. Correction of the foot will enable a longer stride and more propulsion from the forefoot. In some people, an orthotic to correct the foot can totally correct the knee overload.

**(b)** In those with good anatomy, the inflamed lesion must be settled and then quadriceps loads are required, within pain tolerance. Rehabilitation is started with low loads and the repetitions are incremented up to 30, at which stage the load is increased and the numbers reduced, gradually increasing until '30 reps' are reached once more. This incrementation is repeated until the expected competitive loads are reached. Pyramids (see Glossary) can be used as an alternative, but again within pain tolerance. Muscles and tendons need time to adapt. The quadriceps and kicking ladders can be added (see Chapter 20).

**(c)** Surgery may be required in certain cases (see individual problems below).

## Lower patellar pole syndrome

### Findings

As for General findings, plus:

Type 1    Palpable tenderness on the superficial surface, whilst the knee is bent or straight, usually central, but often para-central of the patellar tendon origin.

Type 2    Tenderness to palpation with the knee straight but not with the knee bent; seems to be more related to the deep surface of the patella, near the tendon origin. This is probably a Hoffa's fat pad impingement.

### Cause

Type 1 is a strain of the patellar tendon origin. There is possibly some anomaly within this diagnosis in that it responds to superficial treatment with physiotherapy or steroid injection, but MRI scanning of the more severe, recalcitrant cases shows fatty degeneration or disruption of the deep surface of the patellar tendon, equivalent to a tendinosis. Type 2 is a fat pad impingement.

### Investigations

None are clinically required unless there is failure to progress. Real-time ultrasound scan and MRI will show bony avulsion, tendinosis or a tendon cyst, and the MRI may show oedema within the fat that lies just deep to the patella (Fig. 11.14). Doppler ultrasound will show neovascularization on the deep surface.

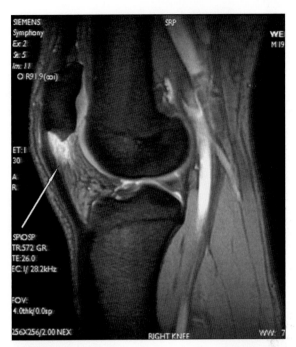

**Figure 11.14 •** MRI shows tendon changes in the patellar tendon origin. The oedema may be secondary to this tendon damage or reflect changes in Hoffa's fat pad. Clinically, the tendon is sore to palpation in flexion and extension; the fat pad only in extension.

 Caveat

In children, an early X-ray for Sinding–Larsen–Johansson syndrome, an apophysitis, is advisable (Fig. 11.15).

### Treatment

As described in General findings, plus:

Type 1    Treatment for inflammation with electrotherapeutic modalities and cortisone injection to the superficial tender areas whilst the knee is bent. Massage techniques to organize chronic scar tissue. Eccentric quadriceps exercises with feet plantar flexed and heels supported on a raised board, progressing to drop squats [19]. A patella tendon brace may help some people. Sclerosis of the neovascular tissue under guided Doppler ultrasound [20]. Surgical

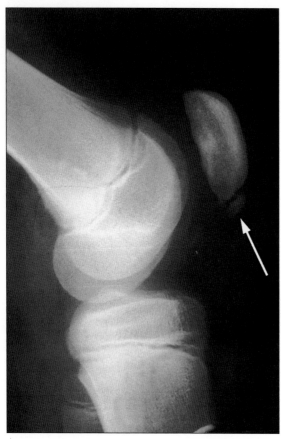

**Figure 11.15** • Sinding–Larsen–Johansson apophyseal lesion (*arrow*).

debridement of the tendinosis [18]. See comment.

Type 2    Cortisone beneath the lower border of the patella to its inferior surface and Hoffa's fat pads whilst the knee is straight. Physiotherapeutic modalities probably cannot reach this area. Surgical excision of the trapped and inflamed fat pad can be curative.

## Sports

(a) In all sports, the power of quadriceps activity must be reduced, as described in General findings above.

(b) Particularly seen in jumpers, volleyball, basketball and weight training.

(c) The injury may take several months to settle and requires graduated loading, with eccentric knee bends, whilst the heels are supported on a raise. Follow this with the Knee ladders (see Chapter 20). In spite of this, the patient often returns to sport too soon.

## Comment

Physiotherapy modalities do not seem successful. Cortisone often produces a pain-free knee within days but rehabilitation to full recovery will still take several weeks to months. The deep surface of the tendon does seem to have the same degenerative yellow look as seen in Achilles tendons. Neovascularization of this tissue, which is seen with a Doppler ultrasound, may be required for healing and may be the cause of pain. Whether neovascularization is required for long-term healing or whether it or the accompanying nerves should be ablated for pain relief and to allow rehabilitation (often over 12–24 months) remains to be seen.

# Sinding–Larsen–Johansson syndrome

## Findings

As described in General findings above, but is usually found in children aged 10–15 years; that is, before skeletal maturity is achieved. There is local tenderness over the lower patellar pole on palpation and resisted quadriceps.

## Cause

An apophysitis at the lower patellar pole caused by too much quadriceps loading.

## Investigations

X-ray the knee to visualize the separate ossification centre (see Fig. 11.15).

## Treatment

Reduction in quadriceps loading, by using low loads, high repetitions and, very occasionally, a cast for 2 weeks in order to rest the apophysis.

## Sports

(a) Pain and limping must be the guide to monitoring the condition (see Chapter 20: How much training?).

(b) Gymnastics – use the ladder principles. Step 1: maintain training on parallel or asymmetric bars and balance routines, plus general abdominal and upper body conditioning. Step 2: walkovers. Step 3: when the patient can run, increment the loads into vaulting using a landing pit. Step 4: build into vaults but 'roll out' the landings. Step 5: plan sessions so as not to have vault and floor routines on the same day. Finish the session with vault or floor routines but roll out the landings. Step 6: as for step 5 but now 'spot' the landings.

(c) Kicking games (football or rugby) – move the player to a position where less kicking is required, such as from fly half to wing three-quarter, and do not take free or place kicks until better.

(d) Jumping sports – reduce jumping until pain-free.

## Comment

This responds, like any overload injury, to a reduction in load, but an apophysis takes longer than expected to heal. Parents and coaches should be warned of this. In my experience ultrasound, interferential and laser do little to help.

# Patellar tendinopathy and tendinitis

## Findings

As described in General findings above. In addition, there may also be a history of pain at rest, improving after movement, which, as it settles with anti-inflammatory treatment, is probably from the peritendinitis. Alternatively, there may be a history of pain, better at rest, worse with loads, which may be from a tendinopathy [21].

## Cause

Inflammation of the paratenon, or degeneration of the patellar tendon, possibly following micro-tears from quadriceps overload.

## Investigations

If pain and tenderness are in the central tendon, look for a tendon cyst with diagnostic ultrasound or MRI (Fig. 11.16). Both can show degenerative changes, and possibly a tear in the deep surface at its origin from the lower pole.

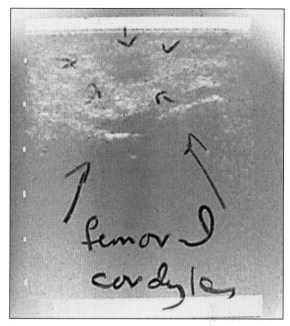

**Figure 11.16** • Ultrasound scan showing patellar tendon cyst.

## Treatment

(a) Tendon cyst – curette out and then quadriceps rehabilitation (see Chapter 20).

(b) Peritendinitis – electrotherapeutic modalities to settle inflammation, peritendinous cortisone. Massage techniques to limit and organize adhesions and scar tissue. When the peritendinitis is pain-free, rehabilitation to the underlying tendon using the quadriceps ladders should be started (see Chapter 20).

(c) Deep surface tendinopathy – eccentric quadriceps work and knee bends with the heels supported on a raise are reported to work, but controlled quadriceps rehabilitation with weights and the knee ladders (Chapter 20) will be required to rehabilitate to sport. If not progressing then surgical exploration of the deep surface [18], or neovascular ablation [20], should be tried (see also the comment for Lower patellar pole syndrome, above).

(d) See also in this chapter, general treatment for overload.

## Sports

Because the injury is caused by powerful, explosive, quadriceps contractions, or eccentric work from landings, such as from volleyball, triple jump, high jump, etc., and also kicking, where the support leg is often affected, the number of games played should be limited, and set piece kicks should be avoided. The injury may require a considerable time to rehabilitate, so early diagnosis and a reduction in training loads is most successful, but surgery and treatment of neovascularization may be required.

## Comment

Central cysts are rare, but accompany mid-tendon pain. Otherwise, the tendon can be as troublesome as the Achilles to settle in the long term. The cortisone breaks the pain cycle if it is caused by the peritendinitis, so permitting rehabilitation of the tendon lesion underneath, but the loading of the tendon must be controlled. The timing of surgery and the role of neovascularization (and precisely what it does) is open to debate, and it does not guarantee a rapid recovery.

## Osgood–Schlatter disease

### Findings

As described in General findings with overload problems, above, plus: tenderness and sometimes local bony and/or soft tissue swelling over the tibial tubercle. Local palpation of, and kneeling on, this area are painful.

### Cause

An overload of the patellar tendon's insertional apophysis at the tibial tubercle; occurs in children, especially during the growth spurt.

### Investigations

A lateral X-ray of the knee or real-time ultrasound show apophyseal widening of the tibial tubercle (Fig. 11.17) and fragmented non-union in the skeletally mature (Fig. 11.18).

### Treatment

(a) As described in General findings above, but this condition, particularly, requires a reduction in quadriceps loads.

(b) Interferential to calm inflammation may help, and occasionally a cast, to rest an active child, is required for about 2 weeks.

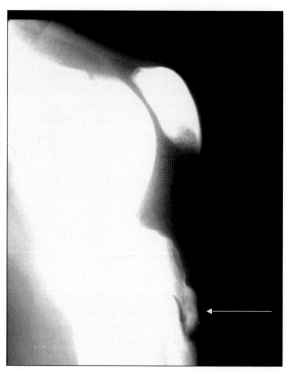

**Figure 11.17** • An 'Osgood–Schlatter' is an avulsion of the developing tibial apophysis. This apophysis is maturing but still shows a diastasis.

(c) Treat any overpronation and posterior tibialis weakness, if it exists.

### Caveat

**This lesion can present in older teenagers or adults as a fragmented, non-union of the apophysis, and surgical removal of these fragments is required [18] (see Fig. 11.18).**

### Sports

The child is often talented, playing school, club, county or junior international, and maybe several different games on the same day. Try to discover the child's sporting ambitions, not the parents' or coach's! Stop minor or less important sports, and less important fixtures, and reduce the amount played. Stop the child from taking all the free and penalty kicks, and even move, for instance, the fly half to wing three-quarter. If the child aches after the game, but is better by the

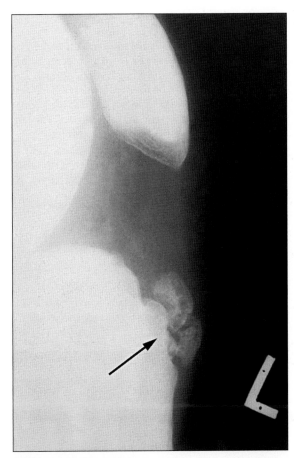

**Figure 11.18 •** Fragmented non-union of the tibial tubercle in a skeletally mature individual.

next day, then this amount of exercise is within his tolerance. If the child limps during the game, or the next day is painful in normal life, then a reduction of exercise is required. Talented sports children need to be kept with their peers, and there are no long-term side effects, apart from a large tubercle, so judicial reduction in training of the quadriceps, and therefore the number of games played, is the management strategy.

## Comment

This condition is very common in the talented child, but also in the child with overpronated feet who has to overload the knee to gain propulsion from this functional 'soft' foot. This second child needs orthotics and encouragement, as their running skills will improve with orthotics.

# Patello-femoral osteoarthritis

## Findings

As described in General findings above, plus:

(a) Clarke's sign is positive (see Glossary).
(b) The bulge test may be positive (see Glossary).
(c) Grating of the patello-femoral joint on passive and active compression.
(d) The patella facets are tender to palpation.
(e) Long-standing maltracking of the patella from overpronation, and/or varus or valgus knees, may be contributory (see Part 2B: Maltracking of the patella).

## Cause

Degenerative changes in the patello-femoral articulation, possibly from old trauma, maltracking, or constant overload.

## Investigations

(a) Lateral and skyline X-ray of the patella may display osteophytic lipping (see Fig. 11.4). MRI can show early chondral cartilage thinning, subchondral oedema and osteochondral defects.
(b) Arthroscopy.

## Treatment

(a) There is a synovial, capsular, inflammatory element that responds to NSAIDs and electrotherapeutic modalities, such as shortwave diathermy and interferential.
(b) Correct any maltracking at the feet and any functional valgus/varus at the knees. A patella brace may help but can increase patello-femoral compression, and the pain.
(c) Reduce heavy loads but maintain quadriceps strength with static quadriceps exercises, straight leg raises or isometrics.
(d) When dynamic exercises are introduced, use low loads, high repetitions, and during quadriceps ladders the ski sit may be omitted (see Chapter 20).
(e) Avoid heavy impact activities and full knee bends.
(f) Hyaluronate injections may be effective.
(g) Arthroscopic trimming of fimbriated chondral cartilage.

## Sports

High loads, especially eccentric, such as downhill running and jumping should be avoided. Low load, high repetition exercises improve quadriceps and the joint (see Part 1C: Intra-articular swelling, Osteoarthritis of the knee). Doubles tennis loads the knees less than singles. Care should be taken with full squats in weight-lifting, and deep bends in field hockey and squash. A higher saddle than normal should be tried when cycling in order to limit the extent of knee flexion, and lower gearing than that required for cardiovascular and muscle training should be used.

## Comment

The articular cartilage reduces bony damage, so conservative preservation of this cartilage should be exhausted before surgical trimming is contemplated. Quadriceps exercises should be maintained to tolerance because weak quadriceps exacerbate the problem and total rest is detrimental [22].

## Stress/fatigue fracture of the patella

### Findings

As described in General findings, plus:

**(a)** The stress fracture has a history of developing localized pain with quadriceps loads.

**(b)** It is tender to palpation over the mid-patella, between the upper and lower poles, usually on the medial or lateral side rather than centrally.

**(c)** The fatigue fracture breaks under muscular loads without external trauma, or without previous warning pains.

**(d)** If the fatigue fracture completes, there is loss of quadriceps function and a tender, palpable, horizontal line, or a palpable, horizontal gap.

### Cause

A rare lesion, caused by overload of the quadriceps mechanism that stresses the patella across the femur, such as a sudden, whipped extension of the knees (as in the Fosbury flop to clear the bar), or persistent overload with a bent knee.

## Investigations

X-ray (Fig. 11.19), but a bone scan or MRI should be undertaken if a stress fracture is suspected, as, before the fracture completes, the X-ray is often normal. The stress fracture is sore on quadriceps loading and on local palpation. The site of tenderness is often at the edge of the patella and in the horizontal mid-portion. The tenderness may start to extend across the patella.

### Caveat

A vertical defect is probably a bipartite patella (Fig. 11.20) and note Haswell's lesion (see Glossary).

## Treatment

**(a)** Reduction in quadriceps loads, for the stress lesion, until pain-free, then introduce the knee

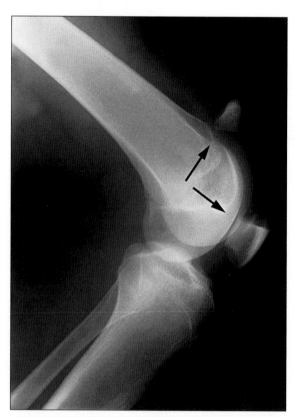

**Figure 11.19** • A fractured patella that occurred at take off at the high jump.

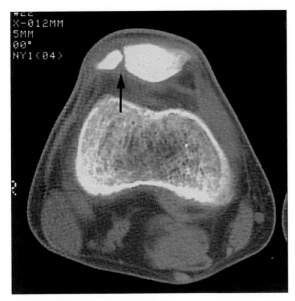

**Figure 11.20** • A bipartite patella.

# Quadriceps expansion

## Findings

As described in General findings above, plus there is local tenderness to palpation over the superior aspect of the patella – centrally, laterally or medially.

## Cause

Micro-tears of the quadriceps attachment to the patella, but graduation to a full tear of the insertional tendon may occur (see Chapter 10: Ruptured quadriceps).

## Investigations

None are clinically required but, if the symptoms persist, MRI and possibly ultrasound may localize the lesion (see Fig. 10.3) An X-ray may show Haswell's lesion (see Glossary) or a bipartite patella, which may be more prone to problems with the quadriceps tendon insertion at the bipartite fibrous union.

## Treatment

(a) Reduce quadriceps loads.
(b) Electrotherapeutic modalities to settle inflammation and/or cortisone injections, localized to the tender point.
(c) Modalities to release scar tissue, such as frictions and cortisone.
(d) Quadriceps ladders (see Chapter 20).
(e) Surgical suture where there is a small dehiscence.

## Sports

(a) Mainly in weight training and weightlifting, with deep knee bends. Beware anabolic steroid abuse.
(b) Occasionally from kicking, or checking to stop, with a deep knee bend.
(c) Hockey, squash, tennis and badminton produce problems by stopping fast with the knee bent, as in stretching out over one leg to play a shot.

## Comment

Most of these injuries settle with appropriate reduction in loads. Cortisone may break the pain cycle to enable rehabilitation to take place. I have seen only one case come to surgery and this professional soccer player had a tear visible on MRI.

ladders but do not include ski sits (see Chapter 20). If the bone scan remains hot but the knee is pain-free, one must proceed with caution.
(b) Immediate surgical repair of the fractured patella.

## Sports

Although a patient of mine with a positive bone scan returned, pain-free, to field hockey, he suffered a fracture when taking-off on the high jump some 6–9 months later (see Fig. 11.19). Reported as occurring during the whip of the legs into extension in Fosbury flop high jumping, and reported in a fast bowler at cricket, and in skiing [23].

## Comment

A rare injury that is more common in adolescents [23]. Perhaps fatigue fractures have had previous minor symptoms, and a bone scan should be performed earlier if there is localized patellar tenderness.

# Rectus femoris tear

Acute pain in the thigh, with a palpable lump in the mid-thigh from the ruptured, contracted muscle end (see Fig. 10.2). Bruising may be present (see Chapter 10).

## Prepatellar bursa (housemaid's knee)

### Findings

A pre-patellar, fluctuant swelling is palpated, with an underlying normal knee.

### Cause

Trauma, usually frictional, between the patella and the ground. The problem is usually seen in 'kneeling professions', but may be acute and produce a haembursitis.

### Investigations

Clinically, none are required, though aspiration, diagnostic ultrasound and MRI will display the lesion.

### Treatment

(a) Knee pads for kneeling activities.
(b) Masterly inactivity. Just leave alone, or ice application as required.
(c) Aspiration.
(d) Hydrocortisone and electrotherapeutic modalities to settle inflammation.

### Sports

Rarely caused by sport, but Canadian canoeists and those undertaking three-position shooting may have problems that can be prevented by the use of polystyrene padding, cut to shape, to kneel on.

### Comment

Treat only if acute or painful; aspiration and intrabursal steroids work rapidly but the bursal swelling still tends to recur.

## Deep infrapatellar bursa or deep inferior pretibial bursa

### Findings

As described Part 2C: General findings with overload problems, plus there is tenderness to palpation around the tibial tuberosity, but it is behind and on either side of the patellar tendon in the skeletally mature individual, and this area may appear swollen.

### Cause

Although a bursa can exist between the skin and tibial tuberosity (pretibial bursa) in patients who kneel frequently, a bursa that may become inflamed exists between the insertion of the patellar tendon and the tibia, especially in those who have a large tubercle. It extends between two sections of Hoffa's fat that slide over each other during normal function [24].

### Investigations

None are clinically required, but ultrasound clearly shows the bursa and the movement of Hoffa's fat pad (Fig. 11.21) and ultrasound will show a fragmented tibial tubercle, which X-ray or CT will delineate further, if surgery should be considered (see Fig. 11.18).

### Treatment

Treat conservatively with electrotherapeutic modalities to settle inflammation and injection of cortisone into the bursa. Surgery to a fragmented tibial tubercle if present and failing to respond to treatment. Rehabilitate through the quadriceps ladders (see Chapter 20).

### Sports

No sport is particularly prone to this injury.

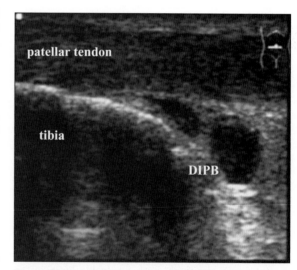

**Figure 11.21** • The deep and superficial elements of Hoffa's fat pads move over each other during flexion and extension of the knee; an inflamed swollen bursa can be created between these two surfaces.

## Comment

A rare problem, which responds well to injection and not so well to electrotherapy. One of my runners with this problem felt that repeated, passive, full-flexion stretching of the knee cured him.

# Hoffa's fat pad syndrome

## Findings

(a) There is a history of a recently increased amount of running, and cases often present in fun runners after their first half marathon.

(b) There is pain at the anterior aspect of the knee, with local tenderness to palpation on either side of the patellar tendon. The fat pad may be described by the patient as swollen, and this may be apparent. It is better seen with the knee straight.

(c) There may be palpable tenderness over the lower patellar pole when the knee is straight but not bent (see Part 2C: Lower patellar pole syndrome).

(d) The entry portals for arthroscopy pass through these fat pads and may remain tender and sensitive for many weeks after surgery.

(e) The fat pads may become immobile and painful after major, multiple ligament disruption of the knee.

## Cause

Not synovial swelling, but oedema of the extra-articular fat pads in the front of the knee. These act as shock absorbers and may become painful and swollen, after increased running.

## Investigations

None are clinically required, although MRI shows the arthroscopic entry portals and, possibly, an inflamed, superior, fat pad impingement under the patella (see Fig. 11.14).

## Treatment

(a) Modalities to settle increased circulation and swelling, such as ice.

(b) Electrotherapeutic modalities to settle inflammation, such as ultrasound.

(c) NSAIDs and, rarely, hydrocortisone.

(d) Surgery to the superior portion [18] if it is repeatedly inflamed from an impingement between the patella and the femur (see Part 2C: Lower patellar pole syndrome).

## Sports

Mainly found with long-distance running, but some fast, step and check games on hard pitches, such as hockey, netball and squash, may cause the problem to flare up.

## Comment

Almost all settle with rest, NSAIDs and ultrasound, but cortisone injections may be required if time constraints so demand.

# Anterior coronary ligament strain

## Findings

McMurray's test (see Glossary) may be positive, and full-flexion weight bearing, such as the squat position, is painful, with local tenderness to palpation over the tibial plateau anterolaterally or anteromedially.

## Cause

The coronary ligament that tethers the meniscus anteriorly is strained, usually by load bearing, full flexion of the knee.

### Caveat

**The possibility of meniscal tears should be considered.**

## Investigations

None are clinically relevant if the signs do not immediately suggest a meniscal tear. If the pain fails to settle with treatment, then investigate with MRI for possible meniscal tear.

## Treatment

Avoid full squat positions. Anti-inflammatory measures, such as cortisone injections or electrotherapeutic modalities.

## Sports

The injury has often been caused in a fall or stumble, although usually the player can run or play through the pain, but full squats must be avoided.

## Comment

An athlete played a full season of elite sport with this injury, just by avoiding full knee squats, and the injury settled with time. It can be quite responsive to cortisone injections but, in my experience, it is unresponsive to electrotherapeutic and massage modalities.

# Part 3 **Medial knee pain**

## PART CONTENTS

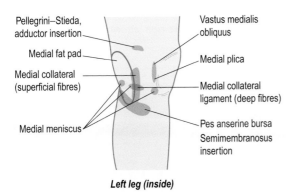

Pellegrini–Stieda, adductor insertion — Medial fat pad — Medial collateral (superficial fibres) — Medial meniscus — Vastus medialis obliquus — Medial plica — Medial collateral ligament (deep fibres) — Pes anserine bursa Semimembranosus insertion

*Left leg (inside)*

## Medial collateral ligament (superficial fibres)

(Sometimes known as the tibial collateral ligament.)

### Findings

There is a history of forced abduction of the tibia, during a fall, twist, wrench or blocked adduction.

### Cause

An abduction strain of the knee, strains or tears of the medial collateral ligament. It may be part of a more major disruption, such as O'Donoghue's triad (tears to the medial collateral ligament, anterior cruciate ligament and medial meniscus) [25].

### Grade 1

(a) No bruising.

(b) Passive abduction is painful.

(c) There is tenderness to palpation, usually over the femoral attachment.

(d) The pain is exacerbated by turning over in bed, and lying on one side with the bad leg uppermost.

(e) McMurray's manoeuvre may be painful, without the clunk.

### Grade 2

As for grade 1, but local bruising and puffiness can be seen.

### Grade 3

Bruising, with passive abduction being pain free, or relatively pain free. There may be gapping of the knee joint, even with the knee held straight, and crutches are required as the knee is unstable. There is tenderness over the femoral and tibial attachment.

### Chronic

The findings are similar to the grade 1, but without an acute episode. Examination shows anatomical or functional valgus at the knees and, frequently, overpronation at the feet.

### Caveat

If there is persistent pain over the medial collateral ligament, or indeed if the pain is getting worse, look for calcification or ossification of the ligament, the Pellegrini–Stieda syndrome, which must be rested. Active treatment encourages further calcification. The Pellegrini–Stieda syndrome may also complicate an adductor tendon tear (Fig. 11.22).

### Investigations

(a) Plain X-rays – Segond's sign may be present medially (Fig. 11.23). Valgus stress X-rays, which may require an injection of local anaesthetic

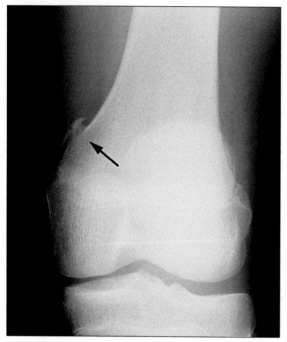

**Figure 11.22** • Pellegrini–Stieda (*arrow*).

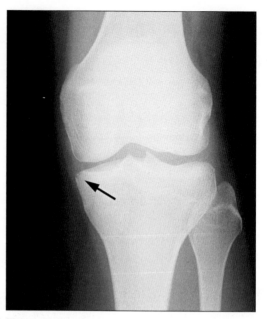

**Figure 11.23** • Segond's sign (*arrow*) small avulsion fracture line.

before the stress can be applied to the joint, show increased valgus gapping of the joint.

(b) MRI shows ligamentous damage, oedema, and also whether internal derangement of the knee joint is present (Fig. 11.24).

## Treatment

### Grade 1

(a) Limit oedema and inflammation with RICE for 48 hours. A pillow placed between the knees, when in bed, will reduce the abduction strains across the knee.

(b) Settle inflammation and organize scar tissue with electrotherapeutic modalities and massage, plus passive flexion/extension of the knees.

(c) Maintain static quadriceps exercises then, when possible, add active knee flexion/extension exercises.

(d) Closed chain knee exercises, with a brace or knee support.

(e) Cross-train, non-impact, e.g. cycling, rowing or swimming, but not breaststroke.

(f) Knee ladders (see Chapter 20).

(g) Add side steps, figure-of-eight runs and cross-over steps before testing for match fitness.

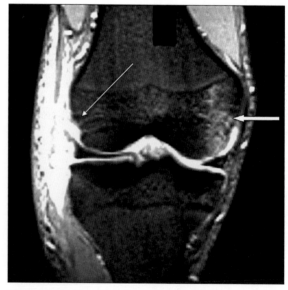

**Figure 11.24** • Grade 2 distraction tear of the superficial fibres of the medial collateral ligament, with the usual contrecoup compression injury on the lateral femoral condyle, showing as bone bruising (*arrow*).

(h) Use a knee support for 4–6 weeks when playing in matches.

## Grade 2

(a) There is a therapeutic balance between immobility, to heal the ligament, and mobility, to maintain joint movement.

(b) A long length, hinged knee brace, with a lockable adjustable hinge range, is most effective as it helps balance mobility and stability.

(c) Maintain static quadriceps. The quadriceps and hamstrings can be worked against a brace (see Glossary: Isometric/isostatic muscle contraction). Straight leg raises and hamstring isometrics are used in the early stages.

(d) Continue as for grade 1– with, and then without, a brace.

## Grade 3

Splint the knee in the acute stage. The ruptured ligaments require surgical repair, preferably within 2 weeks. The knee should be examined to exclude further damage – to meniscus, cruciates and popliteal artery. Rehabilitate as described for grade 2.

## Chronic

Treat as for grade 1, but correct the causes of the genu valgum.

## Sports

This is an important ligament for knee stability. Proprioception is improved by pressure from any support on the skin. A hinged knee brace may be of mechanical value in sports where this is permitted. Problem sports include:

(a) Breaststroke – reduce the frog kick to a narrow wedge kick.

(b) Snow skiers who cannot parallel and have to use edging and snow plough techniques will strain the ligament.

(c) Twisting, turning and checking, at any sport.

(d) Football – side foot kick and side foot tackle.

(e) Martial arts – side, and round the head, kicks.

## Comment

This is a fairly common injury, which I have kept separate from that of the tender, deep fibres of the menisco-collateral ligament, which responds to injections and is tender to palpation along the joint line. The superficial fibres of the medial collateral ligament are tender on the bone of the femur and/or the tibia and should not be injected.

# Medial collateral ligament (deep fibres)

(Sometimes known as the menisco-collateral ligament.)

## Findings

The pain may be sharp and intense, or constant, but is exacerbated by abduction and external rotation of the tibia. The pain is worse on turning over in bed, lying on the side with the bad knee uppermost, and by twisting and turning, including getting into a car and driving with the knee externally rotated. There is no swelling but McMurray's test may be tender without the clunk (see Glossary). There is often loss of some degree of flexion and it is sore to palpation over the mid- to posterior medial joint line [1]. Check for overpronation.

## Cause

Strain or nipping, during external rotation and valgus forces, of the deep fibres of the medial collateral ligament that attach to the peripheral margins of the medial meniscus. The chronic strain is more common in mid- to old age.

## Investigations

None are clinically required, unless a meniscal tear is suspected. A trial of treatment is not out of place.

## Treatment

(a) Correct overpronation at the foot if it is present.

(b) Local cortisone injection to the tender area.

(c) Driving with the foot over the accelerator, and toeing into the brake, rather than with the foot covering the brake and toeing out to the accelerator. Getting in and out of a car with both legs together.

## Sports

(a) This injury is often seen in a middle-aged person who has recently taken up running and has an overpronated foot.

(b) Anyone who runs with a 'windmill' style of running.

(c) Breaststroke.

(d) Golf – reverse pivot, with the left heel on the ground (Fig. 11.25).

## Comment

Although painful, cortisone gives dramatic relief. An overpronated foot, if not corrected, will produce a recurrence. Fairly frequently the presentation has pain over the joint line that is more posterior than this lesion; it seems to settle with cortisone, but over a longer time (such as a few weeks), and there is no obvious meniscal damage.

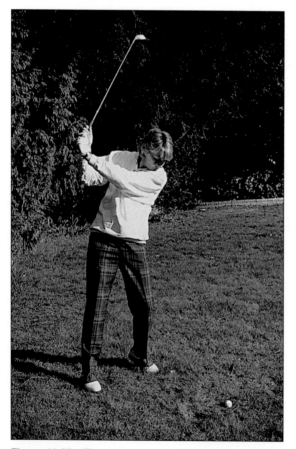

**Figure 11.25** • The reverse pivot, at take away, pushes the weight on the left side; it should be on the right leg. This twist across the bent left knee can injure the deep fibres of the medial collateral ligament (heel down) and the Achilles (heel up), as here.

## Medial meniscal damage

Tenderness along the joint line can be indicative of meniscal, and menisco-collateral ligament, damage, but if this is accompanied by intra-articular swelling then a meniscal lesion is more likely (see Part 1C: Meniscal tear).

## Semimembranosus/pes anserine bursa

### Findings

Type 1 There is a history of recently taking up running, or increase in speed, in a 'shuffle' runner, who often stands with the ipsilateral foot externally rotated.

Type 2 A history of a knee injury, which gradually changes its character during rehabilitation. The pain moves or a new pain appears, located over the semimembranosus bursa.

Both types may, or may not, appear locally swollen and are tender to local palpation over the bursa or hamstring insertions. Resisted hamstrings, with an externally rotated tibia and knee at 30–50° flexion are painful. Check for overpronation and a weak posterior tibialis.

### Cause

The pes anserine (or the semimembranosus, semitendinosus and gracilis) bursa becomes inflamed where these tendons cross the tibia towards their insertions.

Type 1 Running styles may be propulsive (bounding), pushing with the foot and calf muscle, or tractive (shuffle), with the hamstrings pulling the body up and over the foot. If the foot is externally rotated during shuffle running then the pressure over the pes anserine bursa increases and can cause inflammation.

Type 2 The hamstrings work co-actively to decelerate the swing phase and lock the knee ready for loading at impact. When the quadriceps are weak, painful, or the knee is unstable, the hamstrings are worked harder to stabilize the knee at impact, producing a secondary, compensatory injury in the semimembranosus bursa and hamstring insertions.

## Investigations

Observe the running style. MRI or ultrasound may show the bursa, but are not required clinically (Fig. 11.26).

## Treatment

Type 1   Alter the running style to a more bounding style, or correct the externally rotated foot. Anti-pronation orthotics help, and the posterior tibialis must be rehabilitated if it is weak. High knee drills will strengthen the psoas and encourage a higher knee lift during running.

Type 2   Discuss the mechanism with the patient, who must not lock up the knee or foot on impact but learn to roll through the foot, from heel strike to lift off. The patient should try counting, for rhythm, and match the feel of the painful leg to the good side (see Chapter 20).

Treat with electrotherapeutic modalities, such as ultrasound and laser to settle inflammation, and friction and massage for any tenosynovitis. Cortisone injection will calm the bursitis.

## Sports

(a) Usually running – see Cause and Treatment for type 1.
(b) Golfers who increase 'coil' tension or take away by pressing the right foot into the ground may on rare occasions produce this bursitis.

## Comment

The protective mechanism, type 2, is very common and, unless recognized, leads to a muddled pattern of knee pain that inhibits rehabilitation. Indeed, some patients have been arthroscoped, needlessly, because this protective mechanism has not been recognized. A few patients have an enthesitis at the tibial attachment of the medial hamstrings.

# Medial patellar facets

There is anterior knee pain and palpable tenderness under the medial side of patella (see Part 1: Dislocated patella; Part 2B: Maltracking of the patella).

# Vastus medialis obliquus

There is pain on quadriceps exercises and tenderness to palpation over the medial, superior border of the patella (see Part 2C: Quadriceps expansion).

# Medial plica syndrome

A tender medial plica, located over the anterior aspect of the medial femoral condyle, may be flicked on palpation. There are usually other findings of maltracking (see Part 2B: Maltracking of the patella; Fig. 11.12).

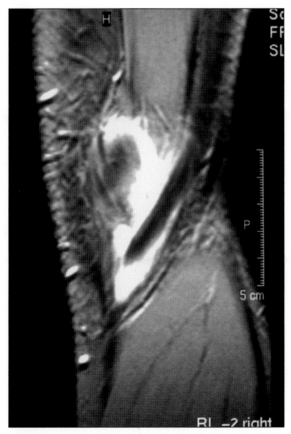

**Figure 11.26** • The pes anserine bursa lying under the semimembranosus, gracilis and semitendinosus tendons is inflamed.

## Pellegrini–Stieda syndrome

Characterized by persistent pain, or pain getting worse with treatment, that occurs after a medial ligament or adductor muscle injury. There is local tenderness, worse on palpation, over the medial femoral condyle (see Tibial collateral ligament; Fig. 11.22).

## Medial fat pad

A pad of subcutaneous fat can be present over the medial aspect of the knee and calf. It is often tender to squeeze or touch, and redder and more painful in cold weather. The knee joint is normal. Therapeutic ultrasound or shock wave therapy may help the discomfort.

# Part 4 **Lateral knee pain**

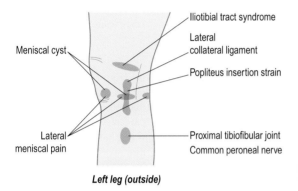

*Left leg (outside)*

## Lateral meniscal tear

There is a catching pain, located over the lateral joint line, which may have an effusion. The joint line may be tender to palpation (see Part 1C: Meniscal tear).

## Meniscal cyst

### Findings

Painful, or painless, firm lump on the lateral side of the knee, over the joint line, that is more prominent in extension than in flexion. There may or may not be symptoms of a meniscal lesion (see Part 1B: Peripheral meniscal tear).

### Cause

Usually associated with an underlying radial tear of the lateral meniscus. It may rarely occur anterolaterally and is uncommon in the medial meniscus.

### Investigations

None are clinically required as this can be palpated clinically, but ultrasound and MRI scan can be used to demonstrate the cyst and any underlying tear (Fig. 11.27).

### Treatment

No treatment is required if this is symptomless, but a trial of cortisone injection into the cyst if it is painful (but there are no other symptoms) may be of benefit. Arthroscopic surgery if there are other symptoms of a meniscal lesion, such as catching and sticking, or an effusion.

### Sports

It does not influence performance unless there are meniscal symptoms.

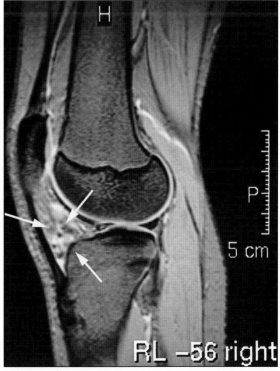

**Figure 11.27** • Anterior meniscal cyst.

## Comment

It is probably worth a trial of cortisone as this may possibly settle the cyst down entirely or produce a painless swelling that the patient finds acceptable, but, if this fails, surgery is required to remove the cyst and, if possible, repair the tear.

# Lateral ligament sprain

## Findings

(a) Acute – pain or laxity to varus stress (see Part 3: Tibial collateral ligament and apply lateral for medial), except that a Pellegrini–Stieda complication is not associated with the lateral side.

(b) Chronic – passive, varus strain, evokes pain over the lateral ligament and, if the capsule is not involved, the knee may have pain-free, full passive flexion and extension. It is locally tender to palpation over the joint line, femoral condyle, or its insertion at Gerdy's tubercle on the tibia.

## Cause

(a) Acute – forced varus injury at the knee, which may have a rotational element, and accompanying capsular or meniscal damage.

(b) Chronic – congenital varus knee (bow legged), often with equino varus feet. Camber running (see Glossary) will produce a varus load on the lower leg.

### Caveat

Look for any accompanying cruciate, meniscal or capsular damage in an acute injury, as the lateral ligament can be a more frequent element of O'Donoghue's triad [1]. If X-ray shows avulsion of the fibula head, this requires early surgery.

## Investigations

None are clinically relevant for grade 1. X-ray (note Segond's sign) if grade 2 or 3 are suspected (see Glossary; Fig. 11.23). MRI may show a ligamentous tear with accompanying oedema, but note that a small pocket of synovium, normally present, suggests a tear when it is in fact intact.

## Treatment

(a) Initially is to reduce the oedema and inflammation – RICE (see Glossary).

(b) Support weight-bearing with a hinged brace, for preference, and non-weight-bearing with crutches.

(c) Electrotherapeutic modalities to settle inflammation and encourage healing, such as ultrasound, laser and interferential.

(d) Organize healing tissue with massage and by maintaining the range of movement with non-weight-bearing extension and flexion, both active and passive.

(e) Cross-train, non-impact, such as cycling, rowing or swimming, but not breaststroke. Build to the knee ladders (see Chapter 20).

(f) Surgical repair of a grade 3 total rupture and major posterolateral corner lesions.

## Sports

(a) Acute – mainly an injury from contact sports, though, occasionally, sudden checking and twisting with the foot locked to the ground, as on artificial surfaces, may cause the strain.

(b) Chronic – usually there has been no trauma. Running and 'straight line' work, which repeat the same strains over the ligament, cause the problem. Thus 'change of direction' sports, which vary these stresses, are less of a problem. However, camber running will produce a varus load on the lower leg and stress the lateral ligament.

## Comment

Lateral ligament injuries are not as common as the medial collateral ligament injuries. If major posterolateral corner damage occurs then the knee is inherently unstable and requires surgery.

# Iliotibial tract syndrome

## Findings

A normal knee, apart from local pain on palpation over the lateral femoral condyle, which is worse when the knee is moved back and forwards at 20–30° of flexion (Noble's sign). The patient may be bow legged, and the iliotibial band tight, with Ober's sign positive. The modified Thomas test may show a tight iliotibial tract (see Figs 22.26, 22.27 and Glossary).

## Cause

The iliotibial tract flicks backwards over the femoral condyle at about 20–30° of flexion, and then forwards as the knee returns to extension. This can cause irritation of the under surface of the iliotibial band, and sometimes to the bursa under this area.

## Investigations

None are clinically required in the presence of a positive Noble's sign (see Glossary), unless the lesion is not responding to treatment, when an ultrasound or MRI scan may show the inflamed bursa.

## Treatment

(a) Settle the soft tissue swelling with RICE (see Glossary).

(b) Electrotherapeutic modalities to settle inflammation and organize scar tissue, such as ultrasound and laser.

(c) Massage, such as frictions, to organize chronic scar tissue. Core stability exercises to the pelvis will decrease pelvic rotation and reduce the tension on the iliotibial tract.

(d) A lateral forefoot wedge may reduce supination at lift off and reduce the pain.

(e) An injection of cortisone into the bursa.

(f) Z-plasty surgery to the iliotibial band at the femoral condyle.

## Sports

This is a rare finding in change of direction sports, being seen mainly in running and cycling. Check whether camber running, downhill running or foot impact with the knee bent [26] are relevant. Check, in runners, for a supinated foot, as this may require an anti-supination orthotic correction. A forefoot wedge for cyclists, either on the pedal or attached to the shoe, may be curative, but is less so in running. Cyclists must have 'play' in their cycle clips or cleats, especially if they cycle with an externally rotated foot, which will be forced into neutral by the cleat and thus tighten the iliotibial band.

## Comment

This is a diagnosis that seems to be missed, and as a result I have seen too many patients with this problem who have been diagnostically arthroscoped. Although it responds well to physiotherapy and injection, surgery may be required to partially divide the iliotibial band.

# Proximal tibiofibular joint

## Findings

There is a history of a traumatic injury, or from a heavy or awkward landing. Examination of the knee joint is normal. Pain is located over the proximal tibiofibular joint and is worse on walking, running and jumping. The pain may travel down the outside of the calf and is exacerbated by local palpation of the joint and translation of the proximal tibiofibular joint.

## Cause

An uncommon capsulitis, acute or chronic, of the proximal tibiofibular joint. Subluxation, anterolateral dislocation, posteromedial dislocation and superior dislocation may occur.

### Caveat

**Consider the differentials of anterior compartment syndrome and spiral fracture of the fibula. The common peroneal nerve, as it winds around the neck of the fibula, may suffer neuropraxia, producing pain, pins and needles or even foot drop [27].**

## Investigations

X-ray to exclude fracture of the fibula, and EMG of the common peroneal nerve if neuropraxia is suspected. MRI may show a cyst (Fig. 11.28).

## Treatment

(a) Rest, and avoid crossing the legs such that local pressure is applied around the joint and nerve.

(b) Support taping or bandaging may control the joint movement.

(c) Impact, or even non-impact events, may be curtailed by pain.

(d) Surgery may be required for any dislocation.

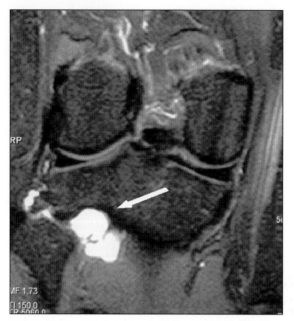

**Figure 11.28 •** This joint was tender to palpation and translation. The knees were in varus and MRI showed a proximal tibiofibular cyst.

## Sports

Triple jump, with its heavy pliometric work, may produce stress across this joint. Taping and support may help, but it may require a lay off from pliometric train-ing (see Glossary: Pliometrics). Otherwise, it occurs by chance in sports where a bad landing or direct trauma can occur.

## Comment

Fortunately a rare condition, as rest is often the only long-term treatment.

## Common peroneal nerve

Pins and needles and numbness over the anterolateral shin, or even foot drop, may occur. There is palpable tenderness around the superior fibular neck when the common peroneal nerve is palpated (see Chapter 12). Its symptoms and signs can be misleading. 'If in doubt check this diagnosis out'.

## Biceps femoris bursa

Posterolateral joint pain, deep to, and associated with, the biceps femoris tendon (see Part 5, following).

## Popliteus tendon insertion strain

Pain on palpation over the femoral condylar notch, at the origin of the popliteus (see Part 5, following).

# Part 5 **Posterior knee pain**

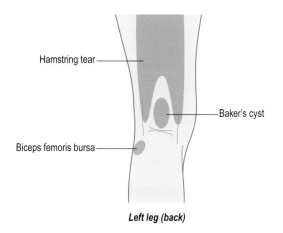

*Left leg (back)*

Labels: Hamstring tear, Baker's cyst, Biceps femoris bursa

## General comments

Posterior knee pain is always difficult to diagnose accurately, so investigations for intra-articular pathology are often required. The gastrocnemius crosses the posterior knee, and its relevance to posterior knee pain is unquantified. Hyperextension can spring the posterior capsule and surrounding structures without major damage.

## Referred pain from the spine and back

Examination for posterior knee pain must include examination of the back. If examination of the knee proves negative, referred pain from the back must once again be considered (see Chapters 2, 5 and 9).

## Popliteal (Baker's) cyst

### Findings

The history is often of discomfort, fullness or tightness behind the knee, rather than pain, and this is worse on squatting. There is a palpable, non-pulsatile, often non-fluctuant swelling behind the knee. This can rupture acutely, giving a swollen calf, thus mimicking a deep vein thrombosis, or leak slowly, causing swelling of the calf or even the thigh (see Chapter 12, Part 2: Leaky knee syndrome). Fluid that is present in the knee may pocket in the back of the knee and in the cyst.

### Cause

The cyst is part of the intracapsular knee space, which can be occupied by an effusion, but a valve-like mechanism in the posterior aspect of the capsule allows fluid to collect posteriorly into the bursa (Baker's cyst) but not escape back (Fig. 11.29).

### Caveat

**Popliteal aneurysm and effort-induced thrombosis.**

### Investigations

Are mainly to establish the cause of a swollen knee, and not to display the popliteal cyst. Ultrasound will display the bursa, whereas MRI will display the cyst and the underlying causative mechanism.

### Treatment

(a) This should be directed at the underlying cause of the swelling. For instance, if the fluid is secondary to early osteoarthritis, an explanation of the cause of the posterior knee discomfort may be sufficient for the patient to tolerate the situation.

(b) Modalities to disperse synovial fluid, electrotherapeutic, aspiration, or injection of the knee with cortisone.

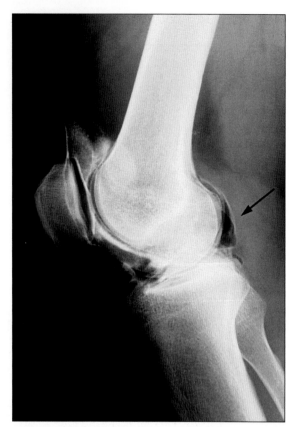

**Figure 11.29** • An arthrogram displays the posterior aspect of the joint from where a Baker's cyst can form (*arrow*).

(c) Aspirate and inject the cyst with cortisone.

(d) Surgical removal.

## Sports

Only full squats are affected because the cyst physically limits knee flexion, but general activity increases the amount of fluid and therefore the patient's awareness of the knee. The cause of the effusion governs the sporting activity.

## Comment

Advice about the nature of the swelling and discomfort is all that is usually required with an osteoarthritic knee; however, injection of the anterior aspect of the knee may give temporary relief. Otherwise direct aspiration and injection of the cyst, under ultrasound guidance, may be required.

## Posterior horn meniscal tear

This often presents with a confusing history of intermittent pain, especially with twisting movements and squatting. An effusion and poorly localizable pain may be the only clinical findings. A diagnostic MRI is required (see Part 1C: Meniscal tear).

## Hamstring tear

There is a history of pain during activity, followed later by discomfort, stiffness, and perhaps bruising along the posterior thigh and behind the knee (see Chapter 9: Hamstring muscle injury).

## Popliteus muscle

### Findings

Diffuse discomfort behind the knee, occasionally with tenderness at the insertion on the lateral aspect of the femur, at the palpable notch. The 'figure-of-four' sign (see Glossary) and resisted internal rotation may be painful (see Fig. 22.5).

### Cause

Strain of the popliteus muscle, which runs from its tendinous origin at the lateral femoral condyle to its muscular insertion along the back of the tibia. The muscle may be injured at the posterior aspect of the knee and, sometimes, strain the tendon at its insertion. It is usually strained in a twisting movement across the knee and, very rarely, the tendon is avulsed.

### Investigations

None are clinically required unless the lesion is failing to respond to treatment, then diagnostic ultrasound scan or MRI. However, neither may be helpful.

### Treatment

(a) Ice, for the muscle, is not advised due to the proximity of the popliteal neurovascular vessels, but may help the insertion.

(b) Electrotherapeutic modalities and, rarely, cortisone to the popliteus origin to settle inflammation.

(c) Massage to organize scar tissue at the origin.

(d) Proprioceptive balancing (see Chapter 20).

(e) Hamstring ladder and knee ladder (see Chapter 20).

## Sports

The injury is usually found in change of direction and contact sports. Many sportspeople play through games, with discomfort and some limitation to performance, whilst it settles.

## Comment

I find this difficult to diagnose with certainty. MRI to exclude intra-articular pathology is often required. Although MRI may show oedema within the muscle, it is often not helpful.

## Biceps femoris bursa

### Findings

There is a history of pain behind, and lateral to, the knee, with sprinting or high heel (heel flick drills). Resisted hamstring testing with a bent knee may be painful, and it is tender to palpation on the medial side of the biceps tendon, near its insertion into the fibula. Examination of the rest of the knee is normal.

### Cause

This is an uncommon irritation of the biceps femoris bursa, at the head of the fibula, close to the insertion and its association with the fibular collateral ligament [28].

### Investigations

MRI or ultrasound may be revealing, but neither is clinically required unless progress is not being made.

### Treatment

Rest from running and/or a cortisone injection to the bursa.

### Sports

Occurs in runners with a short, fast, running cadence that encourages fast flexion at the knee. Encourage lengthening of the stride and increased drive from the calf and forefoot.

### Comment

Cortisone and lengthening of the stride are usually effective. In my experience, electrotherapeutic and massage techniques have not improved the healing time.

## Intra-articular pathology

If in doubt about the cause of posterior knee pain then investigate further for possible intra-articular pathology.

## Popliteal artery entrapment syndrome

Patients with exercise-induced calf pain, or pain behind the knee, must have their peripheral pulses checked. Their calves should then be exercised and the pulse rechecked at the onset of pain, if possible with a Doppler recorder. If there is any doubt about the arterial integrity then refer to a vascular specialist (see Chapter 12, Part 2; Fig. 12.8).

## References

1 Shelbourne KD, Nitz PA. The O'Donoghue triad revisited. Combined knee injuries involving anterior cruciate and medial collateral ligament tears. Am J Sports Med 1991;19:474–477

2 Maffulli N, King JB. Letter. Anterior cruciate ligament injury. Br J Sports Med 1998;32:266

3 Shelton WR, Barrett GR, Dukes A. Early season anterior cruciate ligament tears. Am J Sports Med 1997;25:656–658

4 More RC, Karras BT, Neiman R, Fritschy D, Woo SL, Daniel DM. Hamstrings – an anterior cruciate ligament protagonist. Am J Sports Med 1993;21:231–237

5 Hull ML. Analysis of skiing accidents involving combined injuries to the medial collateral and anterior cruciate ligaments. Am J Sports Med 1997;25:5–40

6 Ettlinger CF, Johnson RJ, Shealy JE. A method to help reduce the risk of serious knee sprains incurred in alpine skiing. Am J Sports Med 1995;23:531–537

7 Webb J. Rugby football and anterior cruciate ligament injury. Br J Sports Med 1998;32:2

8 Stanitski CL, Paletta GA. Articular cartilage injury with acute patellar dislocation in adolescents. Am J Sports Med 1998;26:52–55

9 Sallay PI, Poggi J, Speer, KP, Garret WE. Acute dislocation of the patella. Am J Sports Med 1996;24:52–60

10 Maenpaa H, Lehto MUK. Surgery in acute patella dislocation – evaluation of the effect of injury mechanism and family occurrence on the outcome of treatment. Br J Sports Med 1995;29:239–241

11 Boynton MD, Tietjens BR. Long-term follow-up of the untreated isolated posterior cruciate ligament-deficient knee. Am J Sports Med 1996;24:306–310

12 Videman T. Experimental models of osteoarthritis: the role of immobilization. Clin Biomech 1987;2:223–229

13 Husskinson EC, Donnelly S. Efficacy of and patient satisfaction with intrarticular injections of sodium hyaluronate (Halgen) in the treatment of osteoarthritis of the knee. Rheumatology 1999;38:602–607

14 Henning CE, Yearout KM, Vequist SW, Stallbaumer RJ, Decker KA. Use of the fascia sheath coverage and exogenous fibrin clot in the treatment of complex meniscal tears. Am J Sports Med 1991;19:626–631

15 Arroll B, Ellis-Pegler E, Edwards NA, Sutcliffe G. Patello-femoral syndrome. Am J Sports Med 1997;25:207–212

16 McConnell J. The management of chondromalacia patella: a long-term solution. Aust J Physiother 1986;32(4):215–223

17 Maenpaa H, Lehto MUK. Surgery in acute patella dislocation: evaluation of the effect of injury mechanism and family occurrence on the outcome of treatment. Br J Sports Med 1995;29:239–241

18 King J. Patella dislocation and lesions of the patella tendon. Br J Sports Med 2000;34(6):467–470

19 Cannel LJ, Taunton JE, Clement DB, Smith C, Khan KM. A randomised clinical trial of the efficacy of drop squats or leg extension curls exercises to treat clinically diagnosed jumper's knee in athletes: pilot study. Br J Sports Med 2001;35(1):60–64

20 Hochsrud A, Ohberg L. Ultrasound guided sclerosis of neovessels in painful chronic patella tendinopathy. Am J Sports Med 2006;34:1738–1746

21 Read MTF, Motto S. Tendo Achilles pain: steroids and outcome. Br J Sports Med 1992;26:15–21

22 Sallay PI, Poggi J, Speer KP, Garrett WE. Acute dislocation of the patella. Am J Sports Med 1996;24:52–60

23 Teitz CC, Harrington RM. Patella stress fracture. Am J Sports Med 1992;20:761–765

24 LaPrade RF. The anatomy of the deep infrapatellar bursa of the knee. Am J Sports Med 1998;26:129–132

25 Millar AP. Meniscotibial ligament strains: a prospective survey. Br J Sports Med 1991;24:94–95

26 Orchard JW, Fricker PA, Abud AA, Mason BR. Biomechanics of ilio-tibial band friction syndrome in runners. Am J Sports Med 1996;24:375–380

27 Gillham NR, Villar RN. Postero-lateral subluxation of the superior tibio-fibular joint. Br J Sports Med 1989;23:195

28 LaPrade RF, Hamilton CD. The fibular collateral ligament – biceps femoris bursa. An anatomic study. Am J Sports Med 1997;25:439–443

## Further reading

Bruckner P, Khan K. Clinical sports medicine, 3rd edn. New York: McGraw-Hill; 2006

Hutson MA (ed.). Sports injuries: recognition and management, 2nd edn. Oxford: Oxford Medical Publications; 1996

Hutson M, Ellis R (eds). Textbook of musculoskeletal medicine. Oxford: Oxford University Press; 2006

Reid D. Sports injury assessment and rehabilitation. Edinburgh: Churchill Livingstone; 1992

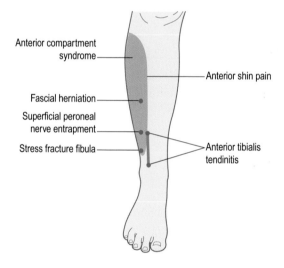

Anterior compartment syndrome

Anterior shin pain

Fascial herniation

Superficial peroneal nerve entrapment

Stress fracture fibula

Anterior tibialis tendinitis

# Lower leg

## CHAPTER CONTENTS

## Part 1 **Anterolateral shin pain**

### PART CONTENTS

## Referred pain

The back should be examined for any evidence of referred pain from the L4/5 segment (see Chapters 2 and 5).

## Stress fracture of the fibula

### Findings

There is pain on running, and, as the lesion worsens, there is also pain on walking. There is typical tenderness to palpation, the site of which is, classically, five fingers (approx. 10 cm) up from lateral maleolus, localized in a 1–2 cm area. This tenderness, together with the history of impact-induced pain, is diagnostic of a stress fracture until proved otherwise. Occasionally, a stress fracture can occur near the proximal neck of the fibula.

### Cause

This fracture is produced in runners, as a result of a supinated foot, bow legs or an internally rotated foot and tibia. The lesion may be more common in those with a low knee style of running, with a windmilling foot action.

## Investigations

An X-ray may show callus and a fracture line (Fig. 12.1) but may be normal, and a bone scan or MRI with marrow oedema will be positive (Fig. 12.2).

## Treatment

(a) Cross-training, with no impact on the legs, for 6–8 weeks.
(b) Achilles rehabilitation ladder (see Chapter 20).
(c) Orthotics (see Glossary).
(d) Strengthen the hip external rotators and the psoas. Core stability training to reduce twisting stresses from the pelvic movements.

## Sports

This is said to be a runner's injury. It occurs generally with a supinated or cavoid foot, but there may be an internally rotated foot, squinting patella and anteverted hip (the miserable malalignment syndrome) (Fig. 12.3). Either the incremental rate of loading must be reduced, to permit adaptation, or the anatomical/functional problems must be corrected. It also occurs in aerobics with astride jumps and 'jumping jacks' onto a supinated foot, when landing on the balls of the feet [1].

## Comment

This is less common than a tibial stress fracture. Pain five fingers up from the tip of the lateral maleolus is invariably a stress fracture, and can be treated as such without further investigation.

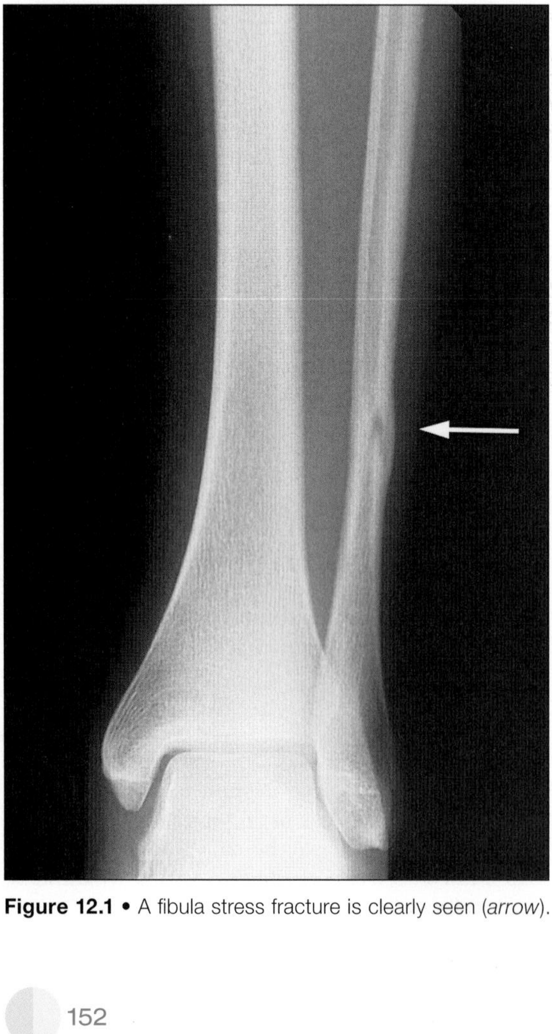

**Figure 12.1** • A fibula stress fracture is clearly seen (*arrow*).

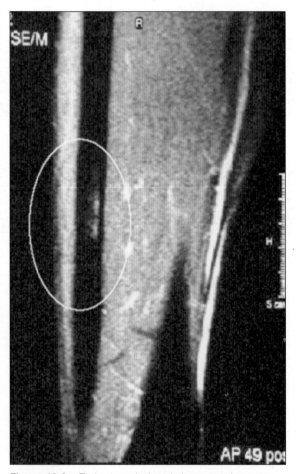

**Figure 12.2** • Early stress lesions in bone are shown on MRI as medullary oedema.

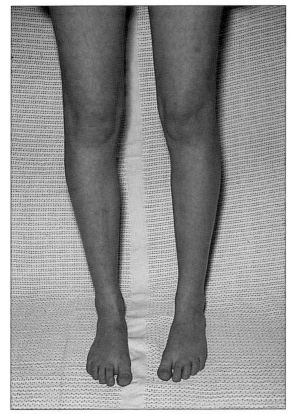

**Figure 12.3** • The miserable malalignment syndrome produces tracking problems in the lower limb that cause problems from the ankle to the hip and to the back.

hallucis and extensor digitorum longus muscles are involved. Some people walk, or march, with their toes and foot pulled upwards, and this overworks the anterior compartment muscles. Shorter soldiers, who have to maintain the same long stride length as their taller companions, are prone to this condition. Others have had pronated feet for a long time and have adapted to the problem by internally rotating the foot, and then using the dorsiflexors of the foot to prop up the arch and stabilize the first ray. Those with anterior compartment problems counteract overpronation by overworking the tibialis anterior muscle.

## Investigations

X-ray to exclude a stress fracture, but a three-phase bone scan may show muscle and exclude bony changes with exercise. MRI post exercise has proved unhelpful. Anterior compartment pressure studies are the investigation of choice. Sometimes, if the patient repeatedly moves his or her foot up and down for several minutes, it will reproduce the compartment pain.

> ### Caveat
>
> All the differentials may have to be eliminated by bone scan, MRI, and EMG. Compartment pressure readings are interpreted differently, depending on whether continuous or interval monitoring is used, and, for some, the rate of fall after exercise is important (see Glossary: Compartment pressures).

# Anterior compartment syndrome

## Findings

The history is as for the posterior compartment, but relating to the anterior compartment (see Part 2: Posterior compartment syndrome). The anterior compartment is often bulky, looking muscle bound, and, when the symptoms are acute, there may be tenderness to palpation. The diagnosis can frequently be established in the consulting room by making the patient repeat rapid dorsiflexion movements of the feet whilst lying on the couch.

## Cause

See Posterior compartment syndrome, but affecting the anterior compartment, between the tibia, fibula and interosseous membrane. The tibialis anterior, extensor

## Treatment

Orthotics, core stability and a reduction in loads and/or a surgical fascial split of the anterior sheath.

## Sports

(a) Running – the shuffle type of runner will often have worn a hole in the top of the shoe, from the big toe pulling into dorsiflexion and rubbing into the shoe.

(b) Untrained cross-country skiers, from pulling the ski forwards with the foot.

(c) Sit-up exercises, undertaken with the toes wedged under a bar to keep the feet down and provide leverage.

(d) Marching – possibly from smaller individuals having to stride out, with their feet emphasizing dorsiflexion, as part of a marching style. To overcome this problem, the armed forces have stopped sorting platoons by size, with the smallest in the middle.

## Comment

It is not that common in sport, in spite of being well described, but perhaps more common in the armed forces. Correction of the cause is often successful, but a fascial split returns the athlete to sport rapidly. Pressure studies carried out during the rest phase from injury may be negative. The compartment test exercise should copy the individual's exercise pattern [2]. The history of exercise-induced pain is an important diagnostic indicator.

## Tibialis anterior tendinitis

Pain on resisted testing of the tibialis anterior and local tenderness over the lower anterior compartment. Crepitus may be present (see Chapter 13, Part 2: Tibialis anterior tendinopathy and synovitis).

## Anterior shin pain

### Findings

The pain is similar to the anterior compartment syndrome, but with the tenderness lying along the anterior tibial border rather than over the muscle (see above).

### Cause

Stress changes on the anterolateral border of the tibia, either adaptive, occurring when the patient takes up running, or caused by stress from the anterior compartment fascial attachment.

### Investigations

(a) X-ray may show thickened, enlarged cortical bone which represents adaptive changes (Fig. 12.4).

(b) A three-phase bone scan may be hot in the blood phase and/or bone phase, with linear increased uptake over the anterior tibia. MRI

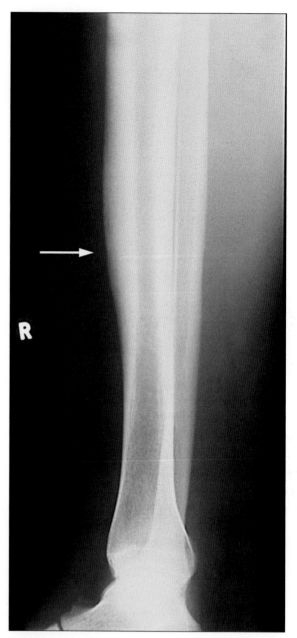

**Figure 12.4** • Thickened cortical bone on the anterior aspect of the tibia. This is not an osteosarcoma but a stress reaction to the recent addition of long runs to this rower's training regime.

can show medullary oedema along the length of the tender bone, and possibly muscle oedema.

(c) Anterior compartment pressures may also be raised, or anterior shin pain may precede the compartment problems.

## Treatment

Reduction in the rate of incremental loading, and possibly a surgical fascial split, especially for patients whose bone scan or MRI shows hot in both blood and bone phases.

## Sports

(See Anterior compartment syndrome.) In some sports, such as rowing, the athletes may run in the winter, and many oarsmen do not run well and have not had impact on their legs all summer. This can produce too rapid an incremental loading of the bones (see Fig. 12.4). The rowing ergo reduces the need for this type of training.

## Comment

This is uncommon, but does seem to be caused by both impact in those who are unaccustomed to running and overuse of the anterior compartment.

# Peroneal muscle strain

This is an uncommon injury, as the tendon usually suffers first. It presents as an ache in the shin, and pain is produced with resisted eversion. It is tender to palpation over the peroneal compartment. There may be crepitus with a tenosynovitis (see Chapter 13). Rarely, a compartment syndrome requiring fascial release occurs.

# Muscle herniation (anterior compartment)

## Findings

This can present as a painless or painful swelling of about 2–4 cm diameter, which is worse on exercise. The hernia is located in the anterior compartment, at about the mid-point. Palpation may reveal a defect in the fascia, usually just below the mid-point of the anterior compartment, and with exercise a tense swelling develops.

## Cause

A defect in the anterior compartment fascia, which is often close to the superficial peroneal nerve, allows the muscle to herniate. The non-tender hernia has room to expand through the defect whereas the painful hernia is starting to strangulate.

## Investigations

(a) If painless, none are clinically required.
(b) If painful, probably none – compartment pressures usually register as normal because the pressure releases through the hernia, and the swelling is visible or palpable.
(c) Ultrasound can help.

## Treatment

None is required if the lesion is painless, but, if painful, a surgical fascial split is required, with care not to damage the superficial peroneal nerve.

## Sports

See Anterior compartment syndrome.

## Comment

Not common. The pit in the fascia can often be palpated when the muscle is not in a flared state. Because the treatment is a fascial split, rather than repair of the defect, there is not much point in measuring compartment pressures.

# Common peroneal nerve entrapment

## Findings

There is a history of pain, numbness, and 'pins and needles' down the outside of the shin. The 'pins and needles' distinguishes this from other local causes. Sensation may be reduced over the anterior compartment and there is local pain on palpation of the posterior lateral surface of the neck of the fibula. The knee joint is normal and the patient may have 'bow legs'.

## Cause

An uncommon irritation of the common peroneal nerve as it swings around the upper fibular neck.

> ### Caveat
>
> **Lumbar disc, problems with the proximal tibiofibular joint (see Fig. 11.28), spiral fracture of the fibula, anterior compartment syndrome, and superficial peroneal nerve entrapment.**

## Investigations

EMG, if severe, but an early neuropraxia may still have a normal EMG.

## Treatment

(a) Check if camber running could be causative (see Glossary). Rest from running and, possibly, even switch to 'change of direction' sports, as these do not constantly repeat the same stresses around the fibula.

(b) Avoid sitting with knees crossed and compressing the nerve, especially with the foot pulled behind the ankle (secretaries).

(c) A lateral forefoot wedge may just reduce supination at forefoot lift off, and so ease the problem.

(d) Surgical release of the common peroneal nerve.

## Sports

Mainly running and jumping, especially triple jump, when the knee may bow outwards on foot impact. The problem is uncommon in change of direction sports.

## Comment

The diagnosis may be a lot harder to make, and the history a lot more confusing, as some patients present with lateral shin and foot pain. There are no pins and needles as such but, rather, a hyperaesthesia. Aggressive palpation of the common peroneal nerve around the fibula neck does not flare these symptoms, and EMG eventually provides the answer as a neuropraxia of this nerve. Although cortisone helps the tarsal and carpal tunnel, I have not been impressed with results of injections in this area. Rest and avoidance of the cause are the best treatments, with perhaps some adverse neural tensioning, although most of my cases have come to surgery.

## Superficial peroneal nerve entrapment

### Findings

Pain, over the lower anterior leg that can spread around the lateral maleolus and outer foot. May have 'pins and needles' and numbness. It is worse with exercise and as the compartment pressure increases. It may come on sitting with crossed ankles, when the pressure of the other leg onto the nerve causes pain. There is very localized tenderness and re-creation of symptoms with palpation over the trigger area.

### Cause

The peroneal nerve is compressed as it passes through the anterior compartment's superficial fascia, but there has often been external trauma around this area causing scar tissue, which traps the nerve.

### Caveat

**Lumbar disc and common peroneal nerve.**

### Investigations

None seem to aid diagnosis. EMG is probably valueless but may exclude a root lesion.

### Treatment

Avoid further external trauma and avoid the causes, such as crossed ankles irritating the nerve further. Cortisone to the trigger area may help, but surgical release may be required.

### Sports

See Anterior compartment syndrome. A stirrup may catch across this nerve when odd riding positions are used.

### Comment

I have usually seen this in office workers who have been sitting with crossed ankles, rather than from sport. In sport it has been in horse riders, either from localized trauma or from the stirrup rubbing over the nerve.

# Part 2 **Calf and medial shin pain**

## PART CONTENTS

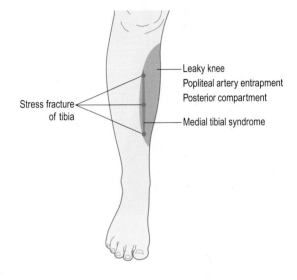

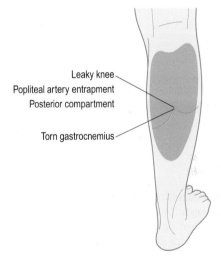

## Referred pain

The back must always be examined for evidence of referred pain from the L5/S1 segment (see Chapters 2 and 5).

## Torn gastrocnemius

### Findings

Presents with a history of acute pain in the calf, and this is the classical 'who hit me with a ball in the back of the leg' story. The calf then becomes acutely swollen and may bruise extensively. There is pain and tenderness over the medial gastrocnemius or its aponeurosis, and a haematoma may be present (Fig. 12.5). The healing, or less severely damaged, muscle has persistent discomfort, usually over the medial gastrocnemius, although the lateral gastrocnemius can be involved. There is pain on walking, jogging, going up stairs, and standing on tiptoe.

### Cause

Usually an acute episode of a torn medial gastrocnemius but the lesion may be lower, having been caused by a tear of the gastrocnemius/soleus aponeurosis. The normal jump mechanism is for the quadriceps to con-

tract first and, when the knee is almost straight, plantar flexion from the gastrocnemius should follow. If this mechanism is reversed, that is if there is plantar flexion when the knee is bent or when standing on tiptoe with a bent knee, then, on straightening the knee, a tear may occur.

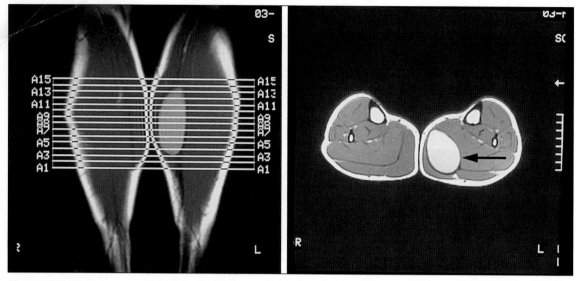

**Figure 12.5** • MRI shows a clearly defined haematoma. This is more easily displayed and aspirated under ultrasound control.

## Caveat

**A calcified haematoma may remain in chronic cases.**

## Investigations

Diagnostic ultrasound displays the haematoma and, in the early stages, blood lying between the muscle bundles. The more chronic cases may lead to a difficulty of diagnosis, for an MRI is normal and investigations are used to exclude other diagnoses. An arthrogram will display a leaky knee syndrome, and Doppler ultrasound will display both the deep vein thrombosis and effort-induced thrombosis. Some experienced ultrasonographers may see diagnostic changes in the muscle.

## Treatment

(a) RICE and crutches.

(b) Early aspiration, under ultrasound control, of any haematoma. This may require repeating weekly for a while (see Fig. 12.5).

(c) A heel raise will rest the gastrocnemius.

(d) Massage techniques, such as effluage, to remove tissue debris and swelling.

(e) Electrotherapeutic modalities to settle inflammation and hasten healing, such as laser and ultrasound.

(f) Gastrocnemius and soleal stretching to prevent scar contraction.

(g) Achilles ladders (see Chapter 20).

## Sports

Sports where acceleration is generated from the plantar flexed foot and a bent knee, such as squash, tennis or a quick single to leg, played off a backward defensive shot at cricket, are particularly prone.

## Comment

Aspiration of the haematoma quickens the rate of healing. Full, pedantic rehabilitation is required to prevent scar tissue and repeat injuries occurring. Chronic calf strain requires pedantic rehabilitation, taking time over the early ladder stages, through to running and pliometrics. This is an injury that, even when apparently better, requires ongoing calf exercises as a recurrence is common.

# Stress fracture of the tibia

## Findings

It is an uncommon injury in change of direction sports and has a history of impact-induced pain, usually from running, but, if severe, the pain occurs on walking or even at rest. The tenderness is on the medial border of the tibia and is localized to a 1–2 cm area and is classically palpated at:

(a) the junction of the lower third and mid-third of the tibia

(b) the junction of the upper third and mid-third of the tibia

(c) the mid-shaft of the tibia.

Occasionally stress fractures appear in other parts of the tibia. So if in doubt, rule a stress fracture out (Fig. 12.6).

There may be bony swelling, localized soft tissue swelling and, if severe, pain on tapping the tibial shaft or resonating under a tuning fork. This lesion is often accompanied by anatomical or functional overpronation of the foot.

## Cause

Repetition of the same load produces cortical subperiosteal stress fractures, either from valgus stress or, most commonly, from valgus and external rotatory stress across the tibia. This external rotation and valgus pressure may be increased by increased external rotation of the tibia, an externally rotated foot with anatomical or functional overpronation of the foot, valgus knees and anteverted hips. Weak posterior tibialis strength is often found with this injury. Broken heel cups and cutaway arches in running shoes will precipitate these strains in the tibia (see Fig. 22.19, 22.20).

## Investigations

(a) None are actually necessary as, clinically, palpation of the tender spot in these three locations is diagnostic of a stress lesion and 'marketable' to the patient.

(b) X-ray can show callus or a lytic area of the stress fracture, where the 'dreaded black line' of the mid-shaft stress fracture suggests non-union, and then completion to a fracture may occur (Fig. 12.7).

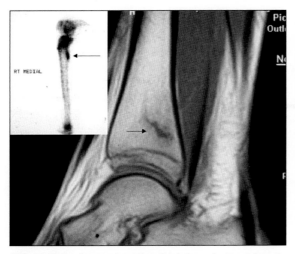

**Figure 12.6** • Scans show that tibial stress lesions occur in less common areas than the classical sites. So if in doubt, rule a stress fracture out.

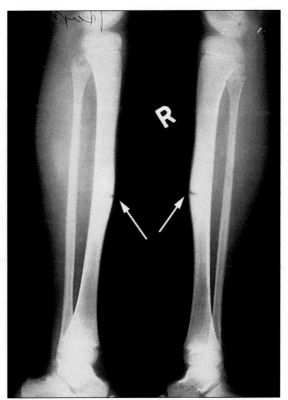

**Figure 12.7** • Bilateral mid-shaft fracture in a ballet dancer, showing the 'dreaded black line' of an impending fracture, which requires surgical nailing. (Mr Justin Howe)

(c) The bone scan is good for displaying an early lesion, especially if the diagnosis is in doubt.

(d) MRI will show the marrow oedema of a very acute lesion but is not as accurate for a cortical lesion, when the lesion is more chronic (see Fig. 12.2).

(e) CT scan will assess the extent of the lesion, especially for mid-shaft stress fractures.

### Caveat

A subperiosteal haematoma from a stress fracture can look like an osteosarcoma on X-ray (see Fig. 12.4). The mid-shaft fracture is usually horizontal, often bilateral, and more common in dancers, where it has been known to fracture entirely (see Fig. 12.7).

## Treatment

Rest from impact for 6–8 weeks, but non-impact cross-training, by cycling, rowing, swimming, etc., will maintain cardiovascular fitness. Correct the biomechanical cause, if relevant; orthotics may be curative. Core stability should be emphasized to prevent anterior rotation of the pelvis and functional valgus at the knees. Start the Achilles top ladder after 6–8 weeks, which will be when walking and jogging are pain-free (see Chapter 20 for ways to increase pace and distance). The mid-shaft fracture invariably requires intramedullary surgical nailing [3], though pneumatic leg braces can be effective in treating non-union [4,5].

## Sports

(a) Athletics – this is a classical, distance-running injury, usually caused by biomechanical problems. However, increasing pace and distance at the same time may precipitate the problem. Switching to lightweight, cutaway-arch running shoes may precipitate overpronation in the well-established runner (see Glossary: Shoes; Fig. 22.19) and the shoe cup (see Fig. 22.20) can break down, ceasing to prevent any excess calcaneovalgus and overpronation. This mechanism is made worse by camber running (see Glossary). Running into the mid-stance phase, as opposed to heel strike, causes the foot to impact into pronation and thus stresses the tibia. The treatment is to encourage heel strike and a longer stride, but note that these patients may require time to strengthen their calf muscles to cope with this new style of running. Hill running and a windmilling action can prevent the foot reaching a supinated heel-strike position so that the impact of foot to ground occurs whilst the calcaneum is in a valgus position.

(b) Aerobics – astride jumps (jumping jacks) and astride bench jumps can force genu valgum and may cause a stress fracture of the tibia. Note these exercise have also been reported to produce fibula stress fractures [1]. Fracture of the fibula is more common in the person with a springy style and supinated foot, and the tibial fracture is more common in the person with a 'knock knee', non-springy style and a pronated foot.

## Comment

This is an extremely common injury, especially in runners, though, because many other sportspeople do their training by running, it appears in a number of sports. Almost all patients have anatomical or functional genu valgum or overpronation of the foot. Attempts to hasten healing include hyperbaric oxygen, low-frequency ultrasound and an infusion of pamidronate. The pamidronate may settle bony oedema, as seen on MRI, because pain-free improvement is rapid.

## Medial tibial syndrome

### Findings

This is impact initiated, but the patient may have good biomechanical function with large calves. The palpable tenderness extends over several centimetres along almost all the medial border of the tibia, and there may be a stress fracture present as well. There may also be anatomical or functional overpronation at the feet.

### Cause

This is not well understood [6] but, fortunately, it is not that common. It may be the same mechanism as for a stress fracture and possibly reflects a gradual adaptation to the loads. However, the loads are just too high, causing periosteal stress either from the attachments of fascia of the posterior compartment or from the elongated muscle enthesis of the posterior tibialis, which in turn causes fibrous thickening [6].

## Investigations

A three-phase bone scan is taken, with an immediate blood flow phase and a delayed blood phase after 2–5 minutes, followed by the bone phase 2 hours after injection. The blood phase being positive indicates that the fascia and muscle attachments are inflamed, whilst the bone scan will show an extensive linear increase in uptake along the tibial border. Pressure studies for posterior compartment syndrome may be of value, for, if they are raised, then fasciotomy will help. MRI can show both soft tissue and marrow oedema.

## Treatment

(a) With mainly the blood-phase positive, or only muscle oedema, try a fascial split.

(b) With mainly the bone-phase positive or mainly bony oedema, try tibial drilling.

(c) Like all overload problems, a reduction in loads, followed by incremental loading when pain-free, can be successful, but takes time for recovery.

(d) Correct overpronation with orthotics for the feet, and increase core stability to prevent pelvic rotation and functional valgus at the knee.

## Sports

Running or dancing, but also in other sports where running is used for training.

## Comment

This problem is often difficult to handle as most patients are too impatient to return to full activities. The problem takes several months to heal under a conservative regimen, so patients proceed to surgery, which can also have quite a delayed recovery time.

## Posterior compartment syndrome

### Findings

(a) Acute – follows a history of trauma, with a tense swelling of the calf, which may be rapidly increasing. There is increasing pain, even without activity, and on compression of the muscle. Eventually the peripheral pulses – dorsalis pedis and posterior tibial – disappear.

(b) Exercise induced – onset of exercise is usually pain-free, but there is increasing pain as the exercise continues. The pain settles when the activity stops. When the syndrome is established the pain may persist for some days after activity. There is no clinical evidence of stress fracture nor of a medial tibial syndrome, both of which have bony tenderness on palpation.

## Cause

It is thought that the muscles swelling within their fascial confines increases the compartmental pressure and gradually reduces the blood supply, producing muscle anoxia. There exist two compartments – the superficial compartment: gastrocnemius, soleus and plantaris, and the deep compartment: flexor digitorum longus, posterior tibialis and flexor hallucis. Some define the posterior tibialis as deep compartment, others as a separate compartment. The acute phase is produced by an acute, post-traumatic bleed. The chronic phase is induced by muscle exercise (usually in runners) causing localized anoxia due to an obstruction of the venous return and/or arterial perfusion.

### Caveat

**As the syndrome becomes established or the athlete continues to run through the pain, so the cessation of activity may not reduce the pain, which can persist for 2–3 days. A rare differential is popliteal artery entrapment syndrome, and sympathetic overactivity. See Reflex sympathetic dystrophy/regional pain syndrome.**

## Investigations

(a) Acute – Doppler ultrasound to assess arterial flow and to observe tissue swelling.

(b) Exercise induced – compartment pressure studies with a split needle catheter (see Glossary: Compartment pressures).

## Treatment

(a) Acute – emergency release of the fascia and debridement of any dead tissue.

(b) Exercise induced
   • RICE (see Glossary) and massage, such as effluage, to reduce the swelling.

- A reduction in running speed and mileage is required.
- Correction of overpronation may unload the posterior compartment and ease the anoxic effect.
- Surgery to release the fascia of one or both deep and superficial compartments.

## Sports

This is a distance running problem, from about 1500 metres upwards, and often also in a ball player or sprinter who has taken up distance running and is still using a fore-foot strike or a strong calf thrust style of running. Alteration to a heel strike and shorter stride length may help. Other repetition activity sports, such as aerobics and trampolining, can be problematical. Speed work in runners may produce some problems. Check for increased pronation, which can be treated.

## Comment

Posterior compartment syndrome often requires surgery, usually of the deep compartment. Some cases will be diagnosed on the history: compartment studies are not always diagnostically accurate because the pressure measurements may well be normal, especially if the athlete has had a few weeks' rest (the problem occurs incrementally). The test exercise before compartment pressure studies should mimic the exercise that produces the problem [2].

## Posterior tibialis tendinitis or muscle strain

### Findings

Tenderness over the medial, deep compartment, close to the tibia, which is worse on resisted testing of the posterior tibialis. This ache may present early in cases of functional overpronation, but it usually does not present alone, being accompanied by the tenderness of posterior tibialis tenosynovitis around the ankle or foot (see Chapter 13, Part 4: Posterior tibialis tenosynovitis). It may also present as part of the medial tibial syndrome (see above).

### Cause

An overload of the posterior tibialis muscle, which may be strained, secondary to overpronation, or the pain may result from a compartment syndrome effect on the muscle. This problem may be seen during the rehabilitation of Achilles tendons. The athlete starts rehabilitation running but instead of running through the foot, via the Achilles, he or she runs with the foot externally rotated to protect the Achilles from load, and so runs in such a way that the posterior tibialis is providing the propulsion.

### Treatment

Correction of technique and corrective orthotics is curative (see Glossary: Orthotics; Chapter 13, Part 4: Posterior tibialis tenosynovitis).

### Sports

This is an injury that is common in the group of anatomical, or functional, overpronators. It is unlikely to be camber or hill running induced, much more likely to be caused by a sudden increase in mileage, pace, bend running, or dancing. Ballet dancers who do not have enough turn out have a tendency to pronate, and may work very hard to restrict their overpronation by firing the posterior tibialis. Walking and edging the foot along the side of a hill, for a long while, can strain the muscle. This injury can be induced during rehabilitation (see Cause above).

### Comment

Probably, the medial tibial stress syndromes, stress fractures and posterior tibial muscle strains have a similar cause of functional overpronation, plus an increase in loading rate to which the tissues cannot adapt.

## Leaky knee syndrome

### Findings

(a) Painless or tense swelling of the calf that usually follows a history of a swollen knee, or Baker's cyst, which seems to have nearly settled.

(b) Semi-acute swelling of the calf but, unlike a muscle tear, painless until the volume of fluid causes discomfort.

(c) There are no dilated superficial veins, as with a thrombosis, but there may be oedema at the ankle.

(d) Homans' sign is negative and the calf is not tender to palpation.

## Cause

The capsule of the knee is not intact, so the synovial fluid leaks out. This occurs with a swollen knee, or Baker's cyst, when the fluid escapes into the calf. If the tear is in the superior pouch, this fluid can be pumped upwards into the thigh by muscle action or joint movement, giving a swelling of the thigh.

### Caveat

**The differential diagnoses include deep vein thrombosis, haematoma in the calf or effort-induced thrombosis, as well as lymphoedema, venous obstruction and systemic problems.**

## Investigations

Doppler ultrasound will exclude deep vein thrombosis. An arthrogram of the knee will display the fluid leak into the calf or thigh. MRI can show interstitial but not intramuscular oedema.

## Treatment

Elevate the leg when at rest and use effluage as a massaging technique. A compression support over the calf may help. The problem is usually self-limiting, healing over time, and only rarely requiring surgery to repair the tear.

## Sports

There is no contraindication to playing any sport, as long as the knee permits.

## Comment

This problem is usually misdiagnosed as one of its more serious differentials. The clue lies with swollen knee problems, and a painless swelling with Homans' test negative.

# Effort-induced thrombosis (Paget–von Schroetter syndrome)

## Findings

An index of suspicion is required to differentiate this from a leaky knee, which has a history of a swollen knee and/or Baker's cyst, and a swollen calf. As the leaky knee syndrome appears, so the Baker's cyst settles, because the fluid has leaked from the knee. This lesion presents with a swollen calf, with no history of trauma or tear, and may occur during travel on a long journey from sitting in a cramped position. Homans' sign is positive and the calf is tender to palpation [7].

## Cause

Paget–von Schroetter syndrome. Possibly, from a tear of the internal wall of a vein, sitting for a long time whilst travelling, local trauma, or systemic causes of increased vascular coagularity. It is more common in the upper limbs.

## Investigations

Ultrasound Doppler studies and a venogram.

## Treatment

Anticoagulate.

## Sports

Reported in joggers, skiers, soccer players and kick boxers, but probably not sports related.

## Comment

Rare, but sometimes presents following very long journeys.

# Deep vein thrombosis

Swelling of the calf, which is often uncomfortable and tender to palpation or squeezing. The superficial veins may be dilated and Homans' test is positive (see Glossary). In sports people, it is most likely to occur during long-distance travel. Prophylactic aspirin, elastic stockings, regular walks around the aeroplane and/or plantar flexion exercises should be utilized. When diagnosed, refer urgently for a vascular opinion concerning anticoagulants.

# Reflex sympathetic dystrophy or regional pain syndrome

May occur after trauma, fracture or a sudden forced stretch of the neurovascular bundle, causing sympathetic nerve effects. However, Gebauer et al [8] report a case of chronic exercise-induced leg pain that responded to sympathetic blockade.

## Stage 1

Increased circulation. Oedema. Hot dry skin. Livid colour. Burning, everlasting pain; worse to touch. Often in a stocking distribution.

## Treatment

Intravascular, sympathetic blockade with guanethidine. Sympathetic ganglion block. Peripheral nerve block. Epidural or spinal block with an indwelling catheter. Elevate and treat with NSAIDs. The patient may gently exercise, but no massage. Neuroleptics are required.

## Stage 2

Pale, cold, cyanotic skin. Vasospasm. Sweating. Atrophy of the skin and muscle. Contraction of the joint.

## Treatment

Treat the pain as in stage 1. Unfortunately, the therapy is less effective.

## Stage 3

Irreversible atrophy of bone, muscle and connective tissue. Joint contractures. The skin is cold, pale and dry. X-ray shows osteoporosis, particularly around the joint. Pain may ease when at rest, but movement causes terrible pain. Sympathetic blockade may not work.

## Treatment

Epidural or sympathetic plexus block to try and obtain movement. TENS. Neuroleptics.

## Comment

This may be seen in sportspeople after trauma, but I did see a gymnast who was stretching her hamstring on someone's shoulder when her foot slipped, and this forced stretch produced a reflex sympathetic dystrophy over the next few days. Fortunately, she responded to therapy for stages 1 and 2. Her bone scan showed lack

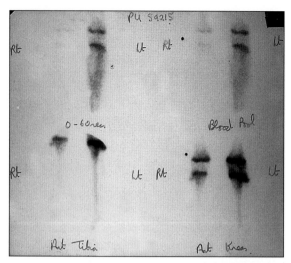

**Figure 12.8 •** A bone scan shows severely diminished uptake in the right leg in the second stage of reflex sympathetic dystrophy in a gymnast.

of circulation (Fig. 12.8). Hot and cold therapy has been recommended.

# Popliteal artery entrapment syndrome

## Findings

There is a history of intermittent claudication in an active young or middle-aged person, which is often unilateral. There are diminished pedal pulses with calf activity or sustained, passive dorsiflexion of the foot. Cramps appear with exercise, which paradoxically may be worse when walking than running. It is worse in endurance events than in stop–start events.

## Cause

Rare, anatomical variations of popliteal artery entrapment, where it is partially compressed by cysts or fibrous bands on the medial head of the gastrocnemius. The variations are often defined into four types depending on the nature of the obstructing band.

## Caveat

Differential diagnosis includes atherosclerotic claudication, venous claudication, and posterior compartment compression syndrome of the calf.

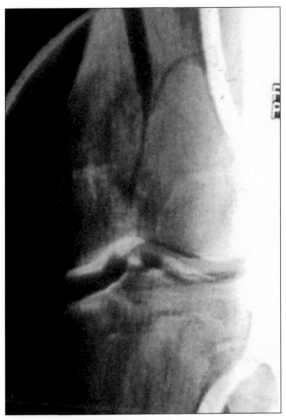

**Figure 12.9** • An obstructed popliteal artery shown on an arteriogram. (Dr Desmond Thomson)

## Investigations

Ultrasound Doppler studies of the dorsalis pedis and posterior tibial arteries before, and immediately after, exercise. Angiography or spiral MRI will define the anatomical variation and help plan management (Fig. 12.9).

## Treatment

In the early stages is to reduce activity, but if this does not improve the situation then surgery to correct the extra-articular obstruction will be required.

## Sports

None are contributory.

## Comment

Fortunately this problem is rare. The history, and a high index of suspicion, are required to diagnose the lesion. This could be called the 'skiving syndrome', as the player avoids hard endurance runs and effort on the pitch but appears to play comfortably in short bursts. Most coaches feel the player is a 'skiver', who avoids hard work, the long runs, and hard work about the pitch, but is happy with the pretty stuff and walking around the pitch waiting for the ball. This attitude of the coach I would consider diagnostic! However, as this is a claudicatory problem, one can understand that long-lasting activity brings it on, whilst short bursts allow the claudication and muscle anoxia to recover before any pain appears.

## References

1  Read MT. Runners stress fracture produced by an aerobic dance routine Br J Sports Med 1984;18(1): 40–41

2  Padhair N, King JB. Exercise induced leg pain: chronic compartment syndrome. Is the increase in intra-compartment pressure exercise specific? Br J Sports Med 1996;30:360–362

3  Orava S, Karpakka J, Hulkko A, et al. Diagnosis and treatment of stress fractures located at the mid-tibial shaft in athletes. Int J Sports Med 1991;12:419–422

4  Batt ME, Kemp S, Kerslake R. Delayed union stress fractures of the anterior tibia: conservative management. Br J Sports Med 2001;35:74–77

5  Swenson JE, Dehaven KE, Sebastianelli WJ, Hanks G, Kalenak A, Lynch JM. The effect of a pneumatic leg brace on return to play in athletes with tibial stress fractures. Am J Sports Med 1997;25(3):322–328

6  Bhatt R, Lauder I, Finlay DB, Allen MJ, Belton IP. Correlation of bone scintigraphy and histological findings in medial tibial stress syndrome. Br J Sports Med 2000;34(1):49–53

7  Gorard DA. Effort thrombosis in an American football player. Br J Sports Med 1990;24:15

8  Gebauer A, Schultz C, Giangarra C. Chronic exercise-induced leg pain in an athlete, successfully treated with sympathetic block. Am J Sports Med 2005;33(10):1575–1578

## Further reading

Bruckner P, Khan K. Clinical sports medicine, 3rd edn. New York: McGraw-Hill; 2006

Hutson MA (ed.). Sports injuries: recognition and management, 2nd edn. Oxford: Oxford Medical Publications; 1996

Hutson M, Ellis R (eds). Textbook of musculoskeletal medicine. Oxford: Oxford University Press; 2006

Reid D. Sports injury assessment and rehabilitation. Edinburgh: Churchill Livingstone; 1992

# Chapter Thirteen

# Chapter Thirteen

13

# Ankle

## CHAPTER CONTENTS

## Part 1  General ankle pain

### PART CONTENTS

### Referred pain

Ankle pain may be referred from the back, common peroneal and superficial peroneal nerves, and the patient will often have a history of 'pins and needles', hyperaesthesia and numbness (see Chapters 2, 5 and 12).

### Comment

One patient whom I saw had had a fall and was unsuccessfully treated for ankle pain over several months. Examination of back movements whilst she was sitting produced ankle pain and no back pain. Her ankle was pain-free on examination. Manipulation of her back rendered her pain-free. When the back is tested with the patient standing, the peripheral joints may be stressed as well, and so produce pain. If the back is tested whilst sitting, then the peripheral joints are unlikely to be stressed.

## Capsulitis of the talar joint

### Findings

(a) There is a history of trauma to the ankle followed by synovial swelling of the ankle joint, infilling the posterior aspect of the joint bilaterally and allowing ballottement of the fluid.

(b) Passive ankle flexion, extension and talar translation hurt in a capsular pattern, but trauma to the ankle usually disturbs the ligaments and tendons as well so that, clinically, there will be accompanying signs from these to confuse the diagnosis.

(c) Inflammatory disease has no history of trauma, therefore no individual ligamentous signs are found, but there is likely to be a capsular pattern of pain accompanied by systemic stigmata.

### Cause

Sprain of the talar joint capsule and its ligamentous thickenings. Inflammatory joint disease.

### Caveat

If there is no history of trauma, consider the diagnoses of gout, osteoarthritis, rheumatoid (adult and juvenile) arthritis, spondylarthropathies, reactive arthropathies and infective arthropathies. Avascular necrosis/idiopathic talar oedema occurs in the older patient.

### Investigations

X-ray for fractures or joint disease and perform the appropriate blood tests, if required. MRI will show an ankle effusion, possible bony trauma (bone bruising) and surrounding soft tissue swelling, and is the investigation of choice.

### Treatment

(a) RICE (see Glossary) and crutches.

(b) Electrotherapeutic modalities to settle inflammation, such as interferential and pulsed shortwave diathermy.

(c) NSAIDs.

(d) If systemic causes are suspected, then diagnostic aspiration of the joint, which must be sent for culture and crystal microscopy.

(e) Injection of cortisone to settle capsular inflammation, via either the anterior or posterior approach.

(f) Isometrics to the posterior tibialis and peroneals, to maintain strength.

(g) Balancing or wobble board exercises, for proprioceptive skills.

(h) Non-impact cross-training, such as swimming, cycling or rowing routines.

(i) Achilles ladders, when impact is permitted (see Chapter 20).

### Sports

Following injury, most ankles will require supporting for 4–6 weeks after reaching match fitness.

### Comment

If this is a traumatic inflammatory lesion then early cortisone injection settles it and permits earlier rehabilitation. However, if possible, take an aspirate before the injection, for culture and polarized light microscopy. Though a bone scan can be the watershed investigation separating bone and soft tissue injuries, MRI, and especially MRI arthrogram, is the most definitive investigation for the majority of ankle lesions.

## Osteoarthritis of the talar joint

### Findings

The history may indicate trauma in the past, previous surgery or just a gradual onset of pain. Examination shows a swollen joint whose cause may be bony, soft tissue or synovial effusion, or all three. There is pain on weight-bearing, and with passive flexion, extension and translation of the talar joint. The range of dorsiflexion and plantar flexion is often restricted physically by osteophytes and the reduced joint space; this produces a hard end feel to passive movement. The posterior tibialis and peroneal muscles are often weak.

### Cause

The cause is degenerative, or post-traumatic osteoarthritis of the talar joint, which frequently is accompanied by subtalar and mid-tarsal osteoarthritis. The osteoarthritis often follows a Pott's fracture, or gross, long-standing overpronation.

## Investigations

X-ray is usually sufficient and cost-effective to define the problem, but CT or MRI scanning can display early chondral cartilage narrowing and subcortical cysts not seen on X-ray (Figs 13.1 and 13.2).

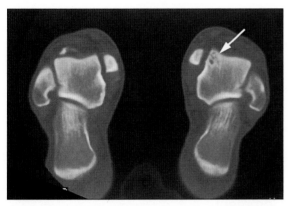

**Figure 13.1 •** A CT scan shows the osteochondral defect in the talar dome of the patient in Fig. 13.4.

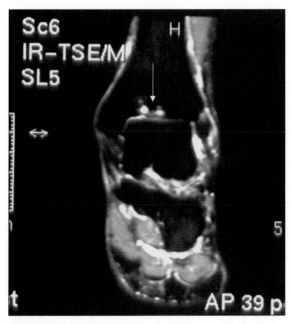

**Figure 13.2 •** MRI shows that damage can occur in the tibial plafond rather than the talar dome.

## Treatment

(a) Electrotherapeutic modalities, such as interferential and pulsed shortwave diathermy, to settle soft tissue inflammation and pain.

(b) NSAIDs.

(c) Intra-articular injection of cortisone for relief of the capsular pain.

(d) A heel raise will increase functional dorsiflexion, which may allow pain-free walking.

(e) The foot may require a firm supportive orthotic if subtalar and mid-tarsal joints are also involved.

(f) Sodium hyaluronate injections (see Glossary).

(g) Surgery to arthrodese the joint or joints (a triple arthrodesis).

### Caveat

**The patient adapts to a limited dorsiflexion of the ankle by pronating through the foot. Therefore, blocking pronation with an orthotic may make osteoarthritis of the talar joint worse. A heel raise may be a better solution, unless the subtalar and mid-tarsal joints are involved, because they do require supporting with an antipronation orthotic.**

## Sports

(a) Avoid impact sports to limit further degeneration, if possible.

(b) Limited dorsiflexion may also require a change of technique for non-impact sports, such as skiing, where a heel raise will increase the functional range of dorsiflexion and, thus, the knee bend required to ski properly.

(c) Swim, row, or cycle for aerobic fitness, but the seat height may have to be adjusted to accommodate the limited range of ankle movements.

## Comment

Osteoarthritis of the ankle severely alters activities, so individual adjustments in technique, and playing aspirations, need to be discussed thoroughly with the patient.

## Osteochondral defect

### Findings

There is a history of an ankle injury, without a fracture, in which the bruising and swelling often occur on both the medial and lateral aspects of the ankle. The most usual presentation is of long-standing ankle pain, failing to settle after the appropriate treatment of a ligamentous and capsular injury (see Capsulitis of the talar joint). Weight-bearing, to some degree, is painful, and swelling of the joint may be present. There is variably pain on dorsi- or plantarflexion, but pain on talar translation is invariably present. The injury may produce a loose body.

### Cause

This often follows a severe sprain of the ankle but may represent a compression stress fracture caused by overuse. Osteochondral lesions are usually in the talar dome (Fig. 13.3), and only rarely in the tibial plafond (see Fig. 13.2). They can be graded for surgical purposes through 1–5.

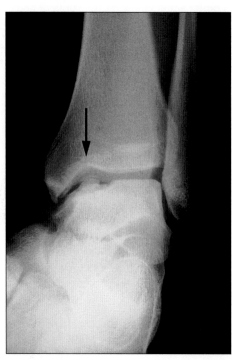

**Figure 13.3** • Osteochondral lesions can be seen on X-ray, but the X-ray is often normal.

### Investigations

(a) Anteroposterior and lateral X-ray are often negative.

(b) Bone scan is the cheapest watershed diagnosis; a positive scan is invariably from an osteochondral defect (Fig. 13.4).

(c) CT or MRI scan display the site and grade of the lesion, and MRI is the investigation of choice (see Figs 13.1 and 13.2).

### Treatment

Grades 1 or 2  Reduce impact and allow time to heal.
Grades 3–5  Surgery.

### Sports

Training should be non-impact: cycling, rowing, swimming or using other non-impact gym equipment. Maintain balance and calf strength. Build up to running via the Achilles ladders, after impact is free of pain (see Chapter 20).

### Comment

Chronic ankles may be unstable, have bony damage or soft tissue injury. Management of chronic ankles is helped by a stress X-ray, as the unstable ankle with no obvious damage is often missed. If the X-ray is negative, for both talar instability and bony damage, then a bone scan, or preferably an MRI scan, will differentiate between a bony or soft tissue lesion. If the ankle has

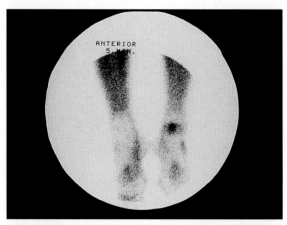

**Figure 13.4** • A hot bone scan indicates the problem in this patient with a normal X-ray. MRI would have shown this lesion.

no bony damage and is stable, mobilize the ankle, possibly with manipulation under anaesthetic, and an injection of hydrocortisone to the talar joint. The chronic soft tissue lesions of the ankle tend to produce adhesions if they have not been rehabilitated properly, in which case manipulation, often under an anaesthetic, is the only way to re-establish ankle range.

## Loose body

### Findings

There is a history of intermittent, catching pain that can abruptly come and go and may be combined with other symptoms from an osteochondral defect, talar joint capsulitis or footballer's ankle.

### Cause

Osseous or chondral fragment within the talar joint, usually following trauma.

### Investigations

(a) X-ray is often the most accurate (Fig. 13.5).

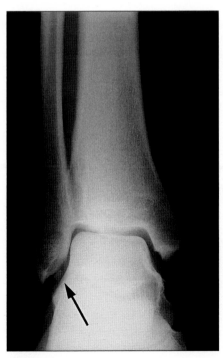

**Figure 13.5** • A loose body between the lateral maleolus and talus (*arrow*).

(b) CT scan is effective, but can miss the lesion if the slices are too wide.

(c) MRI is not good at showing cortical bone, and non-visualization of a loose body on MRI does not exclude the diagnosis. However, all can miss the loose body but may show the defect from where the loose body originated.

(d) Arthroscopy.

### Treatment

Arthroscopic removal of the loose body.

### Sports

Rehabilitate via the Achilles ladder (see Chapter 20). Cardiovascular fitness should be biased to non-impact cross-training for future protection of the joint.

### Comment

The intermittent history of catching pain, without instability, is almost pathognomonic of a loose body.

## Footballer's ankle

### Findings

There is a history of rest pain, better with activity. Inspection and palpation show thickened, swollen, soft tissues around the ankle, with no synovial swelling, unless a loose body is in the joint or the capsule is inflamed. There is a stiff, limited joint range.

### Cause

Chronic minor trauma to the ankle, from both sprains and direct trauma (kicked), which heals with thickening and calcification of the soft tissues, osteophytes and loose fragments.

### Investigations

X-ray and MRI show extracapsular soft tissue swelling and calcification (Fig. 13.6).

### Treatment

(a) Electrotherapeutic modalities, such as ultrasound and laser, to settle inflammation.

(b) Massage and mobilizations, such as frictional massage, to release scar tissue.

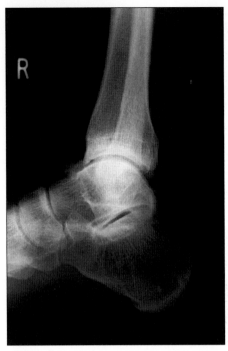

**Figure 13.6** • Extra-articular calcification and osteophytes, and early joint space narrowing, in the so-called 'footballer's ankle'.

(c) Ankle mobilizations and electrotherapeutic modalities, such as interferential, pulsed shortwave diathermy and ultrasound, to warm and mobilize scar tissue.

(d) Proprioceptive rehabilitation.

(e) Achilles ladders (see Chapter 20).

## Sports

Invariably soccer, but the patient can play sport with this ankle, because the pain improves with activity. They may prefer strapping or an ankle support, plus shin pads with ankle flaps. Pre-match NSAIDs may help.

## Comment

This is a stiff ankle caused by soft tissue damage and has a history typical of soft tissue lesions, i.e. mainly worse at rest, better on the move. As such, physiotherapy and mobilization help, and an injection of steroid or local anaesthetic is rarely required.

# Syndesmotic strain

## Findings

This lesion presents as a severe ankle injury, with the patient attending accident and emergency centres. There has been an injury severe enough to disrupt the distal tibiofibular syndesmosis, but it has not fractured a bone. There is often a history of acute trauma that, at the time, had medial and lateral bruising, and a capsulitis of the ankle, but the X-ray showed no apparent fracture. This ankle sprain takes longer to heal, and the patient often presents with chronic ankle pain at a soft tissue or sports clinic, with a history of a severe acute injury in the past, but still having pain on pushing off into acceleration. Initially, all stress testing across the ankle may be positive, but, in the chronic case, the syndesmotic (syndesmal) stress test, or external rotation stress test, is positive [1] (see Glossary).

## Cause

This is a severe ankle injury where the medial maleolus, and possibly talar ligaments, have withstood the force, but the distal tibiofibular and interosseous ligaments are disrupted.

 Caveat

**May have a proximal fibular fracture. The force comes in at the ankle and leaves near the knee. The X-ray should show the whole length of the fibula.**

## Investigations

MRI in the acute stage shows an effusion tracking up between the distal tibia and fibula, within the syndesmosis. Later, an X-ray might show ectopic calcification in the interosseous ligament (Fig. 13.7) [2].

## Treatment

(a) Cast or plastic boot, ankle brace for stability.

(b) Electrotherapeutic modalities to settle inflammation, such as ultrasound, laser and interferential.

(c) Massage techniques to organize scar tissue.

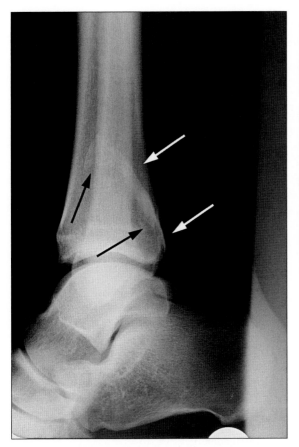

**Figure 13.7** • A syndesmotic ankle injury showing calcification in the osseous ligament and behind the tibia.

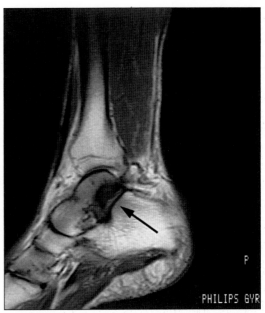

**Figure 13.8** • MRI showing decreased signal in the talus and around the subtalar joint from avascular necrosis or idiopathic oedema of the talus.

**(d)** Proprioceptive rehabilitation.

**(e)** Achilles ladders (see Chapter 20).

**(f)** Surgery, if the lesion remains unstable or there is a widened, distal, tibiofibular diastasis.

## Sports

None are particularly prone to this injury.

## Comment

Usually the trauma is high enough to produce an ankle fracture, which is the frequent result. The syndesmotic strain is, therefore, uncommon, often missed at the acute stage and will present as chronic ankle pain. The stability of the ankle governs the decision as to whether surgical screwing of the tibiofibular syndesmosis is required. The syndesmotic lesion takes longer to heal, can show ectopic calcification, and causes a persistent low-grade discomfort [1–3].

# Avascular necrosis and idiopathic oedema of the talus

This is usually from non-sporting causes, catabolic steroids, alcohol and barbiturates, but it may occur after trauma, and in scuba diving – from the nitrogen gas bubbles, the 'bends' (Fig. 13.8). However, idiopathic talar oedema presents in the older individual and all its features are similar to this condition. The pain and MRI changes, if treated early enough, settle with an infusion or oral administration of pamidronate. A plastic walking boot can ease the discomfort whilst healing takes place.

## PART CONTENTS

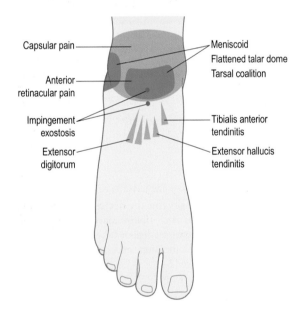

Capsular pain — Meniscoid
Flattened talar dome
Tarsal coalition

Anterior
retinacular pain

Impingement
exostosis — Tibialis anterior
tendinitis

Extensor
digitorum — Extensor hallucis
tendinitis

## Tibialis anterior tendinopathy and synovitis

### Findings

The patient presents with pain, which may travel up into the tibialis anterior muscle and down to the tendinous insertion at the medial cuneiform and first metatarsal. There may be palpable crepitus, and there is tenderness to palpation, over the tibialis tendon. The pain is worse with resisted dorsiflexion of the foot.

## Cause

(a) A tendinopathy or tenosynovitis of the tibialis anterior muscle and tendon. A tendinopathy is uncommon and usually occurs at the musculotendinous junction. The injury may be at the insertion, under the anterior retinaculum of the ankle joint, and, occasionally, low over the musculotendinous junction. It is not a common injury.

(b) The mechanisms are similar to the anterior compartment syndrome, but usually this is a more acute overload (see Chapter 12).

(c) This injury often appears secondary to a foot or ankle problem, because the patient is wary of impact onto the unstable or damaged foot. The patient uses the tibialis anterior, long extensors, posterior tibialis and peroneals to lock up and stabilize the foot at impact. The tibialis anterior and extensor digitorum are not accustomed to this work and suffer an overload and/or rubbing injury as the tendons stand out from the foot and rub into the shoes.

(d) Occasionally it is caused by a shoe with the laces tied up too tightly, which then rubs against the tendon.

(e) The foot must be held into dorsiflexion to hold the body for 'inclined bench sit ups', and the tibialis can be overloaded. This mechanism may apply during other exercises.

## Investigations

None are clinically required but ultrasound and MRI will reveal the lesion.

## Treatment

(a) RICE.
(b) Electrotherapeutic modalities to calm inflammation, such as ultrasound and laser.
(c) Massage techniques to release adhesions, such as frictions.
(d) Steroid to the synovial sheath, or the enthesis, to settle inflammation, and reduce adhesions.
(e) The use of padding either side of the tendon, where it bows out across the dorsum of the foot, will take the shoe pressure off the tendon.

(f) A supportive orthotic may help the mechanism as in Cause (c), above.

## Sports

(a) Avoid inclined or ordinary sit-ups with the feet under a bar, or held by a colleague, for leverage.

(b) Inexperienced cross-country skiers may concentrate on sliding the ski forwards by dorsiflexing the foot and toes.

(c) 'Shuffle runners', who do not thrust from the forefoot to achieve lift-off, may have to dorsiflex their toes and feet faster to clear the ground at take-off.

(d) Step aerobics and hill running may lead to increased dorsiflexion of the foot and toe.

## Comment

It is not common in sport, but quite frequent as part of a protective mechanism, as mentioned above. A major help is to lengthen the stride and relax the foot during the lift-off and carry phase, and work on psoas strength to improve the knee carry.

## Extensor hallucis tendinopathy and synovitis

See Extensor digitorum longus tendinopathy, but note a weak, painless muscle may be caused by L5 nerve palsy.

## Extensor digitorum longus tendinopathy and synovitis

### Findings

Pain in the anterior compartment of the lower leg and/or under the anterior retinaculum at the ankle, which is tender to palpation and worse with resisted toe extensors. There may be audible and palpable crepitus. The skin over the tendons may be red and sore. Examination of the inside of the shoe near the toes often reveals a hole or pit that is being worn away by the dorsiflexed hallucis. Weak painless extensors of the toes are likely to be caused by L5 nerve palsy.

### Cause

Overuse of extensors of the toes, or rubbing of the extensor tendons by the shoes. These muscles are used either to protect an unstable foot or ankle, when they lock up together with the calf, posterior tibialis and peroneals, producing a solid foot at impact, or when they try and do the work of the posterior tibialis and hold up the long arch of the foot. This occurs in inexperienced runners who run and impact into the midstance phase, which collapses the longitudinal arch. The dorsiflexors can be overused by shuffle runners, who dorsiflex the foot and toes in the swing phase (see Tibialis anterior tendinopathy and synovitis, and Anterior retinacular pain).

### Treatment

As for tibialis anterior tendinopathy and synovitis, but applied to the extensor tendons.

### Sports

As for Tibialis anterior tendinopathy and synovitis.

### Comment

Some of these runners will wear a hole in the top of their running shoe, from the big toe nail pulling up into the shoe during the swing phase of running. Lacing up the shoes too tightly does not allow room for the tendons to bridge the joints without rubbing into the shoe. Padding either side of the affected tendon will distribute the pressure points away from the tendon itself. This can be sufficient to relieve the problem as it is very difficult to change this particular running style. An orthotic which helps to reduce pronation also reduces the need for the supporting muscles to lock up, which is the patients' way of preventing overpronation, especially in an externally rotated foot.

## Impingement exostoses

### Findings

The pain is worse at the end range of active and passive dorsiflexion movements of the ankle, and sports that increase ankle dorsiflexion – landing from jumps and vaults, stretching for a drop shot – will indicate this in their history. There is local tenderness to palpation.

### Cause

Exostoses form from forced dorsiflexion and impingement of the anterior tibia onto the distal talus and talonavicular [4] bones.

## Investigations

Lateral X-ray of ankle and foot (Fig. 13.9) is the cheapest and most available investigation, but ultrasound, CT and MRI may show the lesion.

## Treatment

Reduce dorsiflexion activities until the pain is tolerable. A heel raise may help by producing a slightly plantar flexed, neutral position of the ankle, and thus a greater range of functional dorsiflexion becomes available. Surgical removal is rarely required, though it can prove successful in recalcitrant cases [5]; however, surgery is advised for the navicular fragment in highly symptomatic cases [4].

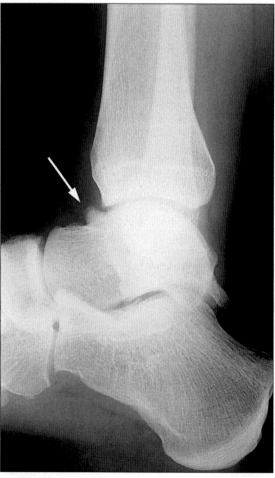

**Figure 13.9** • An impingement exostosis in a gymnast (*arrow*), whose X-ray also shows a Stieda process from the posterior talus.

## Sports

Though the impingement occurs in squash and badminton, whilst 'grubbing up' a drop shot, it is particularly seen in gymnastics, where over-rotating forward landings or under-rotating backward landings produces increased dorsiflexion at the ankle. The coach may help by lifting the gymnast to aid the under-rotation, or use a landing pit, whilst the injury is sore. Adjustment of mat height, higher for forward landings, lower for backward, may be possible during training. This injury may be part of the footballer's ankle (see Part 1: Footballer's ankle).

## Comment

These exostoses develop over time, often without problems, and may be seen by chance on an X-ray. However, they may be acutely traumatized and can fracture, which is when the pain appears. Management is to see them through this phase, limiting training to the pain-free elements, such as asymmetrical bars with no dismounts, and limit the number of causative landings per training session for gymnasts.

## Anterior meniscoid of the ankle

### Findings

A persistent pain after an ankle injury, which is worse on active and passive dorsiflexion of the talar joint. There is tenderness to local palpation at the anterior, superior lateral, or superior medial corners of the talus.

### Cause

This is a name given to a mesh of vessels and connective tissue that lies over the front of the talar joint, and is contiguous with the synovium of the talar joint. It becomes hypertrophied and inflamed after injury or chronic impingement.

**Caveat**

Osteochondral lesion and impingement exostosis. Navicular stress fractures can appear tender to palpation over the talus and therefore can be misdiagnosed.

## Investigations

None are clinically required unless therapy has failed, when a bone scan may be hot in the blood phase and MRI shows oedema and swelling in this area.

## Treatment

Injection of cortisone into the meniscoid and, if this fails, surgical debridement [6].

## Sports

May be undertaken, as there is no long-term damage, but plantar and dorsiflexion of the ankle will flare the lesion. NSAIDs may help.

## Comment

Although surgery has been discussed, none of my cases have come to surgery, as all have responded well to one or two cortisone injections and correction of foot biomechanics.

# Anterior retinacular pain

## Findings

The superficial tissues are puffy, red, and tender to palpation over the anterior retinaculum. Resisted isometric testing of the foot and toe extensors are pain-free.

## Cause

Caused by compression of the anterior retinaculum, by a boot or shoe, whilst the extensor hallucis, extensor digitorum longus, or tibialis anterior are being used.

## Investigations

None are clinically required.

## Treatment

Release the pressure of the shoe, as this is often produced by tying the laces into the eyehole that is highest and widest; therefore, do not lace the shoes up to the top eyelet holes. Soft padding under the tongue of the shoe lessens the pressure of the shoe. Electrotherapeutic modalities to settle inflammation, such as ultrasound and laser. NSAIDs.

## Sports

See Tibialis anterior tendinopathy and synovitis.

## Comment

Modern shoes are being cut higher. The top eyelet holes are being placed further round the side of the shoes and rubbing is occurring more frequently over the retinaculum.

# Tarsal coalition

Bony or fibrous fusion of the talus, calcaneum, or cuboid limits mid-foot movement and requires more range from the talar joint (see Chapter 14).

# Flattened talar dome

This problem may limit ankle dorsiflexion and produce impingements, meniscoid or capsular pains (as discussed above). It may increase pronation, but an anti-pronation orthotic will increase the dorsiflexion problems at the ankle so a heel raise orthotic is required. A lateral X-ray reveals the problem.

## Part 3 **Lateral ankle pain**

### PART CONTENTS

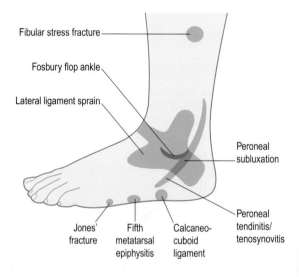

Fibular stress fracture

Fosbury flop ankle

Lateral ligament sprain

Peroneal subluxation

Peroneal tendinitis/tenosynovitis

Jones' fracture

Fifth metatarsal epiphysitis

Calcaneo-cuboid ligament

## Sprained ankle: lateral bruising

See Acute lateral ligament sprain and Chronic lateral ligament sprain. If the bruising appears more towards the toes, see Calcaneocuboid ligament sprain and also Chapter 15.

## Sprained ankle: lateral and medial bruising

### Findings

(a) A history of an inversion sprain accompanied by plantar flexion, with rapid swelling. Bruising appears on both sides of the ankle, though, if only the capsule is strained and there has been no ligamentous tear, bruising can be absent.

(b) The ankle is tender to palpation over the anterior talofibular ligament, middle talofibular ligament or calcaneofibular ligament.

(c) Talar translation is painful, as is passive plantar flexion. If anterior translation is painful, it suggests that a combined lesion of lateral ligaments with a capsulitis or posterior tibiofibular ligament damage has occurred.

(d) Possible capsular signs from the ankle joint; extension and flexion hurt.

(e) Calcaneotibial compression test is positive (Fig. 13.10) (see Glossary).

(f) Bruising is lateral, posterior and medial.

(g) There is often an effusion of the ankle joint.

### Cause

The ankle ligaments are sprained or partially torn by an inversion and forced plantar flexion movement, so that the posterior capsule and posterior tibiofibular

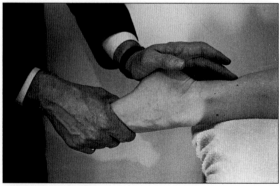

**Figure 13.10** • The calcaneotibial compression test whipping the foot into plantar flexion.

ligaments are damaged as well, plus the tissues at the posterior aspect of the ankle joint are compressed and traumatized. There may also be a traumatic capsulitis present.

## Investigations

A patient who has been able to bear weight after the injury is unlikely to have a fracture but because, clinically, this lesion is more difficult to distinguish from a fracture, it may be worth an X-ray. A request should be made that the presence of an os trigonum or stieda process be reported. Because they are normal variants, these are often not reported, but they can cause ongoing problems and can even fracture.

## Treatment

(a) As for unilateral swelling, but electrotherapy for the ankle joint, such as interferential and shortwave diathermy, will help.

(b) Cortisone injection of the back of the ankle joint and posterior calcaneotibial space to settle tissue oedema. The injection may require repeating.

## Sports

No sport is particularly causative, but these problems are common during training or returning to the sport after the injury:

(a) Kicking, especially with the foot plantar flexed, as in the drive and volley. This problem persists after the acute phase has settled, until the injury has healed entirely. Strapping to limit plantar flexion may help.

(b) A sudden stop to change direction, as in field hockey or squash, which forces the posterior aspect of the calcaneum upwards against the tibia, is painful.

(c) The accelerated, plantar flexion movement required for jumping is painful.

(d) Dancing on pointes causes problems.

## Comment

All may require an injection at the posterior aspect of the ankle to reduce inflammation and speed recovery. This injury takes more time to heal than unilateral bruising, often becoming a chronic ankle problem (see Part 5: Posterior ankle pain.).

# Acute lateral ligament sprain

## Findings

(a) A history of an inversion sprain with rapid swelling, which may or may not bruise laterally, or, if mild, pain but no swelling.

(b) It is tender to palpation over the anterior talofibular, and possibly the middle talofibular and/or calcaneofibular ligament.

(c) Distraction of the ankle joint by passive inversion and plantar flexion stresses the anterior talofibular ligament, and passive inversion and dorsiflexion tests the calcaneofibular ligament.

(d) Compression of the talus against the fibula is pain-free, but this test will be painful with a fracture of the fibula.

(e) If anterior translation is painful, it suggests a combined lesion, with capsulitis or posterior tibiofibular ligament damage, has occurred.

(f) Bruising is lateral and concentrated around the ankle and mid-foot, but will track up the leg.

## Cause

An inversion sprain of the foot, with a sprain, partial tear, or tear of the ankle ligaments. The anterior talofibular ligament (ATFL) is damaged in plantar flexion and inversion, and the posterior calcaneofibular ligament during dorsiflexion and inversion.

## Investigations

None are clinically required if the patient can weight bear, or compression (not distraction) of the talus on the fibula or tibia is pain-free, as a fracture usually hurts in these circumstances (see Fosbury flop ankle). X-ray will exclude a fracture, and MRI arthrogram will expose a torn ligament as well as inflammation.

## Treatment

(a) RICE for 48 hours, plus non-weight-bearing crutches.

(b) Compression can be specifically applied beneath and behind the lateral maleolus by using orthopaedic felt under the strapping.

(c) NSAIDs.

(d) Electrotherapeutic modalities to settle inflammation, such as laser and ultrasound.

(e) Massage techniques to remove tissue debris and to organize fibrocytes, such as effluage and frictions.

(f) Non-weight-bearing flexion, extension, inversion and eversion exercises. The non-injured ankle may be worked at the same time as this seems to give a feedback to the damaged side. Tracing the alphabet with the toes gives a full range of movement.

(g) Weight-bearing as soon as possible, with support, but note that the first few paces hurt and then the pain eases up with continued walking. However, the pain returns after walking when the patient stands still or rests.

(h) Support the ankle, initially with a pressure pad, beneath the fibular and over the calcaneum, and use an adjustable elastic bandage, tubigrip, elasticated anklet or ankle brace [7].

(i) Cross-training should be non-weight-bearing, such as swimming, rowing or cycling, and raising or lowering the bicycle saddle will increase the ankle range of movements.

(j) Proprioception should be trained by performing one-legged balancing exercises at home whilst brushing the hair, cleaning the teeth, answering the phone, etc. This requires the ankle to balance the body rather than the brain to concentrate on balancing. Balancing with the eyes shut and on a wobble board increases the coordination required.

(k) The movement and rhythm of the good leg may be used to educate the damaged ankle to perform normally. Counting from 1 to 9 will provide a good rhythm.

(l) Isometrics will maintain the strength of the posterior tibialis and peroneal muscles.

(m) Follow the Achilles ladders and, after the sprinting stage, the kicking ladder, figure-of-eight cutting drills and sidestep routines may be added (see Chapter 20).

(n) Surgery is required if the ankle is unstable, but this is usually assessed later [8].

## Sports

Change of direction sports should not have too high a sole on the shoe because this leads to ankle instability. Use a support for about 6 weeks after returning to games. Evidence from basketball is that prophylactic ankle braces, or taping, is of value in preventing injury to the ankle [7]. Straight line sports must follow the Achilles ladders, whilst change of direction sports must add sideways movements, such as sidesteps and cutting manoeuvres (see Chapter 20).

## Comment

This is a very common injury, for which it is important to give home proprioceptive exercises so that rehabilitation is done frequently; too many feel that 20 minutes, three times per week, on a wobble board is all that is required. Rehabilitation is little and often, several times a day. The major problems are instability, with weak peroneals, or later a chronic stiff ankle that has not been rehabilitated properly. There is evidence that prophylactic strapping is of benefit [7].

## Chronic lateral ligament sprain

### Findings

Type 1  Painful or painless inversion, weak peroneals and poor balance.

Type 2  The inversion range is increased and is often pain-free. The peroneals may be either strong or weak. The patient complains of recurrent sprains or weakness of the ankle.

Type 3  There is tenderness to palpation over the relevant lateral ligament, with a thickened appearance of the soft tissues. Inversion is limited and painful.

### Cause

All have a history of previous inversion injury of the ankle, or repetitive injuries.

Type 1  Weak peroneals and proprioceptive dysfunction.

Type 2  Unstable ankle joint, from a partial tear of the lateral ligaments.

Type 3  Adhered scar tissue, from poor rehabilitation, producing a stiff ankle joint.

**Caveat**

**Osteochondral fracture of the talus, meniscoid of the ankle, and posterior impingement.**

## Investigations

(a) X-ray of the ankle for osteoarthritis, osteophytes, footballer's ankle and osteochondral lesions.

(b) Stress the talus and mid-foot into inversion, and X-ray for talar tilt or talar translation, which is positive in type 2 (Fig. 13.11). Minor talar tilt is often not reported but can produce a quite considerable functional deficit. If translation is used to measure instability, 6 mm is the acceptable maximum of movement. If surgery is considered then an MRI arthrogram will evaluate the problem further, displaying the relevant tears.

(c) If the X-rays in (b) above are normal then an MRI arthrogram will exclude an osteochondral lesion (see Figs 13.1–13.4), a meniscoid, and chronic ligament tear.

## Treatment

Type 1   Proprioceptive exercises to enhance balance, such as balancing on the affected leg or using a wobble board (see Acute lateral ligament sprain), plus peroneal isometrics. Follow this with rehabilitation through the Achilles ladders.

Type 2   Strapping, or preferably bracing, of the ankle. Surgery will be required if this remains unstable [7]. Proceed to the Achilles ladder for rehabilitation.

Type 3   Manipulations and mobilizations of the ankle. Cortisone injections to the joint, via a posterior approach, frictions to the scar tissue and, if no progress is being made, then manipulation under anaesthetic followed by immediate rehabilitation using the Achilles ladders (see Chapter 20).

## Sports

Change of direction sports need an ankle support for 6–8 weeks after return to sport, but if the ankle is unstable then a support brace should be used for longer, if not always. Surgery might have to be considered. Rehabilitation includes figure-of-eight, sidesteps, cross-over steps and court drills for racket games (see Chapter 20).

## Comment

Stress X-ray is the vital first investigation for the chronic ankle. After this has been performed, MRI arthrogram has superseded other investigations, but can still miss a loose body and so CT scan and arthroscopy will still have a place in undiagnosed chronic ankle problems. I feel that peroneal and posterior tibialis weakness to manual testing is in fact a dysfunction rather than a genuine weakness, because the apparent weakness picks up so rapidly, within 2 weeks with proper rehabilitation.

## Calcaneocuboid ligament sprain

Pain occurs on stressing the mid-tarsal joint, with palpable tenderness over the calcaneocuboid joint line (see Chapter 15).

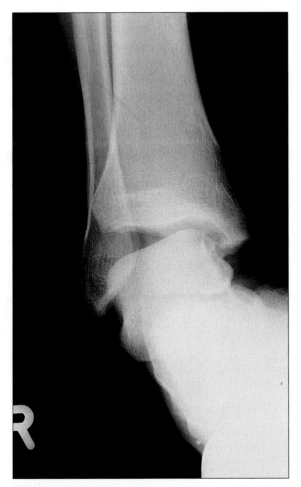

**Figure 13.11** • Stress views of the ankle show talar tilting due to torn and lengthened lateral ligaments.

## Peroneal tenosynovitis

### Findings

There is tenderness over the peroneal tendons around the lateral malleolus, and possibly over the proximal tip of the fifth metatarsal. Swelling of the synovial sheath may occur. Resisted eversion is painful and passive inversion may be painful. There may be pain around the back of the lateral malleolus and the peroneal muscle may be painful (see Chapter 12).

### Cause

Synovitis of the tendon sheath, tendinopathy or partial tear of one or more peroneal tendons. More traumatic forces may produce complete rupture of the tendons. The most common problem is a strain of the tendon from an oversupinated foot or recurrent inversion injury (see Peroneal subluxation). However, recurrent inversion sprains may produce partial tears that require surgical repair, as will ruptures from acute trauma. It is not as common as one would expect, for it seems that an acute inversion sprain is not resisted by the peroneals to an extent that damage occurs, and, therefore, the injury damages the ankle ligaments. The strain can occur with overcorrected antipronation orthotics, walking to edge the outside of the foot, as in hill walking along a mountain side, or broken heel cups in a supinated foot. Occasionally, a high-cut shoe will rub the peroneal retinaculum and sheath producing a tenosynovitis.

### Investigations

None are clinically required for a strain. Ultrasound and MRI show the tendinopathy, synovial fluid, and partial or complete tear.

### Treatment

(a) RICE.
(b) Electrotherapeutic modalities to settle inflammation, such as ultrasound and laser.
(c) Massage techniques, to prevent adhesions in the tenosynovitis, such as frictions.
(d) Cortisone to the synovitis.
(e) Correct any dysfunctional orthotics or broken shoes.
(f) Peroneal isometrics.
(g) Proprioceptive balancing.

(h) Tape or brace the ankle with a hinged plastic boot.
(i) Surgical repair of the tendons.

### Sports

Check that the heel cups of the shoes are stable (see Glossary: Shoes). Worn heels, from heel strike, can increase the amount of supination, which will stress the peroneals. Use of strapping or an ankle brace if 'fell walking' with a lot of edging, or whilst running on rough ground, will give support. Use strapping or an ankle brace for a chronic tendinopathy.

### Comment

This is an uncommon injury, as it is more common for the peroneal muscles to become weak or dysfunctional, rather than develop a tendinopathy or synovitis. Note, during rehabilitation of the ankle ligaments, peroneal muscle pain may occur in the lateral compartment of the lower leg.

## Peroneal subluxation

### Findings

There is a history of a click or flick, plus or minus pain, over the lateral malleolus, and a feeling of insecurity of the ankle. Subluxation of the tendon is reproduced with resisted eversion of the foot and can be seen, and palpated, as the tendon jumps forward onto the lateral malleolus.

### Cause

The peroneal tendon subluxes anteriorly from its groove behind the lateral malleolus.

### Investigations

None are clinically required if this is felt manually, but this subluxation may be visualized on ultrasound.

### Treatment

Minor episodes may be restrained with padding and strapping over the fibula, which functionally deepens the peroneal groove. Perhaps orthotics, to correct over-supination, may help. If these measures cannot control the tendon then surgery to deepen the peroneal groove is required [9].

## Sports

(a) Rehabilitate through the Achilles ladders, but, after the sprinting stage, add figure-of-eights and shuttle run drills. Sidestep and cross-over drills should be started as early as possible (see Chapter 20).

(b) Karate and soccer – some kicks with the outside of the foot may cause problems.

## Comment

Not common but sometimes traumatic. If minor, it is worth a try with conservative padding before considering surgery.

# Flat foot impingement syndrome

## Findings

A pronated foot with calcaneovalgus that is often severe. Pain is experienced anterior and inferior to the fibula and is worse on passive eversion and dorsiflexion.

## Cause

With an excessively pronated foot, especially from calcaneovalgus, the fibula impinges onto the calcaneum or anterior talus. Sometimes a pes planus will also suffer this problem, but a pes planus is a normal variant whereas overpronation is pathological.

## Investigations

None are clinically required, or effective.

## Treatment

Local steroid to the area will give rapid relief, but correction of the overpronation, with an orthotic and proprioceptive exercises, is required for long-term control.

## Sports

Check that the heel cups of the shoes have not broken, thus increasing pronation. Camber running, or edging in hill walking, may precipitate the problem (see Glossary: Shoes).

## Comment

This is a localized presenting area of pain in a chronically overpronated foot, which usually occurs when activity is increased.

# Fosbury flop ankle

## Findings

There is pain on compression, but not on distraction of the fibula and talus.

## Cause

Impingement between the lateral surface of the talus and fibula. If the take-off foot of the Fosbury flop high jumper is planted with too much external rotation then the fibula is driven onto the talus, causing impingement and bruising of the articular surfaces.

## Investigations

None are clinically required in a high jumper with the above clinical signs; however, if in doubt, an MRI may show bone bruising and exclude other diagnoses.

## Treatment

Alter the technique to reduce external rotation of the take-off foot. Electrotherapeutic modalities to settle intra-articular inflammation, such as interferential and shortwave diathermy. NSAIDs.

## Sports

The Fosbury flop style of high jumping requires a reduction in the amount of external rotation of the foot at plant and take off.

## Comment

This was more common when Fosbury flop jumpers tried to get more rotation in their jump, but coaches now seem to be aware of the problem and I have not seen a case of it for several years.

# Subtalar joint

See Sinus tarsi, below.

# Sinus tarsi

Presents with lateral ankle pain, without any other apparent cause, and is possibly worse on subtalar inversion and eversion (see Chapter 14).

# Part 4 **Medial ankle pain**

## PART CONTENTS

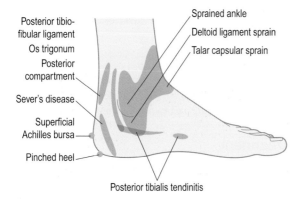

## Sprained lateral ankle

An inversion, plantar-flexed sprain will affect the capsule of the ankle and produce bruising, swelling and discomfort around the medial side as well as the lateral aspect, but the dominant physical signs are from the lateral ligaments (see Part 3: Sprained ankle: lateral and medial bruising).

## Deltoid ligament sprain

### Findings

There is a history of fairly major trauma to the ankle, with tenderness over the deltoid ligaments and on passive eversion of the foot. If there is bruising, check that compression of the talus onto the tibial maleolus is pain-free, as compression pain indicates bone damage may be present.

### Cause

An eversion injury to the ankle, from stumbling on rough ground, a blocked side foot kick, or direct trauma.

This injury requires a fair degree of force, just below that required to produce a Pott's fracture, to damage the strong deltoid ligament.

### Investigations

With bruising, X-ray, as this is a strong ligament and an avulsion from the medial maleolus or a frank Pott's fracture may be present.

### Treatment

Treat any fracture as the priority, but, for ligamentous damage alone, use a cast brace to rest and maintain immobility over 7–10 days. Subsequently, mobilize with crutches, non-weight-bearing, then gradually introduce weight-bearing. Even when non-weight-bearing, active dorsi- and plantarflexion should be maintained, and electrotherapeutic modalities to settle inflammation, plus massage techniques to reduce and control scar tissue, can be added. Management of the injury then follows the regime prescribed for the lateral ligament. A chronic deltoid sprain may require a cortisone injection to release scar tissue and aid mobilization.

### Sports

Repetitive deltoid ligament sprains at a low-grade injury are part of the footballer's ankle (see Part 1: Footballer's ankle; see Fig. 13.6).

### Comment

In the acute phase, it is important to exclude a possible fracture, which might not alter management but defines the extent of the problem. Chronic deltoid ligament pain often does not settle with physiotherapy although it does well with a cortisone injection.

## Posterior tibialis tenosynovitis

### Findings

The patient gives a history of medial calf pain, which may extend around the medial maleolus to the navicular tubercle, or even under the transverse arch of the foot. Swelling over the line of the posterior tibialis may be present, is tender to touch, and crepitus may be felt

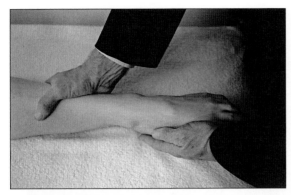

**Figure 13.12** • Resisted posterior tibialis. The foot and toes must be plantar-flexed to prevent tibialis anterior helping this movement.

posterior to the ankle. There may be tenderness to palpation over the navicular tubercle and under the transverse arch. Resisted posterior tibialis is painful and weak (Fig. 13.12). A weak, painless posterior tibialis is dysfunctional, and rarely ruptured (unless there is marked swelling of the sheath) and the problem follows failed ankle rehabilitation or chronic overpronation.

## Cause

The chronic pronated foot does not produce a posterior tibialis tendinopathy as in these cases the posterior tibialis has an inhibitory weakness that avoids stress. Pain appears in the acute or subacute overload of the posterior tibialis tendon, which, in the absence of trauma, is from functional overpronation. It may therefore occur following Achilles injury, when the patient externally rotates the foot to achieve propulsion, unfortunately from the posterior tibialis, but thus avoiding stressing the Achilles. The same happens if the patient normally runs with externally rotated feet, or strives for foot propulsion from pronated feet. Semi-acute collapse of the longitudinal arch, or the avoidance of weight over the first two rays of the forefoot, provokes a protective posterior tibialis activity and overload, especially seen in dancers on pointes. There may be a tenosynovitis, or even a rupture of the tendon.

 Caveat

Stress fracture of the tibia, tarsal tunnel and accessory navicular (Fig. 13.13).

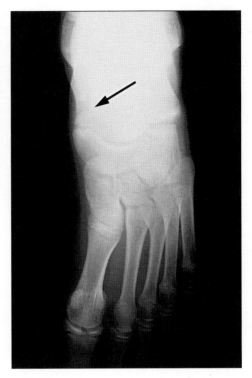

**Figure 13.13** • The accessory navicular forms the navicular tubercle and is joined by a fibrous band to the navicular (*arrow*).

## Investigations

(a) None are clinically required for minor stresses.

(b) X-ray for an accessory navicular (see Glossary), especially in children or adults with localized tenderness to palpation of the navicular tubercle (see Fig. 13.13).

(c) Ultrasound or MRI scan for posterior tibialis tendinopathy, tenosynovitis or rupture, but these investigations could be held in reserve and used if the patient fails to rehabilitate or there is no evidence of posterior tibialis function returning when the pain eases (Fig. 13.14). Note that occasionally the damage is to the tendon element lying distal to the navicular attachment.

(d) In chronic cases, blood should be taken for full blood count, ESR, rheumatoid factor and antinuclear antibodies, as this is a problem that often accompanies systemic inflammatory disease.

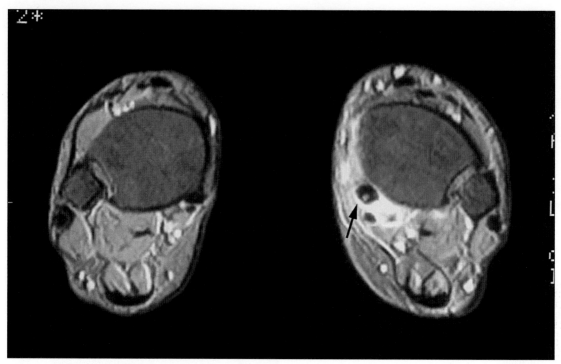

**Figure 13.14** • T2-weighted MRI scan shows oedema around the posterior tibialis and an intratendinous lesion (*arrow*).

## Treatment

(a) Strapping or bracing of the ankle for support.

(b) RICE – beware of the posterior tibial nerve, which can be damaged by ice that is below 0°C (see Glossary: RICE).

(c) Correct any technique that promotes functional pronation. Check the heel cups have not broken in the running shoes (see Glossary: Shoes).

(d) Correct any functional genu valgum (see Chapter 11, Part 2B: Maltracking of the patella).

(e) Corrective orthotics, or orthotics to reduce functional pronation.

(f) Electrotherapeutic modalities to settle inflammation and reduce adhesions, such as ultrasound and laser.

(g) Massage techniques to reduce adhesions, such as frictions.

(h) Cortisone to any tenosynovitis or the navicular insertion.

(i) Posterior tibialis isometrics.

(j) Achilles ladders (see Chapter 20).

(k) Surgical repair of a total rupture.

## Sports

(a) Change of direction sports cause more of a problem, requiring ankle braces and supportive orthotics until the lesion is better.

(b) Running – the foot that is on the higher part of the road will be overloaded if the road is cambered. Rough ground will produce some moments of excess pronation, and uphill running, bend running, sprint start drills and a windmilling style of running can all produce this problem. In fact, the psoas and rectus femoris are often weak in these individuals, so the treatment should include high knee drills to encourage a longer stride, which allows time for the foot to complete its swing phase and impact on the heel in supination. If possible, correct any externally rotated foot style of running or block functional pronation with orthotics. Stop hill running until recovered.

(c) See maltracking of the patella and tibiocollateral ligament pain in the knee (see Chapter 11, Parts 2 and 3).

(d) Fell walking – edging the outside of the boot for a long time when walking along slopes.

(e) Rolling over pliés at ballet – dancers without full turn-out should be permitted to reduce turn-out. They are never going to make professional ballet dancers so they should be permitted to dance, and enjoy themselves, without getting hurt. Correct the technique to eliminate 'fishing the foot' for demi-pointe work because this fault overloads the posterior tibialis strength.

## Comment

Posterior tibialis problems epitomize sports medicine, where the anatomy can promote overpronation and an inhibitory weakness, or the technique can cause a functional overpronation, with overuse of the posterior tibialis in trying to correct the problem. The orthotic 'corrects' the anatomy of the first and minimizes the skill fault in the second. Running must be taught, because it is a skill. These faults, which start at the foot, may then transfer stresses onto the knees and so the patient presents with knee pain rather than foot pain. Tenosynovitis improves dramatically with cortisone to the sheath, allowing rehabilitation of the muscle tendon, which is often inhibited by pain. The presence of an accessory navicular suggests the injury will take longer to recover.

## Flexor hallucis tenosynovitis

### Findings

Pain is present at the posterior medial aspect of the ankle, at the site of the musculotendinous junction, and sometimes on the medial aspect of the heel and arch of the foot (see Chapter 14). Resisted great toe flexion is painful and weaker. The tendon ruptures rarely, but, in this case, resisted toe flexion is weak and painless, unless an adhesive tenosynovitis has developed around the rupture; in these cases pain is present and hides the diagnosis.

### Cause

Strain of the flexor hallucis, from sprinting or bounding, but it is most commonly seen in dancers especially ballet, from pointe work.

### Investigations

Clinically, none are required, unless failing to progress, when real-time ultrasound or an MRI will display the tendon, a synovitis of the tendon sheath or a rupture.

### Treatment

(a) Electrotherapeutic modalities to settle inflammation, such as ultrasound and laser.

(b) NSAIDs.

(c) Cortisone to settle the inflammation of the synovitis.

(d) Massage techniques to reduce adhesions, such as frictions.

(e) Passive toe flexion and extension exercises to reduce adhesions.

(f) Isometric toe curls against the other foot or therapist.

(g) Block starts, initially with hands resting on a desk then hands resting lower down, say on a bench, and finally block starts with the hands on the floor.

(h) Achilles ladders (see Chapter 20).

(i) Surgery is required if a rupture is present. Ruptures are found, usually, in ballet dancers.

### Sports

(a) Ballet – rest from pointes and large jumps.

(b) Running – the insertion of a forefoot bar allows the forefoot to roll through without the great toe reaching the ground. As this bar is lowered, so the toes will work more into contact with the ground, until the forefoot bar can be removed for normal drills.

### Comment

Not a common lesion, except in dancers. It may present as a medially placed, plantar fasciitis, or indeed may be the actual cause of pain, in some types of so-called plantar fasciitis.

## Tarsal tunnel syndrome

### Findings

There is pain over the medial ankle, radiating to the sole of the foot, and sometimes up into the calf. The pain may wake the patient at night, and 'pins and needles', numbness and paraesthesia, worse with walking or dorsiflexion of the foot, may be present. Tinel's test (see Glossary: Tinel's sign) over the posterior tibial nerve is positive, and two-point discrimination may be lost in the foot. Weakness of the intrinsic muscles of the foot may be present. A fusiform swelling may be palpated over the posterior tibial nerve. Overpronation, often gross, is present.

## Cause

Compression of the posterior tibial nerve around the inferior border of medial maleolus, within the tarsal tunnel, which is almost invariably caused by a calcaneovalgus producing marked overpronation of the foot.

## Caveat

Referred root pain from the back, or other causes of neural pain. Check pulses and for diabetes.

## Investigations

(a) X-ray of the foot and ankle to assess bony and arthritic state.
(b) EMG may show abnormalities of the medial and lateral plantar nerves.

(c) Blood tests for systemic inflammatory disease and diabetes.

## Treatment

(a) Correct the pronatory malfunction (see Glossary: Overpronation, Supination/pronation).
(b) NSAIDs.
(c) Perineural steroids can relieve inflammation and reduce the compression on the nerve, as a stopgap, but treatment is to correct the cause.
(d) The patient may require surgical arthrodesis of hind foot if this is deformed and unstable.

## Sports

This is rarely seen in sport, as pronatory problems present early and are treated before the damage is severe enough to cause tarsal tunnel symptoms. It is seen in those with a chronic subtalar problem who take up activities. Skiing boots, whose controls tighten a cable adjustment, may cause compression of the nerve [10].

## Comment

It is not common, and is usually caused by gross, rear foot deformity. Orthoses and shoe heel cup strengthening give long-term help, even after surgery.

# Part 5 **Posterior ankle pain**

## PART CONTENTS

The posterior structures of the ankle are shown in (Fig. 13.15).

## Achilles peritendinitis

### Findings

This is an inflammatory lesion of the paratenon and appears to have a history of rest pain, better with activity [11]. Therefore, the pain is worse first thing in the morning and on sitting, but is better on walking. Runners can 'run off' the pain. The foot 'attitude' is normal as are the Simmonds' and Thompson's tests (see Glossary). Calf stretching and muscle activities, such as rising onto the toes and hopping, are painful. The tendon is tender to touch, and may have audible and palpable crepitus in the acute stage. The tendon may appear puffy and swollen.

### Cause

Inflammation of the paratenon from rubbing by the Achilles tag of a shoe or boot, or from being part of a combined lesion (see Combined Achilles lesion). Following surgery to the Achilles tendon, adhesions may be present and troublesome.

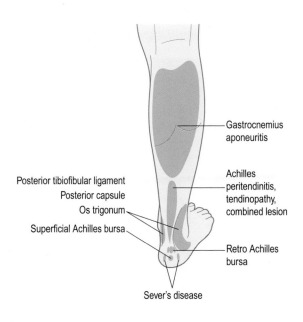

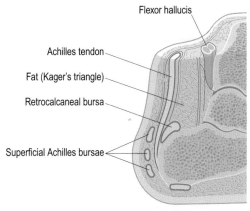

*Achilles tendinopathies*

**Figure 13.15** • Diagram of the posterior structures of the ankle.

## Investigations

Real-time ultrasound will establish whether this is a pure peritendinitis or a combined lesion, but if not available then a trial of treatment is a reasonable approach for this typical history. MRI is a very effective investigation, although more expensive.

## Treatment

(a) Settle the inflammation with peritendinous cortisone using a bent needle, NSAIDs and electrotherapeutic modalities, such as ultrasound and laser.

(b) Prevent adhesions forming with massage techniques, such as cross-frictions.

(c) Rehabilitate via the Achilles ladder, but only the bottom ladder should be attempted before a review consultation with the physician, with no hopping routines until then.

(d) Rehabilitate via the top Achilles ladder (see Chapter 20).

### Caveat

If the history of rest pain has gone, but pain still persists and investigations were not available, then an assumption of an associated tendinopathy should be made.

## Sports

Check that the Achilles heel shoe tag has not been rubbing the Achilles. The apparent cut-away heel tag may still be too high or too rigid. Cut away the tag, or release the tension on the Achilles with cuts either side of the heel tag. These should not compromise the heel cup. Some sports shoes have a lace hole placed slightly on the side of the shoe. This will tighten the heel tag and should not be used (see Achilles tendinopathy and Glossary: Shoes).

## Comment

Unlike methylprednisolone (Depo-medrone) and tri-amcinolone, hydrocortisone acetate causes little subcutaneous atrophy, and mobility and rest pain morbidity are dramatically improved in 1–2 weeks [11,12]. Self-frictions of the tendon with NSAID gel may be required for maintenance. Peritendinous injections do not appear to increase the rupture rate [12], and, if the needle is placed in a tendon, extreme pressure is required to inject. The technique uses a bent needle, which is withdrawn until the injectate flows [13].

# Achilles tendinopathy

## Findings

Typically, there appears to be a history of pain, increasing with activity and better at rest. Active and passive stretching of the gastrocnemius (knee straight, dorsi-flexed ankle) or soleus (knee bent, dorsiflexed ankle) is painful and limited. Resisted plantar flexion, which may require testing by a one-leg heel raise, or hopping, is painful. Passive whipped plantarflexion, tested by calcaneotibial compression, is pain-free (see Fig. 13.10). There may be a palpable swelling in the tendon that moves with the tendon. It is locally tender to compression. The attitude (see Fig. 13.22) and Simmonds'/Thompson's test is normal (see Glossary).

## Cause

Partial tear (Fig. 13.16), myeloid, myxoid, hyaline degeneration of collagen fibres (Fig. 13.17) or cystic degeneration (Fig. 13.18). Ageing is a factor, but the cause is possibly attritional, from vibration shock at

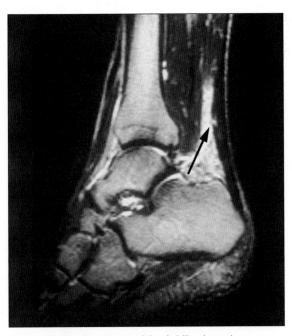

**Figure 13.16** • Partial tear of the Achilles (*arrow*).

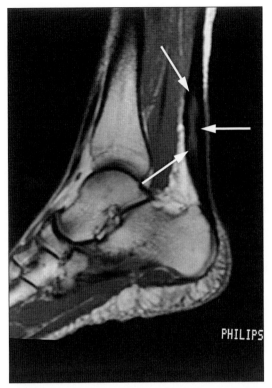

**Figure 13.17** • Degenerative tendinopathy within the Achilles tendon seen on T1-weighted MRI.

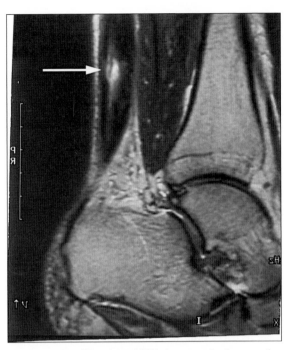

**Figure 13.18** • T2-weighted MRI shows cystic degeneration (*arrow*).

impact, overpronation or incoordination between the quadriceps and calf muscle. EMG studies suggest that the quadriceps straightens the knee before the calf plantar flexes the foot, and movements that stress this mechanism or that encourage plantar flexion, whilst the knee is bent, may promote Achilles attrition [14,15].

## Investigations

Diagnostic ultrasound scan and MRI scan can expose the extent of the lesion and display degenerate cysts. Ultrasound confirms the function of the tendon (Fig. 13.19), as scanning the passively moved tendon may show a rupture that is not visible in the static phase. The upper limit of a normal tendon diameter is considered to be 0.5 cm.

## Treatment

**(a)** A heel raise in the shoes will reduce the load on the Achilles tendon.

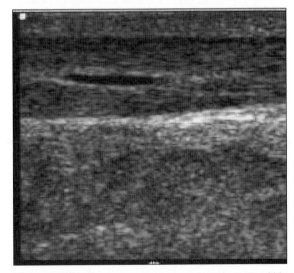

**Figure 13.19** • Scans may show asymptomatic cysts within the Achilles tendon, as displayed by ultrasound.

**(b)** Orthotics, if overpronation is contributing to a 'side to side' distortion during movement [16,17].

**(c)** Achilles ladder (see Chapter 20), and/or repetition of eccentric 'heel drops'.

**(d)** A cyst, sometimes called 'red degeneration', which can be seen on scanning should be curetted out.

**(e)** Surgery or percutaneous needling to longitudinally split the tendon fibres and encourage vascular neogenesis.

**(f)** Sclerosis or disruption of new vessels under Doppler ultrasound guidance.

## Sports

**(a)** Athletics – a sudden increase in speed, or distance, may create too much load for the tendon. Camber running encourages lateral movement of the calcaneum and bowing of the tendon. Repetition sprints, with too little recovery time, can fatigue the quadriceps, causing an upset in calf/quadriceps coordination. Uphill running may produce overload of the Achilles.

**(b)** Hill walking and climbing – when climbing using the forefoot, the heel may drop too low, increasing the forces on the Achilles. However, by using 'high heels', i.e. finding a rock to support the heel, or zig-zagging up the hill using the sides of the foot, this problem is prevented.

**(c)** Cricket – very often an Achilles tendon tears when a back foot shot is played to mid-wicket, and a quick single is run. The weight is on the ball of the back foot activating the calf and then the knee straightens for the run, upsetting the calf/quadriceps coordination.

**(d)** All sports – sudden acceleration from a bent knee position and a plantarflexed foot.

## Comment

It is the tendinopathy, a degenerative lesion, that delays healing, and this damage may cause later rupture. Whether surgery, with longitudinal splitting, encourages invasion of new blood vessels to repair tissue or whether, post surgery, the patient accepts a longer rehabilitation is still debatable. Certainly, a patient with a tendinopathy can go all the way up the Achilles ladders, play four games and break down again – so it is difficult to project when full recovery has occurred. Ultrasono-graphic monitoring may help. Vitamin C encourages the formation of collagen from fibroblasts in vitro; however, collagen neogenesis is still the problem in vivo, though early stem cell research suggests that nearly normal tendons may be regenerated (see Combined Achilles lesion).

## Combined Achilles lesion

### Findings

A history of both peritendinitis and tendinopathy, with elements of rest pain and exercise-induced pain (see Achilles peritendinitis and Achilles tendinopathy). Therefore, exercise pain will still be present once the rest pain has settled with treatment.

### Cause

An Achilles tendinopathy, combined with a surrounding peritendinitis.

### Investigations

Diagnostic ultrasound can show thickening of the tendon and the tendinopathy, with increased echogenicity surrounding the tendon from a peritendinitis. MRI will display the peritendinitis on STIR, T2 and other fat-suppressed sequences (Fig. 13.20). T1-weighted sequences display the tendinopathy to greater advantage.

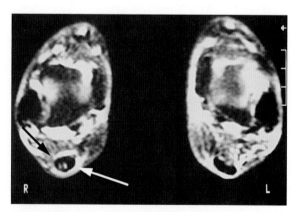

**Figure 13.20** • T2-weighted MRI showing a combined lesion with increased signal around the tendon from the peritendinitis and two areas of degeneration within the tendon.

## Treatment

The paratenon is an inflammatory lesion and responds to anti-inflammatory therapy, whereas the tendinopathy is a degenerative lesion and does not; therefore treatment with anti-inflammatory methods will help only the peritendinous element. Use electrotherapeutic and massage techniques to settle inflammation and prevent adhesions, or cortisone to the paratenon if required, but only whilst a history of morning and rest pain remains. The peritendinitis element usually settles in 1–2 weeks with this treatment, and the history converts to no morning and rest pain, the exercise pain becoming dominant. Then start the Achilles ladders, eccentric loads and stretching for the tendinopathy (see Achilles tendinopathy). Self-massage, physiotherapy or ultrasound to the peritendon during rehabilitation will limit adhesions. Possible longitudinal splitting of the tendon for the non-progressing lesion and surgical strip of the paratenon if it becomes chronic and stenotic. Sclerosant injections to, or disruption of, areas of neovascularization [18,19].

## Sports

See Achilles tendinopathy.

## Comment

This is the most common lesion of achillodynia. The pain of the paratenon will stop rehabilitation, and produce pain and dysfunction with daily activities. So, after this element has been treated, rehabilitation can be tolerated. Apart from stretching, rehabilitation should be minimal until clinical review 1–2 weeks after any cortisone injection, so that the extent of any underlying tendinopathy (Fig. 13.21), and therefore the type of rehabilitation, can be assessed. Doppler ultrasound shows new vessels on the deep surface of the tendon. Injection and obliteration of these vessels seems to relieve pain but tendon eccentric exercises are still required for a considerable time [18]. Equally, some early results suggest that a large volume (20 mL) of normal saline injected under the paratenon will strip the paratenon and produce relief from pain. The question still arises as to whether neovascularization is necessary for repair or just a painful side effect, and whether the treatment is producing pain relief by destroying the accompanying nerves, rather than obliterating the new vessels [19].

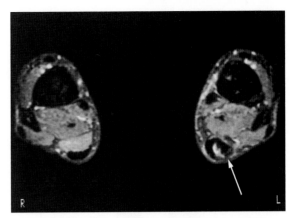

**Figure 13.21** • A combined lesion on T1-weighted MRI with nearly full-thickness tendinopathy.

## Ruptured Achilles

### Findings

(a) The prone-lying foot attitude is vertical, whereas the normal foot has a degree of plantar flexion (Fig. 13.22).

(b) If the patient lies prone, with the knee bent, the ruptured Achilles foot will lie horizontal, whereas the normal foot lies with 20–30° of plantar flexion.

(c) Simmonds'/Thompson's squeeze test is positive (see Glossary).

(d) There may be a palpable gap in the tendon.

(e) The patient cannot rise on tiptoe, although passive dorsiflexion may be pain-free.

(f) The calcaneotibial compression test is negative (see Fig. 13.10; Glossary).

### Cause

Extrinsic cause – the tendon being cut by a knife, glass, etc.

Intrinsic causes – acute overload of the Achilles, possibly during an uncoordinated movement between the quadriceps and calf muscles, particularly if the calf muscle is actively working whilst the knee is bent [14,15]. The rupture may occur apparently de novo, or following existing degeneration or partial tear of the tendon, which may have been asymptomatic. It is more common in sedentary workers [14,20,21]. Partial rupture of the Achilles can occur and is treated as a tendinopathy (see Fig. 13.16). Fluoroquinolones may increase the rate of rupture.

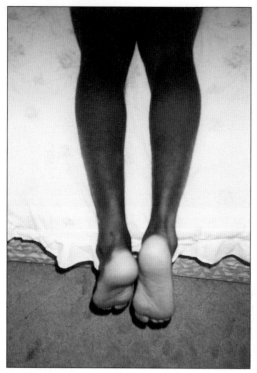

**Figure 13.22** • A ruptured Achilles on the left with vertical attitude of the foot.

## Investigations

None are clinically required if the signs are recognized, but real-time ultrasound or MRI will confirm the injury, especially if the consultation is several weeks after the rupture and adhesions are changing the signs.

## Treatment

**(a)** Surgery is advisable for sportspeople, the repair being stronger than with cast bracing.

**(b)** Cast or brace the foot into equinus, and gradually move the foot towards neutral by readjusting the brace.

**(c)** Postoperative rehabilitation, via the Achilles ladders (see Chapter 20).

**(d)** Partial rupture may be treated initially as an Achilles tendinopathy.

## Sports

See Achilles tendinopathy. Most results suggest that the damaged Achilles and calf never recover full strength. A surgical repair achieves the best return of power and athletes can return to sport. Stem cell transplants at this time may have a future. Achilles rehabilitation should be maintained even after a full return to sport.

## Comment

This diagnosis is still missed too frequently because too much emphasis is put on Simmonds'/Thompson's test, which can be made to produce plantar flexion by squeezing the posterior tibialis muscle. The prone-lying foot attitude is a very good indicator (see Fig. 13.22). Ultrasound is relatively cheap and should be used if there is any doubt as to the diagnosis. Late surgical repair may be undertaken, but the best results are obtained when performed within the first 2 weeks.

## Retro Achilles bursa

### Findings

There may be a history of pain at night and in the morning, initially feeling better with activity but then becoming increasingly painful. There is painful, reduced, active and passive dorsiflexion of the ankle. Active plantar flexion is painful and there may be palpable tenderness bilaterally over the bursa, which may be slightly swollen.

### Cause

Inflammation in the bursa. The bursa is bounded by the Achilles insertion below (the middle one-third of the calcaneum), the upper one-third of calcaneum in front, the overlying Achilles tendon behind, and the fat pad cranially (see Fig. 13.15). The bursa may be flared by a large calcaneum, possibly from calcaneovalgus or an overlying Achilles lesion. It may be part of Haglund's syndrome.

 Caveat

**Retro Achilles bursae can be associated with seronegative or seropositive arthropathies.**

### Investigations

Though it may be diagnosed clinically, ultrasound displays the bursa very well. If the bursa recurs, or does not settle, then a full blood count, ESR, autoimmune profile, HLA-B27 and rheumatoid factor should be performed.

## Treatment

(a) Steroid injection of the bursa.
(b) Electrotherapeutic modalities to settle inflammation, such as ultrasound and laser.
(c) Treat any accompanying features of Haglund's syndrome (see below).
(d) Treat any systemic cause.
(e) Remove, or alter, a tight heel cup or 'Achilles tag' from the shoes, and consider a heel raise which moves the tendon away from the calcaneal boss.
(f) Use a gel second skin.
(g) Avoid Achilles stretching exercise and 'heel drops' (see Chapter 20: Achilles ladders).

## Sports

See Achilles tendinopathy.

## Comment

Perhaps more common than expected, and a surprising number are associated with systemic inflammatory problems.

## Superficial Achilles bursa

### Findings

Pain is located over the bursa, which lies between the skin and the calcaneum. It is locally tender to palpation and the pain may be worse in the morning, better on the move, then worse with increased activity. Active and passive dorsiflexion of the foot is painful. Resisted plantar flexion is pain-free. The pain is worse in shoes, and the bursa may be red and swollen. It may be part of Haglund's syndrome (see below).

### Cause

Inflammation in the bursa that lies between the posterior aspect of the calcaneum and the skin, which is generally rubbed by the shoe (see Fig. 13.15).

### Investigations

None are clinically required but the bursa is well seen on ultrasound.

## Treatment

(a) Electrotherapeutic modalities to settle inflammation, such as ultrasound and laser.
(b) Cortisone injection into the bursa.
(c) Correct the heel rub from the shoes by fitting grips at the side of the heel, which will hold the shoe but stop rubbing of the posterior aspect. Skin gels, slick plaster with soap or two pairs of socks can prevent rubbing between the shoe and skin.
(d) Check if any calcaneovalgus needs correcting.
(e) Check the heel cups of the shoes are not too hard nor cut at an angle.
(f) See Haglund's syndrome (below).

## Sports

Make certain the shoes fit comfortably and are correct for the sport.

## Comment

Steroid injections will settle the bursitis rapidly, but the cause must then be corrected to prevent a recurrence. Silicone gels are very effective in preventing rub from the shoes.

## Haglund's syndrome [22]

### Findings

There is a large, thickened, superficial Achilles bursa, known as a 'pump bump', caused by shoe rub. There is also an inflamed retro Achilles bursa (see Retro Achilles bursa and Superficial Achilles bursa).

### Cause

A combination of retro and superficial Achilles bursae, produced by a protuberant, superior boss of the calcaneum rubbing against the shoe and Achilles tendon.

### Investigations

A weight-bearing X-ray can be used to record the angle of the calcaneum and to assess the relevance of the superior calcaneal boss in causing pressure on the overlying structures.

## Treatment

(a) Treat as for superficial and retro Achilles bursae.
(b) Use soft heel cups, and even sandals, to prevent local rubbing.
(c) Surgical removal of the calcaneal boss or a calcaneal osteotomy.

## Sports

Obviously, this syndrome is better with a sport that uses no shoes or sandals. Surgical correction has to be considered for other sportspeople.

## Comment

Fortunately this is rare. It is still better to adjust the shoes, rather than the individual, if at all possible.

## Posterior tibiofibular ligament

The posterior tibiofibular ligament is a thickening of the posterior capsule – see below.

## Posterior capsule

### Findings

There is a history of an impingement mechanism, such as an inversion sprain of the ankle with plantar flexion, a foot forced into plantar flexion by kicking a ball or having the kick blocked, a sudden stop, which drives the heel into the ground, or a sudden drop onto the heel, such as an unforeseen step down, missing the kerb or a step. The ankle is swollen, with bruising on its lateral, medial and posterior aspects. Standing on tiptoe is painful and the calcaneotibial compression test is positive (see Fig. 13.10 and Glossary). A soccer player can side-foot and chip the football, but is not able to drive or volley the ball.

### Cause

A compression injury between the calcaneum and posterior aspect of the tibia that bruises the structures that lie at the back of the ankle.

### Caveat

Os trigonum (see Fig. 13.23) or Stieda process (see Fig. 13.9).

## Investigations

X-ray to exclude an os trigonum and a Stieda process of the talus, which may be fractured. Kager's triangle may be distorted on X-ray (see Fig. 13.15). An MRI will show the oedema at the back of the ankle, but the expense of this investigation is hardly justified.

## Treatment

This is as for bilateral bruising of lateral ligaments of the ankle (see Part 3: Sprained ankle: lateral and medial bruising):

(a) Electrotherapeutic modalities to settle inflammation, such as shortwave diathermy and interferential.
(b) An injection of cortisone around the posterior capsule, posterior tibiofibular ligament and deep structures at the back of the ankle.

## Sports

(a) Ballet and high jump force this abutment of the calcaneum with the posterior structures of the ankle. The dancer should avoid pointes, but may be able to handle quarter and demi-pointes. This impingement problem settles so rapidly with a cortisone injection that high jumpers are not 'out' for long.
(b) Footballers can train, and utilize the kicking ladder (see Chapter 20), with side-foot and chipping, but can build into the drive/volley only as the injury improves. Strapping to prevent forced plantar flexion may help, but it is difficult to apply.
(c) Checking suddenly at field hockey, or stretching for a drop shot in squash and badminton.
(d) Stamping the heel down during a squash shot produces posterior compression. (Yes, some players do this with nearly every shot.)

## Comment

This is often the persistent pain, several months after an ankle injury has occurred, and it may be cured in 2–3 weeks or less with one or two steroid injections into the posterior structures around the talar and subtalar joint. It is often misdiagnosed as an Achilles problem, as both these problems have pain on rising to tiptoe, but achillodynia does not have a positive calcaneotibial compression test.

# Os trigonum/Stieda process

## Findings

Active and passive plantar flexion is painful and the calcaneotibial compression test is positive (see Fig. 13.10 and Glossary).

## Cause

The os trigonum, a separated ossification centre of the talus, is trapped (rather like a nut between the jaws of a nutcracker) between the upper surface of the calcaneum and the posterior tibia during forced plantar flexion. The Stieda process is a fused os trigonum that has produced an elongated posterior element of the talus (see Fig. 13.9).

## Investigations

Lateral X-ray of the ankle shows the os trigonum, but many radiologists consider this a normal variant and make no mention of its existence – so the clinician may have to request that the presence of an os trigonum be reported. Both an os trigonum (Fig. 13.23) and a Stieda process may fracture and become fragmented.

## Treatment

(a) Electrotherapeutic modalities to settle inflammation, such as interferential and pulsed shortwave.

(b) Cortisone to the posterior aspect of the talar joint and around the os trigonum.

(c) Surgery to remove the os trigonum [23] or fragmented pieces.

## Sports

(a) See Posterior capsule.

(b) Ballet dancers and high jumpers will require surgery to remove the os trigonum if this is a persistent problem. Other sports only need the acute episode treating conservatively.

## Comment

Although not common, it can be very problematical for those requiring large degrees of plantar flexion, and surgery is probably the treatment of choice in these cases.

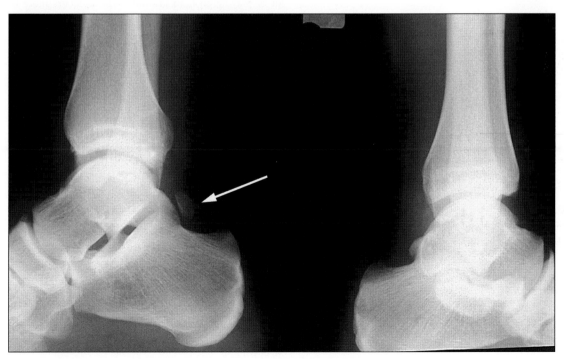

**Figure 13.23** • An os trigonum (*arrow*).

## Lateral process of talus fracture

Snowboarders produce some unusual fractures around the ankle, of which the lateral process of the talus appears to be the most frequent. MRI, CT and a bone scan will display the lesion, but some consider that assessment by CT is most suitable to assess the lesion fully [24]. Although most of these fractures are traumatic, a possible stress fracture may occur in this area [25].

## Sever's disease

### Findings

Pain over the posterior aspect of the calcaneum, but also about 2 cm along the medial or lateral side of the calcaneum, that is painful to palpation in a child who is skeletally immature.

Type 1  Is worse on impact, but heals faster.
Type 2  Is worse on thrust and lift-off of the foot and takes longer to heal.

### Cause

This is not a disease but a calcaneal epiphyseal problem in children.

Type 1  An epiphysitis, from impact of the calcaneal epiphysis.
Type 2  An apophysitis, from the pull of the Achilles.

### Investigations

None are clinically required, and an X-ray is difficult to interpret as the normal epiphysis is irregular and does show some sclerosis (Fig. 13.24).

### Treatment

(a) A heel raise may help type 2 because it reduces the leverage from the Achilles.
(b) Reduce the amount of exercise.
(c) Ensure that the shoes have the best shock absorbability.
(d) If limping during exercise, the child should be removed from exercise.
(e) If the heel hurts after exercise but is better by the morning, maintain the exercise level.
(f) If the heel hurts in the morning, and when walking, then reduce activity by 10–50%.

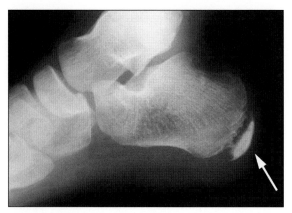

**Figure 13.24** • An X-ray of a child with Sever's disease showing the calcaneal apophysis.

(g) Occasionally a cast brace, for walking, will rest the heel for the 2–3 weeks required for recovery.

### Sports

Type 1 occurs more frequently, and in those running a lot or playing on hard ground. Type 2 occurs more in gymnasts, jumpers and ballet dancers.

### Comment

I have never seen long-term problems with this condition. Children like to play with their peers, so I try to maintain them in activities, but titrate the amount of exercise against pain. I have seen a very irregular calcaneal epiphysis following a fall, and this needed cast bracing and a very long time to settle, suggesting that it was probably a traumatic epiphyseal fracture.

## Flexor hallucis tenosynovitis

Pain from the flexor hallucis may be felt immediately behind the medial maleolus, and sometimes in its muscle, which lies just behind and adjacent to the ankle joint. Injury is particularly associated with ballet dancers and the tendon may rupture (see Part 4).

## References

1 Boytim MJ, Fischer DA, Neumann L. Syndesmotic ankle sprains. Am J Sports Med 1991;19:294–298

2 Taylor DC, Englehardt DL, Bassett FH. Syndesmosis sprains of the ankle: the influence of heterotopic ossification. Am J Sports Med 1992;20:146–150

3 Miller CD, Shelton WR, Barrett GR, Savoie FH, Dukes AD. Deltoid and syndesmosis ligament injury of the ankle without fracture. Am J Sports Med 1995;23:746–750

4 Orava S, Karpakka J, Hulkko A, Takala T. Stress avulsion fracture of the tarsal navicular: an uncommon sports-related overuse injury. Am J Sports Med 1991;19:392–395

5 Niek van Dijk C, Tol JL, Verheyen CCPM. A prospective study of prognostic factors concerning the outcome of arthroscopic surgery for anterior ankle impingement. Am J Sports Med 1997;25(6):737–745

6 Ferkel RD, Karzel RP, Del Pizzo W, Friedman MJ, Fischer SP. Arthroscopic treatment of antero lateral impingement of the ankle. Am J Sports Med 1991;19:440–446

7 Firer P. Effectiveness of taping for the prevention of ankle ligament sprains. Br J Sports Med 1990;24:47–50

8 Liu SH, Baker CL. Comparison of lateral ankle ligamentous reconstruction procedures. Am J Sports Med 1994;22:313–317

9 Kollias SL, Ferkel RD. Fibular grooving for recurrent peroneal tendon subluxation. Am J Sports Med 1997;25:329–335

10 Jackson DL, Haglund B. Tarsal tunnel syndrome in athletes: case reports and literature review. Am J Sports Med 1991;19:61–65

11 Read MTF, Motto SG. Tendo Achilles pain: steroids and outcome. Br J Sports Med 1992;26:15–21

12 Read MTF. Safe relief of rest pain that eases with activity in achillodynia by intrabursal or peritendinous steroid injections: the rupture rate was not increased by these steroid injections. Br J Sports Med 1999;33:134–135

13 Hutson MA (ed.). Sports injuries: recognition and management, 2nd edn. Oxford: Oxford Medical Publications; 1996

14 Arner O, Linholm A. Subcutaneous ruptures of the Achilles tendon. Acta Chir Scand 1959;239(Suppl)

15 Distefano GJ, Nixon J. Ruptures of the Achilles tendon. J Sports Med Phys Fitness 1973;34–37

16 Clement DB, Taunton JE, Smart GW. Achilles tendonitis and peritendinitis: etiology and treatment. Am J Sports Med 1984;12(3):179–185

17 Jones SM, Robertson JA. Presentation to BASM conference, Birmingham. Br J Sports Med 1984;19:53

18 Alfredson H, Ohberg L, Forsgren S. Is vasculo-neural ingrowth the cause of pain in chronic Achilles tendinosis? An investigation using ultrasonography and colour Doppler, immunohistochemistry, and diagnostic injections. Knee Surg Sports Traumatol Arthrosc 2003;11:334–338

19 Ilum Boesen M, Torp-Pedersen S, Juhl Koenig M, et al. Ultrasound guided electrocoagulation in patients with chronic non-insertional Achilles tendinopathy: a pilot study. Br J Sports Med 2006;40:761–766

20 Hooker CH. Rupture of the tendo Achilles. J Bone Joint Surg [B] 1963;35B:360–363

21 Barfred T. Achilles tendon rupture. Acta Orthop Scand 1973;44(Suppl 152):126

22 Rossi F, La Cava F, Amato F, Pincelli G. The Haglund syndrome (H.s.): clinical and radiological features and sports medicine aspects. J Sports Med 1987;27:258–263

23 Marotta JJ, Micheli LJ. Os trigonum impingement in dancers. Am J Sports Med 1992;20:533–536

24 Kirkpatrick DP, Hunter RE, Janes PC, Mastrangelo J, Nicholas RA. The snowboarder's foot and ankle. Am J Sports Med 1998;26:271–277

25 Motto SG. Stress fracture of the lateral process of the talus: a case report. Br J Sports Med 1993;27:275–276

## Further reading

Bruckner P, Khan K. Clinical sports medicine, 3rd edn. New York: McGraw-Hill; 2006

Hutson M, Ellis R (eds). Textbook of musculoskeletal medicine. Oxford: Oxford University Press; 2006

Reid D. Sports injury assessment and rehabilitation. Edinburgh: Churchill Livingstone; 1992

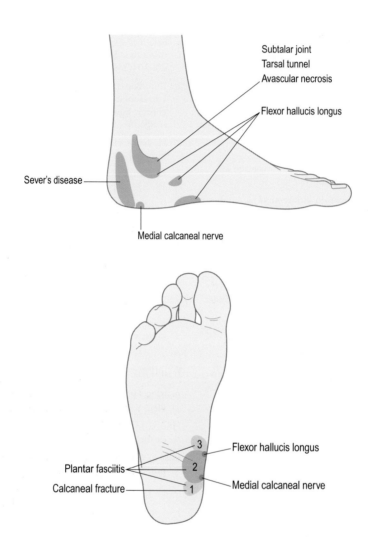

Subtalar joint
Tarsal tunnel
Avascular necrosis

Flexor hallucis longus

Sever's disease

Medial calcaneal nerve

3  Flexor hallucis longus
Plantar fasciitis
2
Calcaneal fracture  1  Medial calcaneal nerve

# Chapter Fourteen

14

# Heel and arch of foot

## Plantar fasciitis

### Findings

Type 1   The inferior surface of the calcaneum is painful, and worse on palpation, but squeezing the rim of the calcaneal fat pad relieves this palpatory pain. It is probably not a true fasciitis.

Type 2   As for type 1, but the pain can also be produced by forced dorsiflexion of the foot and toes, and by rocking up over the balls of the feet and toes at a 45° angle, such as in a sprint start position. There is tenderness to palpation over the calcaneal enthesis of the spring ligament.

Type 3   There is a history of acute or semi-acute pain, often under the arch of the foot, and the tenderness is not under the calcaneum but over the spring ligament, which may be thickened and tender.

### Cause

Possibly plantar fasciitis is a 'catch-all' phrase that may include flexor hallucis and medial calcaneal nerve problems as well. Type 1 is not a fasciitis, but trauma of the fat pad. However, this lesion is often talked of as a fasciitis, so has been included under this heading.

Type 1   Damage to the fat pad of the heel, which presents more often in the elderly. The fibrous stroma separates the fat into compartments so that, during compression, the loculated fat is prevented from spreading and therefore acts as a good shock absorber. When the stroma weakens, the fat pad is less tightly contained and becomes functionally thinner, thus allowing impact to reach the calcaneal periosteum.

Type 2   An enthesitis of the plantar spring ligament.

Type 3   A degenerative lesion within the spring ligament, which may lead to partial rupture.

Caveat

## Caveat

Gout, spondylarthropathies, L5/S1 disc, calcaneal stress fracture, medial calcaneal nerve entrapment and flexor hallucis tendinitis.

## Investigations

Certainly the lesions can be managed without investigation. X-ray may show a spur, which is considered non-causative of plantar fasciitis but it just might reflect the pull on the enthesis (Fig. 14.1). Ultrasound and MRI scans can indicate oedema and show a tendinosis or a tear in the spring ligament (Fig. 14.2), whilst MRI can also exclude a calcaneal fracture. Blood tests (uric acid, autoimmune profile, ESR and HLA-B27) will rule out systemic causes.

## Treatment

Type 1:

(a) An orthosis to squeeze the fat pad, diminish impact and correct calcaneovalgus.

(b) Low Dye strapping to squeeze the fat pad [1], possibly with iontophoresis of acetic acid [2] (see Glossary).

(c) 'Air-soled' shoes, which use the same principle as the stroma of the fat pad, will reduce impact.

(d) Non-impact cross-training, such as biking, rowing or swimming.

(e) Electrotherapeutic modalities to settle inflammation, such as ultrasound.

(f) A trial of cortisone to settle the inflammation in the fat and around the periosteum.

Type 2:

(a) Treat as for type 1.

(b) Use a heel raise, especially a shock-absorbent raise, in the early phase to reduce the tension in the spring ligament.

(c) Cortisone injection to the enthesis.

(d) Stretch and load the enthesis and spring ligament by rocking over the toes, as in a sprint start, or use a foot rocker. This stretch may be maintained at night by a cast that holds the foot dorsiflexed.

(e) Stand on the edge of the stairs, rise onto tiptoe and then drop the heels as low as possible over the edge of the stairs to stretch the spring ligament, and then load it by standing on tiptoe.

(f) Return to running, etc., via the Achilles ladder (see Chapter 20).

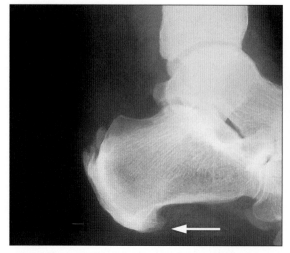

**Figure 14.1** • A plantar fascial spur. This patient also has an Achilles spur. Some people appear prone to entheseal stress lesions.

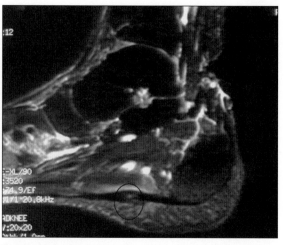

**Figure 14.2** • Type 3 tendinopathy, with a partial tear of the spring ligament.

Type 3:

(a) Electrotherapeutic modalities, such as ultrasound, to settle the inflammation.

(b) Rest, and shorten the spring ligament with a heel raise, and then gradually reduce the height of the heel raise as the injury repairs.

(c) Gradually introduce stretch and load exercises, as in type 2 (d)–(f).

## Comment

This is a troublesome condition that takes several months to settle. Defining the lesion will make rehabilitation and treatment easier. A heel raise, in types 2 and 3, may be made of sheets of paper, reduced by one a day, to gradually stretch out the plantar fascia. I think only types 1 and 2 respond to cortisone and, occasionally, if there is an inflammatory element, type 3. All need rehabilitation afterwards. Type 3 takes an age to repair, and may rupture, when, rather like the biceps tendon, it then gets better! My injection rate fell when I used a shock-absorbent orthotic with edges that squeeze the heel pad, for type 1.

## Medial calcaneal nerve

### Findings

Pain to palpation in a line over the medial inferior calcaneum, and a history of heel pain that is worse on impact. There may be pain at night and at rest. A blunt probe (a closed ball point pen) may be used to palpate small tender areas. If these tender points are then marked on the skin, a straight line, running down the calcaneum towards the sole of the heel, will be outlined.

### Cause

Compression of the medial calcaneal nerve as it passes over the medial side of the calcaneum into the heel pad. Calcaneovalgus encourages this compression, though poorly fitting heel wedges or orthotics may cause irritation of the nerve between the shoe and orthotic. The medial calcaneal nerve may be caught in the scar tissue of the damaged plantar fascia.

### Investigations

As for plantar fasciitis. An EMG is not of value.

### Treatment

(a) Correct any calcaneovalgus with a medial heel wedge or orthotic.

(b) Perineural cortisone around the medial calcaneal nerve.

(c) Treat any accompanying plantar fasciitis.

(d) Surgical release of the nerve from scar tissue.

### Sports

Avoid impact sports until better. Check that the running style and shoes, especially broken heel cups, are not producing a functional calcaneovalgus. Fit the appropriate orthotics (see Plantar fasciitis). Rehabilitate via the Achilles ladder (see Chapter 20).

### Comment

This is, possibly, slightly more common than is usually recognized, and is part of the plantar fasciitis complex. However, in spite of the correct treatment, it takes a while to settle.

## Sever's disease

Pain in a child that is worse with activity and is tender on palpation over the posteromedial or posterolateral calcaneum, along the line of the enthesis (see Chapter 13).

## Flexor hallucis longus

The flexor hallucis longus remains muscular to the level of the posterior ankle joint. Pain is worse when standing on tiptoe and with resisted great toe flexion. Sometimes, tenderness may be palpated just forward of the heel, under the arch of the foot (see Chapter 13, Part 5).

## Subtalar joint

See Sinus tarsi.

## Sinus tarsi

### Findings

(a) The sinus tarsi is the route by which an injection may be placed at the ligament at the neck of the talus, which, when strained, may produce lateral mid-foot and ankle pain.

**(b)** Passive inversion and eversion of the subtalar joint is painful. The range of movement may be reduced and have an obvious calcaneovalgus.

**(c)** Sometimes, a history of trauma and osteoarthritis of the talar and talonavicular joints accompanies this problem.

**(d)** There is frequently pain on impact of the heel, but it may be pain-free at rest.

## Cause

**(a)** Osteoarthritis (OA) of the talocalcaneal joint, from chronic calcaneovalgus or secondary to trauma.

**(b)** Sprain of the ligament to the neck of the talus, at the base of the sinus tarsi.

**(c)** Avascular necrosis or idiopathic oedema of the talus (see Fig. 13.8).

### Caveat

**Fracture of the neck of the talus can occur near its articulation with the calcaneum.**

## Investigations

**(a)** X-rays for degenerative changes.

**(b)** MRI is the definitive investigation, particularly for degenerative OA, avascular necrosis or fracture, although a bone scan and CT may be helpful.

## Treatment

**(a)** Electrotherapeutic modalities, such as shortwave diathermy or interferential to settle inflammation and ease pain.

**(b)** Cortisone injection of the subtalar joint by a posterior, lateral or sinus tarsi approach.

**(c)** An orthotic designed to control subtalar movement.

**(d)** Avoidance of causes for avascular necrosis, such as alcohol, barbiturates, etc. Pamidronate, intravenous or oral, may help.

**(e)** Surgical fusion of the joint for OA, or removal of a talar fracture fragment that has failed to unite.

## Sports

**(a)** Sports that produce impact on the foot prove to be a problem, and may have to be abandoned if chronic changes of OA have occurred.

**(b)** Golfers will not be able to roll over the foot during the follow through, and may have to turn the left foot out, and open the stance, to overcome this problem.

## Comment

Not a common problem. Injection of cortisone, via the sinus tarsi, is the best initial approach, but if the chronic ligament strains have scarred up the joint then manipulation under anaesthetic and injection via the sinus tarsi may be required.

## Tarsal coalition

### Findings

Usually found during investigation of a stiff foot that does not functionally pronate well and has caused tracking knee problems, recurrent ankle sprain or anterior ankle pain. However, ankle pain may be the presenting feature. The mid-tarsal and subtalar joints are immobile.

### Cause

Fibrous, cartilaginous or bony fusion between the calcaneum and the talus, and, sometimes, between the cuboid and calcaneum, limit tarsal range of movement.

### Investigations

X-ray (Fig. 14.3) or CT scan.

### Treatment

Needs to be directed to the secondary affected areas. Pronation partly occurs through the mid-tarsal joint, and this movement is limited by tarsal coalition. A heel raise will allow more movement through the talus and the forefoot, reducing the need for pronation.

### Sports

A stiff foot will reduce the adaptations required for change of direction sports, and running may produce secondary injuries, such as knee tracking problems. The ideal sports for this problem are, therefore, non-impact

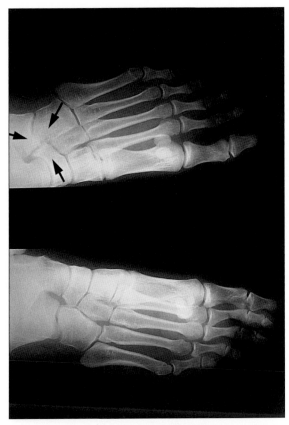

**Figure 14.3** • Tarsal coalition between talus and cuboid, and a bridging of the navicular (*arrows*).

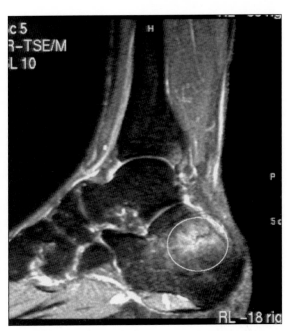

**Figure 14.4** • MRI shows the calcaneal stress fracture with surrounding oedema.

sports, but slowing down the rate of loading in impact sports will allow secondary areas time to adapt.

## Comment

Early advice concerning this problem will help the patient to move to a more appropriate sport.

## Tarsal tunnel syndrome

This syndrome produces heel and arch pain, which is accompanied by 'pins and needles', numbness or weakness. There is tenderness to palpation over the tarsal tunnel (see Chapter 13, Part 4).

## Avascular necrosis/idiopathic oedema of the talus

Subtalar joint pain that is non-diagnostic should have an MRI (see Fig. 13.8). Avascular necrosis often affects the subtalar joint, involving the calcaneum and/or talus. Orthotics may help to stabilize the joint, and a reduction of systemic causative factors, such as alcohol, are advised. It is possible that idiopathic oedema of the talus is a differential diagnosis, or even a synonym. Treatment with a walking boot and intravenous or oral pamidronate (or other bisphosphonates) may be curative.

## Calcaneal fracture

### Findings

Impact pain in the calcaneum whilst standing or walking, and the fracture is locally tender to pressure.

### Cause

From an acute impact, landing on the heel, but it may also present as a stress fracture with an insidious onset.

### Investigations

X-ray if there is a history of acute trauma. If no fracture is visible then MRI scan for a stress lesion (Fig. 14.4). CT may be required to display the extent and healing of the fracture.

## Treatment

A protective cast, with a mid-foot rocker and, later, soft absorbent soles rather than hard shoes.

## Sports

Jumping into the shallow end of a swimming pool is the most common cause of a calcaneal fracture. Continue non-impact sports whilst waiting for the bone to repair.

## Comment

I have seen only one stress fracture of the calcaneum in nearly three decades of dealing with sports injuries, though some colleagues feel it is a reasonably common problem.

## References

1  Hlavac H. The foot book. Mountain View: CA: World Publications; 1977

2  Osbourne HR, Allison GT. Treatment of plantar fasciitis by LowDye taping and iontophoresis: short term results of a double blinded, randomized clinical trial of dexamethasone and acetic acid. Br J Sports Med 2006;40(6):545–549

## Further reading

Bruckner P, Khan K. Clinical sports medicine, 3rd edn. New York: McGraw-Hill; 2006

Hutson M, Ellis R (eds). Textbook of musculoskeletal medicine. Oxford: Oxford University Press; 2006

Reid D. Sports injury assessment and rehabilitation. Edinburgh: Churchill Livingstone; 1992

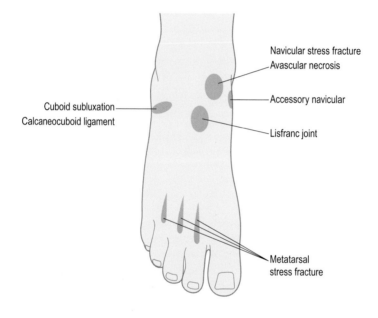

Navicular stress fracture
Avascular necrosis

Accessory navicular

Cuboid subluxation
Calcaneocuboid ligament

Lisfranc joint

Metatarsal
stress fracture

# Mid-foot

## Calcaneocuboid ligament

### Findings

When lateral bruising is found mainly over the mid-foot and tracking towards the toes then, invariably, the calcaneocuboid ligament has been damaged. The lesion is not well diagnosed and treated, and thus often presents as a chronic ankle or foot pain. Rough ground is particularly troublesome, and pain is produced on pronating and supinating the mid- and forefoot, across the mid-tarsal joint. There is tenderness to palpation over the calcaneocuboid joint.

### Cause

Part of the inversion sprain mechanism, but more stress has passed through the mid-tarsal joint, straining the ligaments between the calcaneum and cuboid.

### Investigations

None are clinically required, and MRI in chronic cases may not be diagnostic.

### Treatment

(a) RICE.
(b) Injection of cortisone to the calcaneocuboid ligament.
(c) Electrotherapeutic modalities, such as ultrasound, laser and interferential to settle inflammation in the ligament and joint, are not that successful.
(d) Rehabilitation as for a sprained ankle (see Chapter 13, Part 3: Sprained ankle: lateral bruising).
(e) Soft arch orthotic to rest the joint from pronation.

### Sports

As for a sprained ankle, but twisting–turning sports may require orthotics and strapping of the mid-tarsal joint to reduce the pronation movements through this joint for 6–8 weeks after the foot and ankle are pain-free (see Chapter 13, Part 3).

## Comment

This injury does not seem to improve with physiotherapy, but an injection, just into the joint capsule over the tender area, works well.

# Cuboid subluxation

## Findings

There is no history of an inversion sprain, but there is pain on jumping and landing, and on rough ground. The mid-tarsal joint has pain on passive testing in plantar flexion, as well as in supination and pronation. It is locally tender to palpation over the calcaneocuboid ligament and the cuboid.

## Cause

Pain in the foot of ballet dancers from a subluxed cuboid or strained ligaments [1].

## Investigations

None are clinically required.

## Treatment

Plantar flexing manipulations, pivoting over the cuboid.

## Sports

Ballet dancers may maintain their range of foot movements by self-manipulation of the cuboid.

## Comment

This is well reported, and written up, in dancers [1], but not other sports. Manipulation seems to be corrective.

# Accessory navicular

## Findings

The problems may present as rubbing of the skin over the prominent tubercle or as a posterior tibialis tendinitis (see Chapter 13, Part 4).

## Cause

The unfused ossification centre of the navicular tubercle (or in the adult, with fibrous union) does not withstand loads from the posterior tibialis as well as the fused tubercle. The tubercle is more prominent, or has been made more prominent, by overpronation, and the overlying skin becomes rubbed by the shoe and becomes inflamed.

## Investigations

X-ray, but ask for the presence of an accessory navicular to be reported as it is a normal variant and, therefore, is often not commented upon by the radiologist (see Fig. 13.13).

## Treatment

As for posterior tibialis tendinitis (see Chapter 13, Part 4); however, a supportive orthotic is very important and it may require a permanent orthotic to reduce the loads or alter its prominence. It takes longer to heal than the posterior tibialis enthesitis described in Chapter 13.

## Comment

This seems to present mainly in adolescence, as adults appear adapted to the problem, even when an accessory navicular is visible on X-ray. It is essential to explain to the patient and parents about its longish morbidity (see Glossary: Accessory navicular or os tibialis externum).

# Navicular stress fracture

## Findings

This presents with an acute or insidious onset of pain over the mid-foot, but clinical examination may or may not produce pain on passive, mid-tarsal joint movements. However, it is usually tender to direct palpation over the navicular.

## Cause

A stress fracture of the navicular seems to occur in sprint, jump and interval sprint games, but not in endurance events. Perhaps when the foot is on tiptoe, as in sprinting, the concave surface of the navicular becomes the anvil, to the hammer of the convex surface of the talus, and this impact load produces the vertical fracture in the navicular.

## Caveat

This fracture is often missed. An index of suspicion, or tenderness over the navicular, is reason to investigate further. A bifid navicular is an extremely rare variation.

## Investigations

An X-ray often misses this sagittally placed fracture, and a bone scan, or more particularly a MRI, is the watershed investigation. A CT scan may be required to display sclerosis around the joint or widening of the fracture, which indicate non-union has occurred.

## Treatment

A cast brace and non-weight-bearing for 1 month, if the scans show no widening or sclerosis of the fracture. Follow this with weight-bearing for 1 month in a cast brace. Later weight-bearing rehabilitation through the Achilles ladders, with caution, for up to 3–4 months (see Chapter 20) [2]. If there is widening or non-union of the fracture then a compression screw should be inserted.

## Caveat

The navicular is prone to non-union (Fig. 15.1), so if there is any doubt as to the diagnosis then the clinician should err on the surgical side.

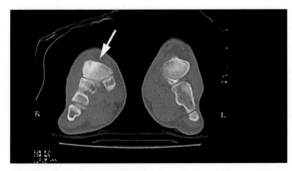

**Figure 15.1** • CT scan showing non-union of the navicular, with sclerosis and separation of fracture.

## Sports

(a) Athletics – seems to occur in sprints up to 400 metres, jumps, and hurdles.

(b) Field hockey – has become more common since the advent of the 'plastic' surface for hockey pitches.

(c) Non-impact cross-training and local muscle strengthening must be maintained.

(d) Impact should be severely limited until the fracture is healed, but it can be introduced somewhat earlier on rebound trampettes.

## Comment

This fracture is often missed. Too often, this injury presents months after its onset, frequently when non-union is established. A negative X-ray does not rule out this injury, and if there is any element of doubt concerning the diagnosis then an MRI or bone scan should be ordered. The morbidity of this problem is excessive, and non-union is common, so a CT scan to assess the problem should be undertaken early. If there is a doubt about non-union then the fracture should probably have a compression screw inserted. Occasionally, the palpable tenderness seems to be over the anterior talar surface, but the problem is likely to be navicular.

# Tarsal coalition

Stiffness of the mid-tarsal joint may be caused by a coalition (see Chapter 14).

# Avascular necrosis of the navicular in young children

Presents with tenderness over the navicular, and limping in the young child (see Glossary: Köhler's disease).

# Lisfranc joint – second tarsometatarsal arthrosis

## Findings

A presentation, in dancers, especially ballet, of mid-foot pain and tenderness over the second tarsometatarsal joint [3].

## Cause

Type 1   A synovitis or ligament strain of this joint; plus a small diastasis can occur.

Type 2   A stress fracture of the proximal second metatarsal.

## Investigations

X-ray may show the expected thickening and sclerosis of the second metatarsal that occurs as an adaptation to the stresses of dancing on pointes, but it does not differentiate the lesion. A diastasis should be looked for on all scans. A bone scan will indicate stress around this joint, and may be more sensitive in this area than an MRI. However, MRI and CT should follow to try to display an oblique fracture, bony bruising or a synovitis.

## Treatment

Type 1   The inflamed joint may be treated with anti-inflammatories, such as NSAIDs, electrical modalities or cortisone, and relative rest. This rest should be in training, avoiding all demi- and full pointe work, plus jumps, but performance can be permitted, as long as progress is being maintained. Some surgeons will consider a screw fixation to stabilize a torn ligament. [3].

Type 2   Should be removed from dancing and might require a cast brace, or even surgery to remove necrotic bone fragments [3].

## Sports

Ballet dancing, where overflexing the forefoot may be contributory.

## Comment

This is one of those under-diagnosed problems, because all dancers expect to have some aches from the Lisfranc joint and are not aware of the extent of the damage they are suffering.

## References

1   Marshall P, Hamilton WG. Cuboid subluxation in ballet dancers. Am J Sports Med 1992;20:169–175

2   Khan KM, Fuller PJ, Brukner PD, Kearney C, Burry HC. Outcome of conservative and surgical management of navicular stress fracture in athletes. Am J Sports Med 1992;20:657–666

3   Harrington T, Crichton KJ, Anderson IF. Overuse ballet injury of the base of the second metatarsal: a diagnostic problem. Am J Sports Med 1993;21:591–598

### Further reading

Bruckner P, Khan K. Clinical sports medicine, 3rd edn. New York: McGraw-Hill; 2006

Hutson M, Ellis R (eds). Textbook of musculoskeletal medicine. Oxford: Oxford University Press; 2006

Reid D. Sports injury assessment and rehabilitation. Edinburgh: Churchill Livingstone; 1992

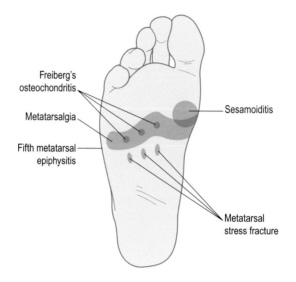

Freiberg's
osteochondritis

Metatarsalgia

Fifth metatarsal
epiphysitis

Sesamoiditis

Metatarsal
stress fracture

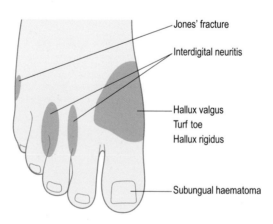

Jones' fracture

Interdigital neuritis

Hallux valgus
Turf toe
Hallux rigidus

Subungual haematoma

# Chapter Sixteen

## Forefoot

### CHAPTER CONTENTS

## Metatarsal stress fracture (march fracture)

### Findings

The history is generally of a gradual onset of pain with activities, although the onset can be acute. The pain is worse on impact, better with rest. There is usually puffy swelling of the forefoot, with local tenderness to palpation over the metatarsal shaft on both dorsal and plantar surfaces. A metatarsalgia and interdigital neuritis may accompany this problem (see Metatarsalgia and Interdigital neuritis).

### Cause

A stress fracture is produced in the shaft of the second, third or fourth metatarsal from too rapid incremental loads. Often seen in army recruits about 3–4 weeks into training.

### Investigations

X-ray (Fig. 16.1); however, as the X-ray can be negative for up to 2–3 weeks, a bone scan or MRI scan should be utilized if there is any doubt.

### Treatment

Rest from impact for 6–8 weeks, but cross-train by exercise such as swimming, biking or rowing to maintain fitness. Use firm shoes or a cast boot to act as a splint, and use the Achilles ladder on return to activity (see Chapter 20).

### Sports

Usually occurs from running, but can occur with walking, marching and change of direction sports.

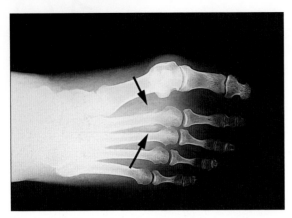

**Figure 16.1** • A march fracture with callus around the second metatarsal.

## Comment

The puffy swelling on the dorsum of the foot and the localized tenderness, especially if present on both dorsal and plantar surfaces, are almost pathognomonic. Repeat X-rays will monitor healing callus but pain is the best guide as to when to return to activities.

## Metatarsalgia

### Findings

**(a)** Pain on standing or walking but, more particularly, on standing on tiptoes or running, when the forefoot impact on the metatarsal heads flares the pain.

**(b)** Tender to palpation over the joint on the plantar surface, and pain may be elicited on passive, dorsi- or plantarflexion of the joint.

**(c)** The foot may have claw toes and be in equinus. This brings the metatarsal heads more prominently in contact with the ground. Overlying skin callus on the sole of the foot may be present.

**(d)** There may be an accompanying interdigital neuritis because the swollen capsule and soft tissue compress the nerve.

### Cause

Impact on the metatarsal heads causes bony bruising, plus joint and soft tissue swelling. A clawed or subluxed metatarsal joint is more prominent. Metatarsalgia in several joints may be a presentation for systemic joint disease, such as rheumatoid arthritis.

## Investigations

X-ray to exclude Freiberg's infraction/infarction in an adolescent, and stress fracture of the metatarsal in an adult. Blood test for systemic joint disease, if relevant. MRI shows both bony and soft tissue problems.

## Treatment

In a normal foot:

**(a)** Rest from impact sports, but train via non-impact cross-training.

**(b)** Electrotherapeutic modalities to settle inflammation, such as interferential, ultrasound and laser.

**(c)** NSAIDs.

**(d)** Fit a metatarsal, transverse arch orthotic proximal to the metatarsal heads, to raise the metatarsal head from impact.

**(e)** Reintroduce impact with a transverse arch orthotic, and increment training into sprints via the Achilles ladder (see Chapter 20).

In the equinus foot:

**(a)** A cast-made orthotic will spread the loads, and silicone pads under the tips of the toes will help them exert pressure on the ground and reduce the force onto the metatarsal heads.

**(b)** If required, chiropody for the calluses.

**(c)** Avoid impact sports.

**(d)** Surgery.

 Caveat

**The diabetic foot and rheumatoid arthritis.**

## Sports

**(a)** Metatarsalgia develops in a normal foot with sprint drills. Sprinting requires forefoot propulsion, and runners who have a low knee carry, such as shuffle runners, are unused to impacting and driving through the forefoot for speed. These drills need to be introduced more slowly so as to allow adaptation and conditioning of the bones and joint.

(b) Stop–start games, especially netball where the sudden stop is mandatory, will impact on the metatarsals.

## Comment

The patient with equinus foot that develops metatarsalgia should consider switching to non-impact sports, but the foot may have adapted over the years, producing large protective calluses. However, these people have often tried something new, or incremented their activity too fast, and only require treatment of the immediate problem and a return to their old technique to which they have adapted.

## Freiberg's osteochondritis/infraction/infarction

### Findings

Should be suspected in an adolescent who presents with local tenderness over the metatarsophalangeal joint, with a history of pain on impact of the foot.

### Cause

An osteochondritis, possibly avascular, of the second or third distal head of the metatarsus. Sometimes known as Köhler's second disease.

### Investigations

X-ray shows squaring of the metatarsal head (Fig. 16.2).

### Treatment

This takes several years to settle, with a transverse arch or metatarsal pad to help. Avoid impact sports and high heels. Well-padded shoes are required. NSAIDs can help, as required. Surgery can have a place [1].

### Sports

Impact sports should be avoided, but the child may try impact games on soft surfaces, or train other skills to pain tolerance until the problem settles.

### Comment

Management is a real problem as it requires a quantum shift from impact to non-impact sport until the problem settles, although the patient may play goal-

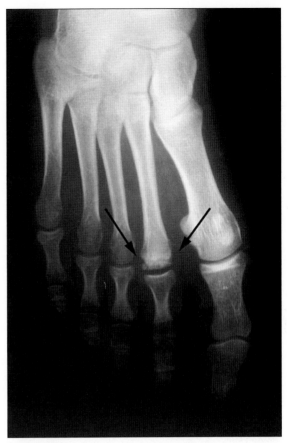

**Figure 16.2** • Freiberg's infraction/infarction with squaring and fragmentation of the second metatarsal.

keeper in team games, for instance. The whole psychosocial, talent and future of the adolescent must be explored.

## Interdigital neuritis

### Findings

The pain is centred between the metatarsal heads and may refer down adjacent sides of the relevant two toes, usually 2/3 and 3/4. There may be pain on non-weight-bearing as well as weight-bearing, which can wake the patient at night. Squeezing the metatarsal heads together provokes pain, and this can be worse in tight shoes, better with bare feet. Factors that provoke the problem, such as increased pronation, metatarsalgia and a march fracture should be investigated (see Metatarsal stress fracture and Metatarsalgia; and Glossary: Overpronation).

## Cause

Irritation of the interdigital nerve as it passes between the heads of the adjacent metatarsals, or a neuroma in this area, known as Morton's neuroma. It is most frequently caused by transverse compression from shoes that are too narrow. The swelling, caused by a metatarsalgia or callus from a stress fracture, will narrow the available space for the interdigital nerve and cause local compression.

## Investigations

X-ray for possible provoking causes, such as a healing callus from a fracture (see Fig. 16.1). MRI may be required for rare soft tissue lesions involving the nerve (Fig. 16.3). Experienced ultrasonographers may be able to detect a neuroma.

## Treatment

(a) Persuade the patient to buy wider and softer shoes.

(b) A metatarsal transverse arch orthotic, just proximal to the metatarsal heads, will lift and separate the heads, though a rise placed over the 4th and 5th metatarsal heads may be effective [2].

(c) Treat any other relevant causes.

(d) Perineural steroid injections seem to reduce any compressive oedema and may be curative.

(e) Surgery for an interdigital neuroma can be considered, but the neuroma tends to reform at the cut end (Morton's neuroma).

## Sports

Avoid impact sports. Cross-training (non-impact) is advised, such as in cycling, rowing or swimming – but the patient may have to pedal the cycle by using the arch of the foot rather than the ball, and may not be able to use a rowing machine because of pressure over the ball of the foot. When walking has become pain-free, jogging and then running may be attempted.

## Comment

Wider shoes and corrective orthotics are often curative, and if corrected early enough prevent a neuroma from forming. Locally placed orthopaedic felt, as a transverse arch elevator, can prove sufficient to widen the interdigital space in the early stages, as long as the narrow shoes that are causing the nerve irritation are changed. Surgical excision of a neuroma may lead to another reforming at the cut end, and I feel this should be undertaken only after all conservative measures have been tried.

## Hallux valgus

### Findings

Painless, but occasionally painful, valgus of the great toe. There will be accompanying findings from the problems that cause this lesion. When painful, all movements of the great toe hurt, and it usually is tender to palpation over the superficial medial aspect where the bursa is inflamed, and this may be red and swollen (the bunion).

### Cause

As part of an anatomical, first ray adductus valgus, or as a secondary effect to overpronation, especially with forefoot varus. The shoe may be too pointed, thus constricting the toes, and it may occur with Morton's toe (second toe longer than the first toe).

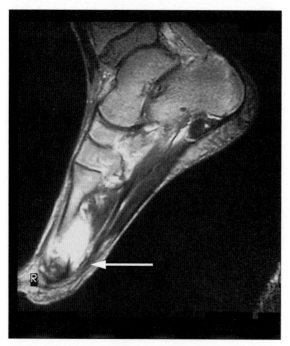

**Figure 16.3** • MRI scan shows an arteriovenous malformation that mimicked interdigital neuritis.

## Investigations

None are clinically required. X-ray can assess the metatarsophalangeal joint for osteoarthritis.

## Treatment

(a) Correction of overpronation. However, in the mobile foot with a forefoot varus, the first ray should be allowed to drop towards the ground. This is achieved by correcting only the hind foot and supporting the longitudinal arch. With a stiff, fixed first ray, correction of the varus deformity with a forefoot wedge in the orthotic is also required.

(b) Press out an area in the shoes to create room for bunions, and use softer, wider shoes.

(c) Gel or anti-blister preparations over the bursa will reduce friction.

(d) NSAIDs, if inflamed and sore.

(e) Electrotherapeutic modalities to settle inflammation, such as ultrasound and laser.

(f) Inject the bursa with cortisone.

(g) Surgery to correct the valgus deformity.

## Sports

(a) Overpronation problems in any sport may be relevant (see Glossary: Overpronation).

(b) Although ballet shoe blocks should hold onto the forefoot, rather than the toes themselves, stress often produces osteoarthritis and valgus deformity at the metatarsophalangeal joint.

## Comment

It is cheaper and less invasive to alter the shoes, rather than the foot, so that early correction of overpronation can be very successful, and may even be so in established problems. Conservative measures should be tried before surgery.

# Subungual haematoma

## Findings

Acute trauma to the toe leaves a throbbing, purplish, painful haematoma under the nail. In the chronic phase the nail is dark brown coloured and 'grows out', leaving normal nail near the base. The nail becomes thickened, ridged and detaches later, with the new nail growing underneath. Because of the differential diagnoses (see the caveat), a history of pain and trauma helps to establish this diagnosis.

## Cause

Driving the foot into the front of the shoe in 'stop–start' games, long-distance running (when perhaps downhill running may cause the problem), or direct trauma that causes bleeding under the toe nail.

## Investigations

None are clinically required, unless a subungual exostosis is suspected.

### Caveat

**Melanoma and subungual exostosis. The discoloration of the melanoma does not 'grow out'.**

## Treatment

Trepanation of the nail, in the acute case. A red hot needle or paper clip can be used to burn through the nail. This immediately releases the haematoma, which is under pressure, and produces instant pain relief. Observation of the chronic staining is required, just to confirm it is moving with the growing nail and is not a discoloration on the nail bed from a melanoma.

## Sports

Padding over the dorsum of the mid-foot allows the laces to be tied tighter, thus holding the foot firm, but leaving room for the toes to be moved and without impacting on the front of the shoe. The shoes should not cramp the toes.

## Comment

Immediate relief is obtained from trepanation, thus a sports medical bag should always contain a needle holder, paper clip and cigarette lighter. The paper clip end is heated to red hot and then a hole is burned in the nail to release the pressure of the blood underneath it.

# Turf toe

## Findings

Red, swollen great toe, often with a subungual haematoma, but there is also pain on all movements of the great toe, including abduction and adduction of the joint.

## Cause

Traumatic arthritis, or even fracture, of the great toe, from driving the foot into the front of the shoe. This particularly occurs on artificial surfaces where the increased friction between the studs and surface permits no slide, driving the toe into the front of the shoe.

## Investigations

X-ray to exclude a fracture. Gout should also be considered.

## Treatment

(a) Preventative. It is best to have 5–10 mm space between the toes and the inside of the shoe, but if the shoe needs to be snug then padding over the arch and forefoot, which enables the laces to be tightened and thus hold the foot firmly, will help.

(b) Inject the great toe joint with cortisone.

(c) Electrotherapeutic modalities to settle inflammation, such as ultrasound and laser.

(d) Splinting, if fractured – the shoe itself may act as a sufficient splint.

## Sports

All those played on artificial plastic surfaces are at risk, although water and sand filling have decreased the deceleration friction, allowing some slide and thus reducing the incidence of the injury.

## Comment

Although often mentioned in American literature, I have not often seen this problem, probably because the pitches are nowadays permitting some slide of the foot.

# Hallux limitus/rigidus

## Findings

Dorsiflexion of the first metatarsophalangeal joint is limited. It may be asymptomatic, but the symptomatic patients have pain, especially on tiptoe, and with running and change of direction sports. The pain, which is worse on dorsi- or plantar flexion of the big toe, is localized to the joint area, which is swollen and may be tender to palpation (see Hallux valgus).

## Cause

Osteoarthritis of the first metatarsophalangeal joint. There may be a congenital tendency. An overpronated foot may prevent full dorsiflexion of the toe.

> **Caveat**
>
> **Gout and sesamoiditis should be considered.**

## Investigations

None are required because there is usually some osteophytic lipping and early osteoarthritis present anyway. X-ray to assess the bony state if surgery is contemplated. Blood test for uric acid should be taken if gout is suspected.

## Treatment

(a) Avoid high heels, which promulgate extension of the toes.

(b) Correct any overpronation.

(c) Widen the shoes, and use a metatarsal bar or a kinetic wedge orthotic.

(d) If painful, use electrotherapeutic modalities, such as ultrasound and shortwave diathermy.

(e) Cortisone injection of the joint if it is inflamed.

(f) Surgery may be required.

## Sports

(a) Runners and joggers will have to shorten the stride length and lift off from the ball of the foot rather than the toe. Running around this problem may be achieved by externally rotating the foot, but this can produce secondary injuries such as overpronation, genu valgum and hallux valgus.

**(b)** The serve at tennis may require a 'jump' to avoid rolling through this joint.

**(c)** Dancers at the start of their career who have this problem should be filtered out, as this will certainly cause problems requiring surgery, which then will not take the stresses of dancing.

## Comment

Steroids are very successful to relieve pain, but alteration of movement patterns that affect the toe, orthotics and adjustment of shoes are vital before surgery is considered.

## Sesamoiditis: fractured sesamoids of the great toe

### Findings

Pain and tenderness over the sesamoids of the great toe, which are not made worse on passive adduction and abduction of the great toe, but may be worse on passive dorsiflexion and resisted plantar flexion of the toe. The forefoot may have increased varus, with functional pronation and an abducted hallux.

### Cause

From impact over the great toe joint, which may be severe enough to fracture a sesamoid.

### Investigations

X-rays should be taken, with specific views for the sesamoids. However, these are small corticated bones where soft tissue oedema and volar plate avulsions are displayed well by MRI, although CT may be required to delineate a fracture.

> **Caveat**
>
> Halluceal sesamoids may normally be uni-, bi-, tri- or quadripartite (Fig. 16.4). Rarely, avulsion of the volar plate, the deep attachment of the sesamoid within the tendon, may occur.

### Treatment

**(a)** Cross-train using non-impact sports, returning via the Achilles ladder (see Chapter 20).

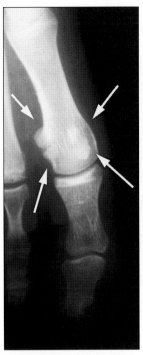

**Figure 16.4** • These sesamoids have not fractured but are quadripartite.

**(b)** Electrotherapeutic modalities to settle inflammation, such as ultrasound and laser. Steroids will ease pain but should not be used if a fracture or avulsion has occurred.

**(c)** Correct any overpronation with orthotics.

**(d)** Perhaps there is a place for surgery if a painful, non-union of a fracture occurs

### Sports

High-impact sports, such as repetition starts in track and field sprinters, lunge drills at badminton, and repetitive jumping/landing games.

### Comment

This is not common, and I personally have seen this condition only in sprinters, badminton players and Aussie rules football players playing on hard grounds (Fig. 16.5).

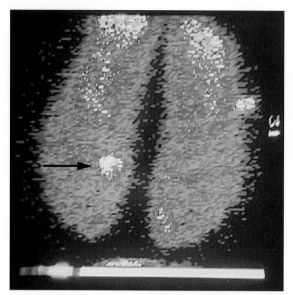

Figure 16.5 • The bone scan shows an increased signal from the sesamoid fracture or bone bruising. MRI and CT will differentiate further.

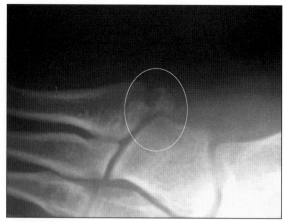

Figure 16.6 • An avulsion of the proximal apophysis of the fifth metatarsal.

## Fifth metatarsal enthesitis

### Findings

Acute traumatic or insidious onset of pain, localized to the proximal end of the fifth metatarsal, that is worse on walking, rough ground and resisted peroneal testing. It is locally tender over the proximal fifth metatarsal head.

### Cause

Apophysitis, enthesopathy or an avulsion fracture of the proximal end of the fifth metatarsal, from overuse of the peroneals.

### Investigations

X-ray of the foot for avulsion (Fig. 16.6) and to exclude Jones' fracture if the injury was traumatic (see Fracture of the proximal shaft of the fifth metatarsal).

### Treatment

(a) Rest from activities.
(b) Wear shoes at all times (except in bed) to act as a splint, or use a plastic walking boot.
(c) Perhaps a cast brace.

(d) Electrotherapeutic modalities to settle inflammation, such as ultrasound, laser and interferential. Cortisone for the enthesopathy, when no avulsion is present.
(e) Check for peroneal weakness, and rehabilitate when the pain permits.

### Sports

Rest from impact, and cross-train with non-impact activities, such as cycling, rowing and swimming. When walking is pain-free, reintroduce running via the Achilles ladder (see Chapter 20).

### Comment

This usually heals without resorting to cast bracing, and the apophysitis in the young is rare.

## Fracture of the proximal shaft of the fifth metatarsal (Jones' fracture)

(a) May present with a history of a sudden pop, or trauma to the fifth metatarsal, and be tender over the proximal metaphysis. These lesions are seen on X-ray and may represent an unfused apophysis, symptomatic sesamoid or non-union, and surgical management may involve shelling out a sequestrum or a compression screw. Take a surgical opinion [3].

**(b)** May involve a fracture across the proximal shaft and is prone to non-union – the Jones' fracture.

**(c)** Spiral fractures of the distal shaft occur in dancers, and may be displaced. They may be treated non-operatively or operatively [4].

## Sports

From discussions I have had with others in this field, it would seem that the injury is becoming increasingly common in professional soccer players but not in other sports. Theories suggest that the habit of soaking the boots before wearing them, so that the boot fits snugly, or wedges – as opposed to studs on the boots – that do not allow rotation of the foot, may be responsible. Certainly a stress lesion also occurs. Soccer players should be MRI scanned for this possibility. This fracture is prone to non-union, so there is a fine line in deciding between rest and surgical screwing of the early stress lesion.

## Oddities caused by the sports shoe

**(a)** *Logo pain.* Plastic logos on the shoes may not stretch as much as leather, so they sometimes cause localized, painful compression of the foot under this area.

**(b)** *Big toe nail.* Some athletes run with dorsiflexed toes, rubbing a hole in the shoe. They are often mid-foot strikers who are trying to firm up the foot for impact by using tibialis anterior and toe extensors to prevent overpronation. Encourage heel strike.

**(c)** *Plantar fascial pain near the arch.* Several insoles are manufactured with the arch support of the shoes rising up too near the heel; thus not matching the shape of the foot arch and causing rubbing of the foot.

**(d)** *Shoe heel tags.* May rub the Achilles causing a peritendinitis. Tags should be soft and easily pulled backwards. If not, cut the tags off, or slit down to the heel cups either side of the tags, but not so close together that the sides can close in again (see Glossary: Shoes).

**(e)** *High sides of the shoe.* These can rub under the maleolus, irritating the tendons of the peroneals or posterior tibialis.

**(f)** *High arch of the foot.* May be rubbed by the shoe lacing on the dorsum of the foot.

**(g)** *Tibialis anterior.* Tendons may be rubbed by too tight a shoe lacing.

**(h)** *Extensor hallucis.* May pull up into the shoe, causing rubbing. Pad either side of the tendon to direct pressure onto this area and away from the tendon.

**(i)** *Shoe nail or stud.* May rub through onto the foot. Unequal wear of the studs can alter the action of the shoe, usually encouraging overpronation.

 Caveat

**Gout, spondylarthropathies, Reiter's, rheumatoid and DISH (disseminated idiopathic skeletal hypertrophy).**

## References

1 Sproul J, Klaaren H, Mannarino F. Surgical treatment of Freiberg's infraction in athletes. Am J Sports Med 1993;21:381–384

2 Hirschberg GC. An effective treatment of Morton's neuralgia. J Orthop Med 1998;20(3):13–14

3 Rettig A, Shelbourne KD, Wilckens J. The surgical treatment of symptomatic non-unions of the proximal (metaphyseal) fifth metatarsal in athletes. Am J Sports Med 1992;20:50–54

4 O'Malley MJ, Hamilton WG, Munyak J. Fractures of the distal shaft of the fifth metatarsal. Dancer's fracture. Am J Sports Med 1996;24:240–243

### Further reading

Bruckner P, Khan K. Clinical sports medicine, 3rd edn. New York: McGraw-Hill; 2006

Hutson M, Ellis R (eds). Textbook of musculoskeletal medicine. Oxford: Oxford University Press; 2006

Reid D. Sports injury assessment and rehabilitation. Edinburgh: Churchill Livingstone; 1992

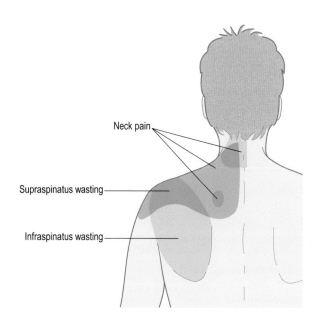

Neck pain

Supraspinatus wasting

Infraspinatus wasting

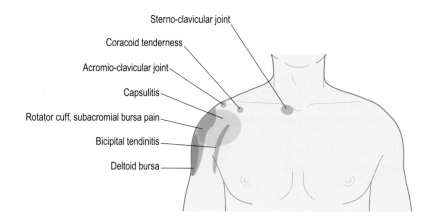

Sterno-clavicular joint

Coracoid tenderness

Acromio-clavicular joint

Capsulitis

Rotator cuff, subacromial bursa pain

Bicipital tendinitis

Deltoid bursa

# Chapter Seventeen

# 17

# Shoulder

## CHAPTER CONTENTS

## Introduction

Movement of the shoulder requires glenohumeral articulation to be coordinated with scapulothoracic movement, which maintains the alignment of the glenoid cavity with the humerus. This coordinated movement is known as scapulohumeral association. During this combined movement, the humeral head rises up in the glenoid to impinge on the inferior surface of the acromion. The elevation of the humeral head is prevented and controlled by the rotator cuff. Damage or malfunction of the rotator cuff allows the humeral head to rise, compressing the rotator cuff and the subacromial space. Thus, as the rotator cuff becomes increasingly damaged or irritated, a vicious cycle is produced. Treatment is directed at breaking this cycle.

Scapulothoracic movement rotates the acromion upwards and away from the humeral head, to avoid impingement, whilst the humeral head is applied to the glenoid, rather like a seal balancing a ball on its nose. The labrum acts almost like a sucker to maintain the close contact of the humeral head into the glenoid cavity. The plane of movement of the scapula is congruent with the posterior thoracic wall; that is, about 20° anterior to the coronal plane drawn between both shoulder joints. Thus movements posterior to this scapulothoracic plane (scaption) will inhibit scapular rotation and encourage impingement (Figs 17.1 and 17.2).

## Mechanical principles applied to management

The patient who has an anatomical or functional dorsal kyphosis will move the plane of scaption in an increased anterior direction. The arc of movement that now lies posterior to this plane has thus been increased, and the possibility of impingement increased. Correction of a

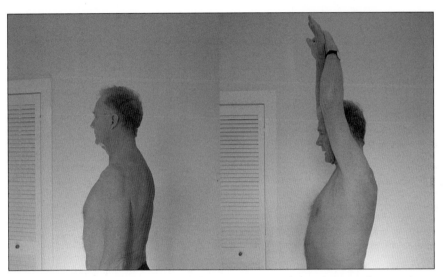

**Figure 17.1** • Circumduction can be completed in the coronal plane because the scapula can move congruently over the chest wall.

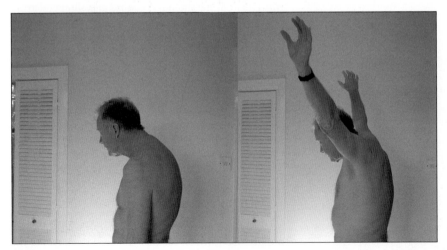

**Figure 17.2** • The anatomical or functional dorsal kyphosis, as shown here, alters the plane of scaption and inhibits scapular rotation in the coronal plane. This encourages subacromial impingment to result.

dorsal kyphosis will decrease the chance of impingement (see Figs 17.1 and 17.2). Equally, a patient who shrugs their shoulder will fix their scapula and limit the range of scapular rotation, causing impingement.

Retraction and external rotation of the shoulder will also be limited by the distance that the scapula can move over the thorax towards the spine. If retraction is increased beyond this limiting point then the posterior movement of the humeral head will be blocked by the scapula, and muscle power or an external force will lever the humeral head in an anterior direction. This movement is opposed by the rather weak anterior capsular ligaments, which, when they fail, will allow subluxation or dislocation of the shoulder.

## Sport

Many weight training exercises will, therefore, produce impingement, such as:

**(a)** wide-placed hands on a bench press, or lateral pull-downs, which limit scapular movement across the thorax

**(b)** too high an elbow position on pectoralis decks, which will cause impingement, and no posterior stop on the machine to prevent excess external rotation will stress the anterior capsule and produce subluxation of the joint.

Throwing and serving at tennis require scapulothoracic rotation first, to point the glenoid to the sky before humeral acceleration takes place. This can be seen in the 'set' position adopted by the tennis professionals just before they hit the serve. The movement is exaggerated by knee bends and lumbar extension (Figs 17.3 and 17.4).

Equally, muscle/tendon damage can occur from concentric overload, too much too soon, or from eccentric overload, decelerating the shoulder after the shot. A sudden block, or loss of resistance to these movements, may produce an acute tear. Rehabilitation requires the re-establishment of scapulohumeral association.

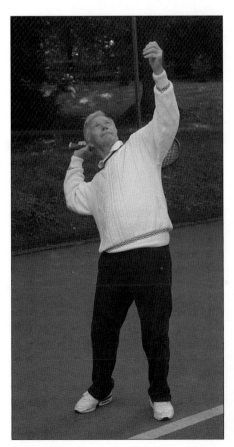

**Figure 17.3** • The scapula has been rotated to allow the shoulder to drop into the set position.

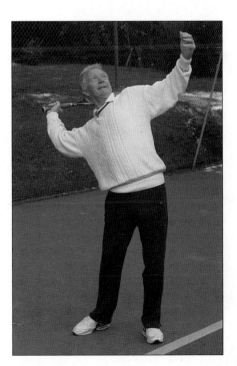

**Figure 17.4** • Scapular rotation has not occurred and this hitting position will cause subacromial impingement.

Trauma to the shoulder may damage the capsule and supporting ligaments and, when more severe, also the glenoid labrum and rotator cuff and cause bone bruising, in addition to straining the other 'shoulder' joints – the acromio- and the sternoclavicular. This instability of the pectoral girdle may be caused in racket and throwing sports by 'front-on' techniques (Figs 17.5 and 17.6). Here, the failure to rotate the upper body forces retraction of the whole pectoral girdle. Thus, this kinetic chain of closely interlinked movement patterns can easily develop secondary injuries that follow on from damage to one element. The disruption in this kinetic chain is referred to as glenohumeral or scapulo-humeral dissociation. Though treatment should be directed at the primary damage, or relief of pain, the injury will recur unless restoration of this normal kinetic function is achieved. It is possible that a fault in this mechanism is responsible for the stress fractures in the clavicle and scapula (Figs 17.7 and 17.8).

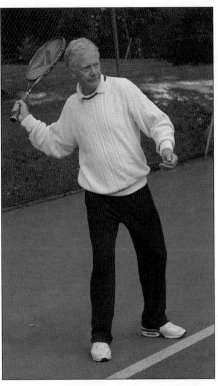

**Figure 17.6** • The player is front-on and has rotated the dorsal spine, which allows full shoulder movement and power to be delivered through the hips and torso.

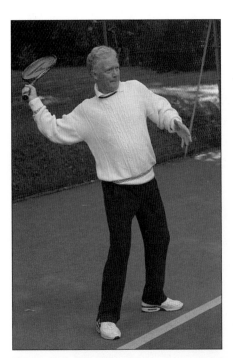

**Figure 17.5** • To achieve power, even more shoulder girdle retraction, as opposed to body rotation, is attempted and this severely stresses the whole pectoral girdle, particularly the anterior capsule, acromioclavicular and sternoclavicular joints. Either dorsal rotation or a side-on position must be used with the shot.

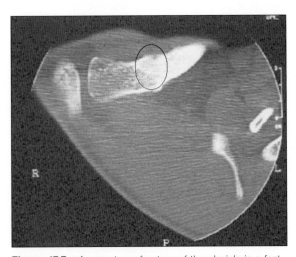

**Figure 17.7** • A rare stress fracture of the clavicle in a fast bowler at cricket. (Dr Philip Bell)

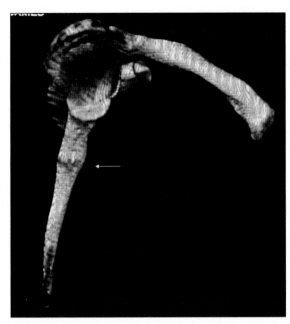

**Figure 17.8** • A rare stress fracture of the scapular in a cricket fast bowler. (Dr Philip Bell)

## Referred pain from the neck

Examinations of the shoulder must rule out referred pain from the neck, particularly from the C5/6 level (see Chapter 3).

## Acromioclavicular joint (shoulder separation)

### Findings

(a) May occur acutely with a fall, but can have a gradual onset.

(b) Classically, pain occurs with overhead work, but carrying heavy weights and lying on the shoulder induces pain that is centred over the acromioclavicular joint.

(c) The patient displays the 'point sign' when they point at the acromioclavicular joint as the site of pain (see Glossary: Point sign; Fig. 22.17).

(d) Referral of pain often radiates up the neck to the ear as well as down into the arm and elbow.

(e) It may hurt to lie prone, resting on the elbows, such as whilst reading a book.

(f) The acromioclavicular joint is the great mimic of the shoulder, so if the diagnostic signs are confusing then a trial injection of the acromioclavicular joint, followed by a review in 7–10 days, is a preferred policy.

(g) Classically, the joint is sore at the end of circumduction, worse on internal rotation and forced adduction across the body, with the shoulder at 90° of abduction.

(h) There is palpable tenderness over the acromioclavicular joint, which may appear swollen and displaced, with an obvious step.

### Cause

The injury is most commonly seen following a fall onto the tip of the shoulder, but it can occur whilst sleeping with the arm pulled across the body, from carrying heavy weights and during overhead work.

| | |
|---|---|
| Grade 1 | Swelling and bruising. No deformity. A tear of the superior ligament but the acromioclavicular joint is stable. |
| Grade 2 | A more extensive tear of the superior ligament, with increased mobility and some subluxation of the joint, but not more than half a shaft thickness. |
| Grade 3 | A tear of the conoid and trapezoid ligaments, with considerable deformity (more than half the shaft distance). There is increased instability of the joint, plus some tearing of the deltoid muscle from the clavicle. |
| Grades 4–6 | Display more severe disruption, with displacement, and are graded by the surgeons with a view to different interventional management plans. |

### Investigations

X-rays of the acromioclavicular joint – both when non-weight-bearing and when weight-bearing, for comparison. X-rays may show subluxation of the acromioclavicular joint, inferior osteophytes, or sclerosis and lysis from osteoarthritis (Fig. 17.9).

### Treatment

(a) Grades 1 and 2. Electrotherapeutic modalities to settle inflammation, such as ultrasound and laser to the ligament. An injection of the acromioclavicular joint with cortisone, especially

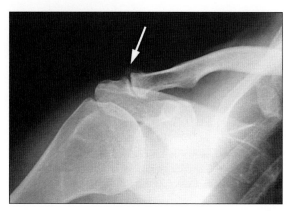

**Figure 17.9** • Superior osteophyte, with superior ligament calcification in the acromioclavicular joint.

for grade 2 lesions. Failure to improve from grades 1 and 2 may require surgical burring of osteophytes or excision of the distal end of the clavicle.

(b) Grade 3. The much larger deformed step, seen in grade 3, in fact causes fewer problems. Ultrasound and laser, and often an injection of hydrocortisone, may help. In the general population it rarely requires stabilization [1]. However, some authorities believe that these should all be repaired in sportspeople [2].

(c) Treatment may vary between the dominant and non-dominant shoulder, a more active approach being taken for the dominant. Rarely, surgical stabilization of the clavicle may be required in elite contact sports, even for the non-dominant arm.

(d) Grades 4–6 require definitive surgery.

 Caveat

Entrapment of the supraspinatus muscle by an inferior osteophyte of the acromioclavicular joint.
Conoid and trapezoid ligament strain.
Impingement of the short head of the biceps by the clavicle, and coracobrachialis origin strain.

## Sports

(a) Usually, there is no problem with 'below shoulder' sports, although carrying heavy weights may flare the acromioclavicular joint.

(b) It is flared by press-ups, overhead weights, overhead badminton shots, volleyball and serving at tennis. As the overhead shot is uncommon in squash, it is the racket game of preference for rehabilitation.

(c) A high take away technique, into adduction of the shoulder, in the backhand at tennis and squash may hurt if this is not accompanied by dorsal rotation.

(d) There can be a problem with contact sports, although many play without problems after the injury has settled [3]. Padding, anterior and posterior to the clavicle, to bring the point of contact away from the acromioclavicular joint may help.

## Comment

Most acromioclavicular joint lesions will be rapidly pain-free following a cortisone injection, and really only grade 1 improves with physiotherapy. Many patients live within the tolerance of the shoulder pain (which may be intermittent) by avoiding causative factors. If the supraspinatus is irritated by an inferior osteophyte then an injection of cortisone, placed behind and under the acromioclavicular joint, may produce relief.

## Subacromial bursitis/inflammation

Inflammation of the subacromial space and/or bursa can exist alone, but it is often accompanied by a rotator cuff injury and scapulohumeral dissociation. Please read the Introduction above.

## Findings

(a) The injury often follows overarm activity, such as throwing, hedge cutting or painting the ceiling, though a fall onto the hand or elbow that drives the humerus up vertically into the acromion is also a common cause.

(b) There is pain from lying on the shoulder, doing one's hair, putting on a coat, driving (hand over the top of the wheel) and reaching into the back seat.

(c) The patient indicates the deltoid area and below as being painful; sometimes the presentation of pain will be over the lateral epicondyle of the elbow, so it can be confused with a tennis elbow. Local anaesthetic into the subacromial space should resolve the diagnostic dilemma.

(d) There may be a painful arc between 80° and 120° (but often only at 180°) with active and passive circumduction, depending on whether the patient shrugs his or her shoulder or not during the test.

(e) Passive and active circumduction may be pain-free, but resisted circumduction at 90° will hurt as the deltoid lifts the humerus into the subacromial space.

(f) Resisted rotator cuff isometrics are pain-free.

(g) The impingement signs are positive (see Glossary).

(h) There may only be a history of not being able to throw, with no positive clinical signs.

## Cause

Compression of the subacromial space between the humeral head and the acromion produces inflammation of the space. This usually occurs because arm elevation is produced at the glenohumeral joint without any accompanying scapulothoracic rotation (see Introduction), but the shape of the acromion may make impingement more likely.

## Investigations

None are clinically required unless failing to respond to treatment. X-ray will assess the shape of the acromion. Ultrasound and MRI can show a subacromial bursitis and rotator cuff damage. The MRI can display labral damage.

## Treatment

Inject the subacromial space with cortisone and local anaesthetic, and at the same time correct any faulty technique to resolve scapulohumeral dissociation and strengthen the rotator cuff.

## Sports

(a) Golf – right shoulder. Correct the flying elbow and too flat a plane of swing (Figs 17.10 and 17.11).

(b) Racket sports – correct the flying elbow (Figs 17.12 and 17.13).

(c) Squash – correct the 'chest front-on position' for the forehand high volley by improving upper body rotation (see a coach).

(d) Throwing – damage is caused by not enough scapulothoracic rotation and upper body turn;

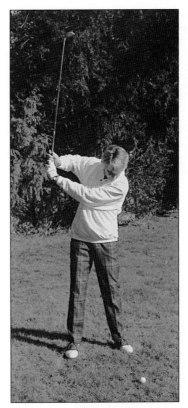

**Figure 17.10** • The 'flying' right elbow at golf.

throw side to underarm whilst troublesome. The player can often bowl at cricket but not throw overarm.

(e) Swim – freestyle. Not pulling far enough back to allow scapulothoracic rotation before the recovery stroke. Too low a position of the elbow during the recovery stroke.

(f) Tennis (serve) – hitting before the 'set' position is obtained so that scapulothoracic rotation has not been achieved (see Fig. 17.4). The patient should try taking the racket directly back to the 'set' position (see Fig. 17.3) by rotating the thorax, with a flexed shoulder that is not externally rotated.

(g) Archery – the draw elbow is taken too high, with the final movement being external rotation of the humerus rather than scapular retraction.

(h) Running – tight shoulders, arms held across the body whilst running with high elbows.

(i) Weights – too wide a grip on the weights bar and working the lifts behind the scapulothoracic

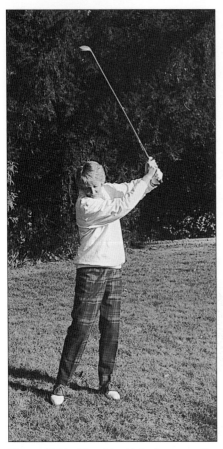

**Figure 17.11** • The 'flying' left elbow at golf.

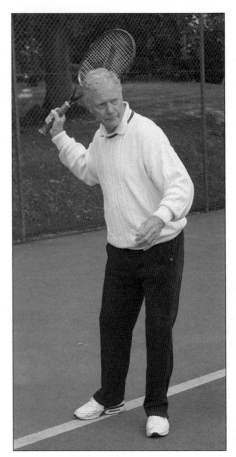

**Figure 17.12** • The normal forehand.

plane (see Introduction), especially with deltoid exercises, does not permit the scapula to rotate fully. Narrowing the grip on the bench press bar will allow the scapulae to rotate further and corrects the problem. 'Flies' and 'pec decks' are worked too close to, or above, the horizontal plane and cause impingement. These exercises should be worked below the horizontal plane.

## Comment

I have used the term subacromial space rather than subacromial bursa as radiology colleagues suggest that ultrasound guidance is required to inject the bursa. Some subacromial bursae are inflamed enough for fluid to be aspirated without ultrasound guidance. For more than 30 years, those patients of mine who have required injections under the acromion without ultrasound-guided techniques have uniformly got better. This sug-

gests that one has injected the bursa, or most likely that injection of the subacromial space is sufficient to settle inflammation in this area. Although physiotherapists treat this injury, I feel the space is best treated with cortisone as an anti-inflammatory. Physiotherapy modalities do not reach the subacromial space in its protected position between the bones. Physiotherapy to the rotator cuff and/or correction of the scapulohumeral dissociation can and should then follow immediately the vicious cycle is broken (see Introduction).

## Subdeltoid bursitis

### Findings

Gradual development of pain over the inferior deltoid area, with pain on active circumduction, but resisted rotator cuff isometrics are pain-free and the impinge-

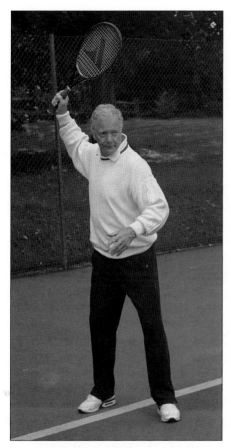

**Figure 17.13** • The flying elbow at tennis.

ment signs are negative. Resisted deltoid action is painful, but at 90° this may stress the subacromial space.

## Cause

Inflammation of the subdeltoid bursa, which may be an extension of the subacromial bursa under the deltoid. It is unusual for the subdeltoid bursa to present as a separate entity.

## Treatment

Treat the subacromial space first, and if this fails then try electrotherapeutic modalities to settle inflammation, such as ultrasound, interferential and laser. Massage techniques such as frictions to prevent intrabursal adhesions can help, as can a locally placed injection of hydrocortisone (under ultrasound guidance) to the subdeltoid bursa.

> ### Caveat
>
> Beware of attrition to the circumflex humeral nerve.

## Sports

(a) Usually, internal and external rotation of the shoulder in the circumducted position, such as a 'front-on' tennis service that is hit wide out from the shoulder.

(b) Carrying or supporting the partner with the elbow at 45–90° circumduction, as can occur whilst dancing and skating.

## Comment

Pain on release of the resisted deltoid may be a subacromial space problem, as this test allows the humeral head to elevate and cause impingement. Generally treat the subacromial space first.

## Rotator cuff injuries

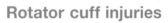

### Findings

(a) Though a fall onto the hand or elbow can cause acute impingement, an acute episode of pain during activity that is followed by weakness suggests a rupture.

(b) Gradual onset of pain referred to the deltoid area, although there may be referral to the elbow or the forearm, and the lesion may be misdiagnosed as a tennis elbow.

(c) Pain, particularly with the elbow elevated above the shoulder, such as when drying hair or reaching forwards or backwards.

(d) Reaching behind the back, towards the dorsal spine.

(e) Acute shoulder pain, getting worse over 4–5 days, suggests the possibility of calcific tendinitis (see below).

(f) The patient indicates the top of arm and deltoid as being where the pain is localized.

(g) There is a painful arc on active movements, and especially on eccentric movement, although passive movement is pain-free (technically) [4] (see Glossary: Drop tests).

**(h)** Pain on resisted internal rotation suggests the subscapularis is involved, whereas pain with resisted external rotation suggests the infraspinatus and, with abduction, the supraspinatus [4]. These may be either weak and/or painful. However, note that the eccentric stabilizing effects of the other rotator cuff muscles (which are technically not involved in the test) may produce pain so that the infraspinatus, acting to stabilize the shoulder, may produce some discomfort on resisted internal rotation.

**(i)** Localized tenderness. Subscapularis anteriorly, supraspinatus over the greater tuberosity; the palpation being made easier with the arm in internal rotation. Infraspinatus – lying prone and leaning on the elbows, as in reading a book, when the posterior humeral head is more tender to palpation than the unaffected shoulder.

**(j)** The impingement signs are invariably positive (see Glossary).

## Cause

Damage to subscapularis, supraspinatus or infraspinatus. Clinically, teres major and minor, which are part of the rotator cuff complex, have not had the signs and symptoms of their injuries well defined. The rotator cuff stabilizes the shoulder and decelerates the shoulder movements to prevent the arm following the ball in a throw. The injury may be a tear, often during eccentric movements, or tendon degeneration from compression of the rotator cuff between the humeral head and acromion causing localized avascularization. The lesion is thus more common in the older person. The other actions of the rotator cuff are to depress and stabilize the humeral head away from the acromion. Rotator cuff damage, therefore, will allow elevation of the humerus, which impinges on the acromion, which inflames the rotator cuff, setting up the vicious cycle as mentioned in the Introduction.

### Caveat

C5/6 neck injury and the acromioclavicular joint, with an inferior osteophyte pressing on the supraspinatus muscle.

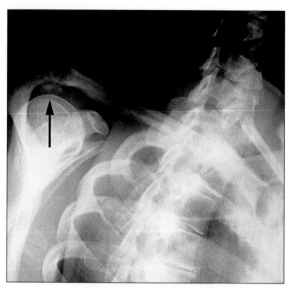

**Figure 17.14** • Calcific tendinitis in the rotator cuff.

## Investigations

**(a)** None are clinically required unless there is failure to progress.

**(b)** Real-time ultrasound can show rotator cuff tears and calcification and is the preferred first-line investigation.

**(c)** X-ray, looking for calcific tendinitis (Fig. 17.14) and, if impingement is a major problem and surgery is being considered, to assess acromial angulation.

**(d)** MRI scan may show supraspinatus degeneration or a localized tear (Fig. 17.15). These are less easy to see in the infraspinatus and subscapularis, which may only show on dynamic views. Dynamic views will particularly display subscapular impingement between the coracoid and humeral head. The MRI may display labral lesions.

## Treatment

**(a)** Treatment is designed to break the vicious cycle, where an injection of the subacromial space calms the inflammation, decreases the pain and allows the rotator cuff to work, even if in a weakened state. A functioning rotator cuff can prevent humeral elevation and the subsequent impingement, which, once again, would irritate and inflame the rotator cuff.

**(b)** Electrotherapeutic modalities to settle

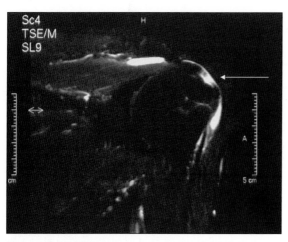

**Figure 17.15** • MRI shows a ruptured supraspinatus (*arrow*) with subacromial space inflammation.

inflammation, such as ultrasound, laser and interferential.

(c) Massage techniques to control and organize scar tissue.

(d) Local injection of cortisone, under ultrasound guidance, into the area of calcific tendinitis. This can be performed successfully without ultrasound guidance by injecting the area that is acutely tender to palpation.

(e) Proprioceptive strapping, to encourage scapular rotation and prevent shoulder elevation during circumduction, i.e. improving scapulohumeral dissociation. The strapping pulls on the skin and this sensation informs the patient of any aberrant movement, such as shrugging.

(f) Isometrics for the rotator cuff.

(g) Isotonics or isokinetics for the rotator cuff.

(h) Throwing, hitting rehabilitation (see ladders, Chapter 20).

(i) Operation to repair any rotator cuff tear. This may be accompanied by debridement of adhesions and debridement of the inferior surface of the acromion, the coracoacromial ligament or the acromioclavicular joint to create more space for the rotator cuff, especially if a mal-shaped acromion is present.

## Sports

(a) Golf – an arm take away with no shoulder rotation injures the left shoulder, particularly the infraspinatus and supraspinatus. The right arm taken flat, but with a flying elbow, compresses the infraspinatus at the posterior aspect of the shoulder.

(b) Tennis – hitting too soon on the serve before the scapulothoracic 'set' position is obtained. This problem is often accompanied by inflammation of the subacromial space (see Fig. 17.4).

(c) All throwing events – if too much power is used, too soon, then the muscles of the rotator cuff may be torn or strained. Many people train their legs to run or kick, but few train their shoulders with graduated exercises, in the off season, to build sufficient strength in the decelerators and stabilizers of the shoulder – the rotator cuff.

## Comment

Although there may be a local area that is tender to palpation, my first treatment is an injection of the subacromial space to break the vicious cycle (see Introduction). This usually settles the pain to a level where physiotherapy and rehabilitation to the rotator cuff muscles may be initiated. Persistent discomfort may require local infiltration, and resistant problems often resolve when the infraspinatus is injected. Some authors suggest three injections and then surgery, but many patients do not want the latter. If only resisted rotator cuff testing is painful then rehabilitation is required. If the impingement signs become positive again during a course of rehabilitation, repeat the cortisone injection to the subacromial space because the still weak rotator cuff has allowed impingement and inflammation of the subacromial space to recur, and the vicious cycle has restarted. Analyse the reasons for giving steroid injections, which have only an anti-inflammatory effect. They do not heal damaged tissue, which requires rehabilitation or suturing. Sometimes the inflammation around the damaged tissue prevents rehabilitation, and this is the justification for administering cortisone. So why three injections, as many authors advocate? One may be more than enough if inflammation is not the problem, and more than three is acceptable if inflammation recurs during rehabilitation. Failure to progress through rehabilitation, or recurrent inflammation of the subacromial space in spite of rest, requires arthroscopic surgery to the space or the rotator cuff, depending upon the findings. Proprioceptive strapping that informs the patient when they are shrugging is very helpful for rehabilitation.

# Calcific tendinitis

## Findings

This may present as a chronic lesion found in a rotator cuff injury that is not settling. Acute calcific tendinitis presents with excruciating pain, which may develop and get worse over 4–5 days. There may be localized swelling and there is always marked tenderness on palpation over the damaged area. The patient does not want to move the arm, and all movements of the shoulder hurt. Resisted movements are painful and non-diagnostic vis-à-vis which muscle is involved (see Rotator cuff injuries).

## Cause

Calcium hydroxyapatite has been deposited in the rotator cuff tendon. This may be found incidentally and be pain-free, or form acutely, producing excruciating pain.

## Investigations

The acute presentation should have an immediate X-ray or ultrasound to confirm the diagnosis; however, if they are not available, the acute localized tender area is indicative. If a shoulder is not progressing with standard treatment and rehabilitation, X-ray or ultrasound should be used (see Fig. 17.14).

## Treatment

(a) Acute. There is excruciating pain on any movement, so a sling and strong analgesia should be prescribed. Cortisone and local anaesthetic may be given, under ultrasound guidance as an intralesional injection or into the local area most tender to palpation. One injection may be curative but the underlying precipitative cause must be treated and rehabilitated.

(b) Chronic. If this is an incidental finding, with no pain, then leave alone. Local friction makes this worse. When painful, intralesional injections of cortisone and local anaesthetic may be curative. If there is recurrent pain then repeat needling of the calcified area and injection with local anaesthetic may release the calcium. Continued pain from the calcified area should be treated with lithotripsy or surgical debridement.

## Sports

These lesions are seen particularly from implemental games, which require shoulder power, or from throwing. Rest from these activities is required in the acute phase. Checks for scapulohumeral dissociation and re-education of this movement are required, perhaps with a proprioceptive taping to prevent shrugging.

## Comment

The finding of calcium by itself does not warrant treatment, which is required only in the painful phase. Acute calcific tendinitis reveals itself by the acute presentation, the intensity of pain description and the painful immobility of the shoulder. This responds well to cortisone injection, but does need resting in a sling and strong analgesia for 48 hours.

# Bicipital tendinosis/tenosynovitis

## Findings

(a) Acute pain with resisted testing or a history of overloaded biceps. There is gradual onset of pain, either referred to the shoulder or down the belly of the biceps muscles.

(b) Passive shoulder internal and external rotation is pain-free.

(c) Circumduction may have a painful arc, but the rotator cuff isometrics are pain-free.

(d) The impingement signs may be positive (see Glossary).

(e) It is differentiated from subacromial space inflammation by positive resisted biceps tests (Yergason's and Speed's; see Glossary).

## Cause

There is attritional degeneration or a partial tear of the tendon, owing to acute resistance of biceps contraction or eccentric overload. Damage is probably created in the bicipital groove, where some impingement on the acromion may contribute to the injury. This lesion is probably overdiagnosed. There may be a partial degenerative tear, with subsequent synovial inflammation and adhesions binding down the tendon, which cause the pain (see Ruptured long head of biceps).

## Investigations

None are clinically required unless the lesion is failing to progress, but diagnostic ultrasound will show synovitis and a partial tear of the tendon very clearly, such that an MRI scan is really not required unless a superior labrum, anterior and posterior (SLAP) lesion is considered.

## Treatment

(a) Electrotherapeutic modalities to settle inflammation of the sheath, such as ultrasound and laser.

(b) Massage techniques to control adhesions, such as frictional massage to the tendon sheath.

(c) Injection with cortisone of the sheath within the bicipital groove.

(d) Isometrics, progressing to dynamic exercises and heavier weights.

(e) Extension and external rotation shoulder stretches, plus extension of the shoulder with pronation of the forearm.

### Caveat

The lesion may well be a partial tear whose integrity is maintained by the adhesions that cause the pain. Local cortisone frees the adhesion and relieves the pain, but exposes the tendon to pain-free loading, which can produce a rupture. Some surgeons in the past have severed the tendon to treat the lesion, relieving the pain, and then treated it in the same way as a ruptured biceps. Patients should be warned of the possible consequence of injection, which may cure the pain but permit a rupture, this having the same curative effect as surgery (see Ruptured long head of biceps).

## Sports

Mainly occurs in those requiring bicipital strength, often weightlifting. Check for anabolic steroid abuse.

## Comment

This diagnosis is often quoted, but any tendon lesion should have pain on resisted biceps testing, which in practice rarely occurs with shoulder pain. It therefore seems to be an overdiagnosed lesion and I believe it is rarer than quoted. The treatment of the subacromial space is preferable when there is no pain on resisted biceps testing. Local bicipital groove or tender point injection should be reserved for the patient with positive resisted pain on biceps testing, or a positive diagnostic ultrasound scan. Sometimes bicipital tendinitis/osis will not heal until the rupture occurs and then it heals to a functional norm, hence the surgical division of the long head of biceps that was utilized in the past.

# Ruptured long head of biceps

## Findings

Bruising over the biceps muscle, with a 'Popeye' shape to the long head of the biceps muscle. Bicipital function is intact but in the early stages may be weaker and painful, although it rapidly becomes pain free. Resisted biceps testing, Speed's and Yergason's tests are painful (see Glossary).

## Cause

Acute, blocked resistance of a bicipital contraction or the end point of chronic bicipital tendinosis. Indeed, chronic bicipital tenosynovitis may not settle until a rupture has occurred, either traumatically or surgically (see Bicipital tendinosis/tenosynovitis).

## Investigations

None are clinically required when a 'Popeye' deformity is visible. Real-time ultrasound confirms the diagnosis. MRI is expensive and not normally required, but should be performed if an associated rotator cuff tear is suspected.

## Treatment

(a) RICE in the acute stage.

(b) Electrotherapeutic modalities, such as ultrasound, laser and interferential to settle inflammation and remove tissue debris.

(c) Massage techniques to remove tissue debris and organize scar tissue.

(d) Allow the long head of biceps to reattach itself, by adhesions, lower down the humerus, but maintain normal elbow movements and add controlled, isometric resistance exercises to the biceps.

(e) Full extension of the elbow must also be maintained, and later full extension of the shoulder, with a pronated forearm.

(f) Add isotonic and isokinetic exercises, to pain onset (see Chapter 20: General muscle ladder).

## Sports

Weight trainers and power lifters should be questioned about anabolic steroid abuse. Biceps curls, preacher curls, upright rowing, rowing machine, etc., may all have to be rehabilitated up to pain onset (see Treatment (f), above).

## Comment

Normal function can return without treatment. I have seen a Commonwealth weightlifting gold medal won by an athlete with a conservatively managed, reattached, long head of biceps.

# Supraspinatus impingement at the acromioclavicular joint

## Findings

Similar to the acromioclavicular joint, but resisted or active movement of the supraspinatus produces pain so that the symptoms may reflect acromioclavicular and/or supraspinatus injury. Tenderness can be just posterior to, rather than on, the acromioclavicular joint, and it may produce actual disuse wasting of the supraspinatus, as well as pain-induced weakness. An X-ray may show an inferior osteophyte from the acromioclavicular joint (see Acromioclavicular joint, Supraspinatus weakness).

## Cause

Impingement of the supraspinatus muscle as it passes beneath the acromioclavicular joint, usually from an osteophyte.

## Treatment

An injection of cortisone is placed behind and beneath the acromioclavicular joint onto the muscle fascia as it passes beneath the joint. An inferior osteophyte, if present, may require surgery.

## Sports

As for the acromioclavicular joint, supraspinatus weakness and rotator cuff injuries (see this chapter).

## Comment

Not common. The patient often indicates that the pain is just behind the acromioclavicular joint; it can do well with conservative treatment, but recurrence is best treated surgically.

# Supraspinatus weakness

## Findings

Weakness and incoordination on active circumduction, and weakness on resisted abduction of the shoulder:

Type 1   As for rotator cuff with a supraspinatus tear.
Type 2   An amyotrophy.
Type 3   Gradual onset of muscle weakness and incoordination, commonly in racket players, with some diffuse shoulder, neck and arm pain. Examination shows both weak and wasted supraspinatus and infraspinatus. Normal passive glenohumeral movements are present, but there may be some discomfort on side flexion of the neck to the opposite side.

## Cause

Type 1   Rotator cuff damage (see Rotator cuff injuries and Supraspinatus impingement at the acromioclavicular joint).
Type 2   Amyotrophy (see Infraspinatus weakness).
Type 3   Damage to the suprascapular nerve as it passes through the suprascapular notch.

## Investigations

See Infraspinatus weakness.

## Treatment

Type 1   See Rotator cuff injuries and Supraspinatus impingement at the acromioclavicular joint.
Type 2   Treat with analgesia in the painful initial stages. Attempt rehabilitation of the muscle as far as possible, when the inflammatory stage has settled down.
Type 3   Surgical release of the nerve at the suprascapular notch followed by appropriate rehabilitation of the shoulder muscles, but see in conjunction with Infraspinatus weakness.

## Sports

Type 1   See Rotator cuff injuries.
Type 2   The patient avoids sport during the painful stage; later, shoulder rehabilitation to its optimum is required.

Type 3   This is seen particularly in racket sports and volleyball. After surgery, type 3 may be rehabilitated back to these sports, but see infraspinatus weakness. If there has been nerve damage then this will take time to regenerate. Do not introduce shot making with a racket too soon, before the rotator cuff strength has returned, otherwise subacromial problems will occur.

## Comment

Damage at the suprascapular notch will affect the nerve supply to both the supraspinatus and the infraspinatus, whereas damage at the spinoglenoid notch affects only the infraspinatus. Not a common lesion, but release of the nerve may help.

## Infraspinatus weakness

### Findings

Type 1   Residual weakness following a rotator cuff tear.
Type 2   Amyotrophy with localized pain and tenderness in the muscle, and a weakness that improves with time.
Type 3   Suprascapular nerve damage, often presenting as gradual weakness and incoordination of the racket or ball control, rather than poorly localized shoulder and arm pain. There is invariably a wasted, weak infraspinatus muscle at presentation.

There are no accompanying glenohumeral signs and surprisingly little functional deficit. There are no abnormal neck signs, although side flexion to the opposite side may provoke some discomfort.

### Cause

Type 1   Rotator cuff damage (see Rotator cuff injuries).
Type 2   Amyotrophy – probably a localized viral neuromyositis.
Type 3   Damage to the suprascapular nerve as it passes around the scapular spine at the spinoglenoid notch, usually in a racket or volleyball player but occasionally with weight training, either because of a traction neuropathy or a cyst compressing the nerve. If the supraspinatus is weak as well, the damage is at the suprascapular notch and not the spinoglenoid notch (see Supraspinatus weakness).

### Investigations

(a) MRI, and perhaps ultrasound, may show a cyst at the spinoglenoid notch that is compressing the infraspinatus branch of the suprascapular nerve.
(b) EMG may show localized denervation or evidence of an amyotrophy.

### Treatment

Type 1   See Rotator cuff injuries.
Type 2   Analgesia for the amyotrophy. Maintain normal activities as far as possible.
Type 3   Surgical release of the nerve if there is a cyst. Increasing the notch size to reduce tension on the nerve seems to help any pain but does not regenerate muscle bulk [5]. This should be followed by appropriate rehabilitation.

### Sports

Outside a ruptured rotator cuff, the gradual onset of infraspinatus weakness is almost entirely a racket or volleyball sport injury. The serve in volleyball may be part of the problem [5]. Release of the nerve entrapment allows rehabilitation and return to sports, but increasing the notch size to reduce traction on the nerve does not seem to alter muscle bulk and function.

### Comment

Neither an amyotrophy nor localized nerve damage are common; however, as one gets better and the other is treatable if there is a cyst present, the clinical diagnosis of the cause should be established and appropriate investigations instituted.

## Dislocations of the shoulder

These fall into two types. One is atraumatic, multidirectional and usually bilateral, and occurs in patients with high ligament laxity scores. Multidirectional, atraumatic instability requires rehabilitation and does badly with surgery. The other is traumatic, unidirectional and can respond well to surgical stabilization.

# Anterior dislocation

## Findings

There is a history of trauma, which has forced the arm into external rotation and abduction. There is pain and an inability to move the arm away from the side. The shoulder appears squared off, with a hollow below the acromion.

## Cause

Trauma to the shoulder, which has caused the humeral head to dislocate anteriorly and inferiorly.

## Investigations

X-ray to exclude a fracture and a Bankart lesion (Fig. 17.16; see Glossary). MRI scan is not required in the initial stages, but if progress is not being maintained then a possible labral tear should be suspected.

## Treatment

(a) Relocation of the humerus, preferably after an X-ray to exclude any humeral fracture.

(b) For 3–4 weeks, support the arm in a sling, in internal rotation, and start isometrics to the rotator cuff.

(c) Maintain hand movements to prevent swelling from a shoulder–hand syndrome and dependent oedema.

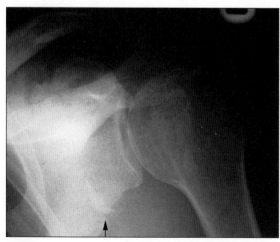

**Figure 17.16** • A Bankart lesion – avulsion of the inferior glenoid margin. (Mr. Basil Helal)

(d) After 3–4 weeks, regain the range of movement, continue isometrics, add isotonics, and then gradually introduce throwing over a short distance to encourage concentric and eccentric muscle activity.

(e) Avoid external rotation in abduction until all subluxation tests are negative (see Glossary: Anterior apprehension test of the shoulder and Relocation test/Jobe's test).

(f) Surgery, if a Bankart lesion or a labral tear is present.

## Sports

See Subluxing shoulder.

### Caveat

A patch of numbness over the deltoid equals damage to the axillary nerve. Swelling in the hand and fingers and loss of pulse equals damage to the artery and axillary plexus, and a fractured humerus is likely to have occurred.

## Comment

Although many surgeons await further dislocation, the young seem to be destined for recurrence and an arthroscopy may reveal a labrum that can be repaired. Hence the dominant shoulder in the young should be considered for repair; the non-dominant may be treated conservatively. One must remember that the young do change their sporting activities as they get older, often giving up the causative sport, and this must influence decision-making for or against surgery.

# Recurrent dislocation

## Findings

There is a previous history of dislocation. The arm jumps out and may be relocated by the patient with a trick move. The arm may be relocated easily or have relocated itself. Apprehension and relocation tests are positive (see Glossary: Anterior apprehension test and Relocation test/Jobe's test).

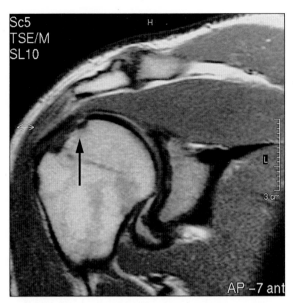

**Figure 17.17** • Hill–Sachs lesion from recurrent trauma between the head of the humerus and the acromion.

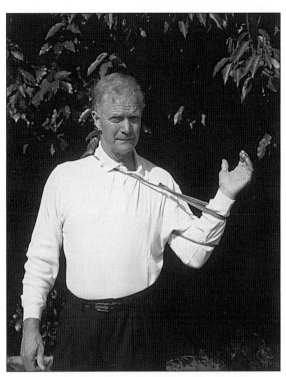

**Figure 17.18** • The non-dominant arm may be strapped to prevent subluxation. The strap circles the forearm and travels behind the shoulder and around the neck to the wrist. If the wrist flies wide, the elbow is pulled downwards. If the elbow flies wide, the wrist is pulled in towards the body. Both mechanisms prevent the dislocation position being reached. I personally won many club veteran squash matches strapped like this.

## Cause

As for anterior dislocation, but when the externally rotated and abducted arm is forced beyond the range of the anterior capsule the arm may dislocate anteriorly and inferiorly, often without pain. There is usually a labral or bony glenoid deficiency.

## Investigations

X-ray to look for a Bankart lesion (see Fig. 17.16) and/or Hill–Sachs (hatchet) lesion (Fig. 17.17) (see Glossary). MRI will show the labral tear and Hill–Sachs lesions, which are more insipient than those that can be visualized on X-ray.

## Treatment

(a) Dominant arm. Withdraw from precipitating events until the shoulder is stabilized surgically. There are several types of repair, and these may vary according to the severity of the pathology.

(b) Non-dominant arm. Avoid the dislocate position and try a restraining strap whilst playing racket sports, until stable (Fig. 17.18). However, if on X-ray or MRI, a Bankart's, labral tear, or Hill–Sachs lesion is present, it will require surgery.

## Sports

See Subluxing shoulder.

## Comment

Surgical stabilization of the dominant arm is invariably required in throwing and hitting sports, and of either arm in rugby players, unless the athlete gives up these sports. Before deciding on a treatment policy for a patient, one must remember that many athletes change or give up their sport as they grow older, and time without a recurrence will allow the capsule to tighten and stabilize the glenohumeral joint.

# Subluxing shoulder

## Findings

(a) The shoulder may jump and catch with some movements.

(b) The patient may talk of a 'dead arm', which may produce 'pins and needles' whilst throwing or hitting.

(c) There can be capsular or rotator cuff signs because of the recurrent stresses, but often a full range of shoulder movement is present. The rotator cuff may be weak, or weak and painful.

(d) Anterior apprehension test is positive (see Glossary).

(e) Relocation test is positive (see Glossary).

(f) With multidirectional instability, where there is a high Beighton–Horan score the sulcus sign is positive for inferior instability, and anterior and posterior draw are increased (see Glossary).

(g) Usually bilateral findings of instability.

## Cause

(a) Previous dislocation.

(b) Hypermobility with congenital ligamentous laxity.

(c) Atraumatic repetitive stretching of the anterior capsule, as in throwing, bowling or serving at tennis.

(d) Weak rotator cuff muscles.

## Investigations

X-ray to exclude Bankart's and Hill–Sachs lesions (see Figs 17.16 and 17.17). With a history of previous trauma consider a MRI scan, which will show any labral deficiency.

## Treatment

(a) Non-dominant unidirectional – rehabilitation of rotator cuff muscles and a shoulder strap restraint (see Fig. 17.18).

(b) Dominant unidirectional – surgery and avoidance of causative mechanisms.

(c) Multidirectional (dominant and non-dominant) – muscle rehabilitation of the rotator cuff and large shoulder muscles, plus reinforcement of scapulohumeral association.

(d) Restriction of activity to avoid subluxing the humerus.

## Sports

(a) All overarm throwing or hitting activities are at risk, but the patient may get away with side arm throwing.

(b) The non-dominant arm can be at risk when it abducts and rotates to check or stop a spin, as in skating or when turning suddenly to chase a ball.

(c) Rugby – diving with the arms outstretched to touch down, the 'fall backwards' tackle with the tackle arm externally rotated and abducted, and propping and hooking in the scrum are all at risk.

(d) Swimming – diving in, butterfly and freestyle are at risk, backstroke particularly. Encourage a high elbow clearance and reduce the length of pull backwards for freestyle until the shoulder is more stable.

(e) Weightlifting – the pectoralis deck (pec deck) may cause a problem when it is used with the elbows level with or above the shoulders, and if there is no stop to prevent the shoulder being forced backwards too far into external rotation, especially when fatigue sets in. There should always be a limiting stop, level with the coronal plane of the shoulders, and the elbows should be held below shoulder tip level.

## Comment

Athletes who present with a strange feeling or popping in the shoulder often do have subluxing shoulders. Proper rest and avoidance of the activity, plus shoulder rehabilitation, is essential. It may mean 2–3 years away from the causative activity. Hypermobility and a high Beighton–Horan score will always cause trouble, and the patient should find another sport!

# Posterior dislocation

## Findings

There is loss of the normal rounded appearance and a limitation of external rotation. The shoulder should be viewed superiorly, and when palpated the humeral head will be noted to lie posteriorly to the acromion. Atraumatic subluxation/dislocation may have a recurrent popping and sliding of the shoulder, without pain, and the patient may be able to perform 'the dislocate' as a trick movement. The posterior apprehension test may be positive and the Beighton–Horan score high (see Glossary).

## Cause

This is an uncommon dislocation of the humerus, posteriorly from the glenoid cavity. It occurs traumatically because the shoulder has been taken too far into extension, but it is more commonly atraumatic in those with multidirectional instability, occurring during functional overstretching.

## Investigations

X-ray with true lateral and axillary views should be requested if there is any doubt, as standard views of a shoulder may not display this lesion.

### Caveat

**Missed diagnosis is common.**

## Treatment

(a) Relocation under general anaesthetic if there has been acute trauma, and if posterolateral disruption of the capsule has occurred then surgery is likely to be required.

(b) Atraumatic cases require training, with biofeedback, of the deltoid posterior fibres. The posterior deltoid fibres hold and relocate the humeral head. Multidirectional instability does not do well with surgery.

## Sports

The butterfly swimming stroke may produce posterior dislocation.

## Comment

This injury is not nearly as common as anterior dislocation. Multidirectional instability tends to present as clicking and can do quite well with biofeedback, but patients probably should be moved out of racket games and rugby, unless they can be rehabilitated.

# Intracapsular ligament tear, SLAP lesion

## Findings

There is a generalized shoulder pain, which disturbs many activities; for example doing one's hair, putting on a coat, driving, etc. There may be a click or catch, and it disturbs sporting activities. On examination, there may be discomfort and limited movement in external, internal and glenohumeral abduction, and possibly a subacromial bursitis is present. A click or jump on the Crank test may suggest a capsular tear, and the active compression test may be positive (see Glossary) [6].

## Cause

Acute traumatic or chronic overuse damage to the capsular ligaments, particularly the Superior Labral, Anterior and Posterior: the so-called SLAP lesion.

## Investigations

The tear may be seen on MRI arthrogram, or not discovered until arthroscopy.

## Treatment

(a) Electrotherapy to settle inflammation, such as shortwave diathermy and interferential.

(b) Functional training and strengthening of the rotator cuff in the non-dominant shoulder, but surgery if not progressing.

(c) Early arthroscopic repair in the dominant shoulder.

## Comment

This lesion often presents as a subacromial bursitis or glenohumeral capsulitis. There may be signs from the rotator cuff. Attempts to calm the inflammation with cortisone and rehabilitate the rotator cuff are valid; however, failure to progress warrants an MRI arthrogram.

# Traumatic capsulitis of the shoulder

## Findings

There is rapid increase in pain around the shoulder and down the arm following a traumatic incident. The arm is stiff and painful at night, hurts to lie on, or whilst doing the hair, putting on a coat or a bra. The pain is eased by resting the arm in a sling. External rotation, internal rotation and glenohumeral abduction are limited and painful on active and passive movements. Resisted rotator cuff testing is pain-free, though it may be damaged as well by trauma, when it produces its own signs (see Rotator cuff injuries).

## Cause

A wrench of the shoulder, or trauma to the shoulder, from forced external rotation.

## Investigations

If major trauma has occurred then X-ray to exclude a fracture or dislocation, and, if not settling rapidly, follow with an MRI to exclude other causes.

### Caveat

**Acute calcific tendinitis and signs of shoulder subluxation.**

## Treatment

(a) NSAIDs.
(b) Intra-articular injection of cortisone.
(c) Electrotherapeutic modalities to settle inflammation, such as interferential and shortwave diathermy, until pain-free.
(d) Isometrics to the rotator cuff.
(e) After 48 hours' rest and NSAIDs, capsular stretching and rotator cuff isometrics should start.

## Sports

(a) Usually traumatic in any sport.
(b) Cricket – a wide open, chest-on style of delivery, with an exaggerated external rotation of the shoulder, may produce an anterior capsulitis. This usually occurs in adolescents trying to bowl too fast. They should be encouraged to slow down, learn to swing the ball and build up pace when they have matured.

Perhaps bowling a 'fast ball' should be limited to a certain number per week in growing children (see Chapter 5: Spondylolysis and stable spondylolisthesis, Sports, (b)).

## Comment

Not that common in its pure form, when it responds rapidly to intra-articular cortisone, but even when pain-free one must recheck the shoulder for signs of subluxation. Early intra-articular injection is very effective. Follow this with shortwave diathermy and interferential whilst the range of shoulder movements is being re-established.

# Atraumatic capsulitis of the shoulder (frozen shoulder, adhesive capsulitis)

## Introduction

Ellis and Remvig [7] point out that authors differ as to whether the lesion should include trauma or be non-traumatic. Some authors define the diagnosis by the volume of the injectate that the cavity can hold, whilst others use clinical signs. They note that many (but not all) reported cases, in fact, had rotator cuff tears and that there was an association with stroke patients, possibly reflex sympathetic dystrophy (complex regional pain disorder), diabetes and Dupuytren's.

## Findings

Stage 1   Diffuse pain in the shoulder, worse when doing one's hair, putting on a coat or bra, and it may wake the patient at night, especially when lying on the shoulder. There may be stabs of pain caused by movements that suddenly pull on the capsule. There is a pain-free inner range, but pain at the outer range of external rotation, internal rotation and glenohumeral abduction in the so-called capsular pattern [8]. Monitored over time, this range of movements becomes reduced. Resisted rotator cuff testing is pain-free.

Stage 2   Limited range of movement, with external rotation limited to 0–5°, internal rotation to the hip pocket and glenohumeral abduction to 30–40°. End of range is pain-free unless forced.

Stage 3 A gradual increase in the range of glenohumeral movements, which are essentially pain-free.

The time span of the lesion may be separated into thirds:

- Stage 1 consists of gradually increasing pain and a decreasing range of movements.
- Stage 2 consists of a very limited range of movement, but is effectively pain-free.
- Stage 3 consists of an increasing range of movement back to normality, almost pain-free.

In total lasting 9 months to 3 years.

## Cause

(a) Ellis and Renvig [7] reviewed the histopathology found by various authors and reported that the majority find angioneogenesis and villous hypertrophy, with the fluid from the joint having a strong fibroproliferative effect. The lesions seem to be concentrated on the capsule, especially anteriorly, rather than the rotator cuff. Thus synovial inflammation and contraction of the shoulder capsule, especially of the lax inferior portion, occurs.

(b) It is more common in the over 40s age group.

(c) This could be a reflex sympathetic dystrophy because it often follows a cervical lesion.

 **Caveat**

**Sometimes the patient develops a greater use of the scapulothoracic range of movement, which gives the appearance of improvement in the condition, whereas the glenohumeral range has actually remained the same.**

## Treatment

Stage 1 Intra-articular injection of cortisone, but, if there is no improvement after four injections, the cortisone is unlikely to help. The injections may be given via a posterior, anterior and then subacromial approach. Concomitant analgesia and NSAIDs should be given. Unfortunately, many so-called intra-articular injections of the shoulder are outside the capsule and Ellis and Remvig

[7] found that authors disagree as to its effectiveness.

Stage 2 Encourage scapulothoracic range of movements and wait for stage 3, or manipulation under anaesthetic, which Ellis and Remvig [7] in their review found to be generally effective.

Stage 3 Therapeutic mobilization and stretching exercises. Manipulation under anaesthetic. Arthroscopic anterior release is sometimes undertaken in the most resistant cases.

## Sports

Not associated with any particular sport, but its consequences are very limiting to any arm-related sports. Maintain general fitness.

## Comment

Physiotherapy in the first stage is useless but effective in stage 3. Intra-articular cortisone can be successful enough to warrant its use, but can also prove ineffective, so that analgesia and advice about the natural history of healing become the treatment of choice. Guanethidine, oral or intra-articular, may have a place if there is a reflex sympathetic element [9]. Manipulation under anaesthetic in stage 2 can be very effective, but may produce a flare so many patients are happy to leave well alone. Biopsy of the capsule shows fibrosis, even after apparent recovery [7]. The range of movement can still be reduced when full function has returned [7].

# Subscapular crepitus

## Findings

Diffuse shoulder pain, sometimes over the posterior thorax, but examination shows pain-free glenohumeral and resisted shoulder movements. Rotation and compression of the scapula on the thorax produces grating and pain.

 Caveat

**The grating may be pain-free, and in that case is probably not the cause of the symptoms. Check then for dorsal, costal and vertebral problems (see Chapter 4).**

## Cause

There is a roughened underside of the scapula, sometimes with an osteophyte pressing against the thorax, which is made worse by a hunched back and shoulders.

## Investigations

None are clinically required, but if failing to improve or suggestive of trauma then X-ray or CT scan to exclude rib or scapula fracture (see Fig. 17.8) and an exostosis. Also consider a bone scan to exclude a stress fracture of the rib.

## Treatment

(a) Relax the shoulder position and retrain the rhomboids to release scapulothoracic pressure.
(b) Electrotherapeutic modalities to settle inflammation, such as shortwave diathermy and interferential.
(c) Occasionally, subscapular injection of cortisone.
(d) Occasionally, surgery to remove any obvious osteophyte.

## Sports

(a) Golf – at the address position, forced straight arms, hunched shoulders and a forced scapula thoracic compression cause pain. Encourage the sit back position and more relaxed arm tension at the address.
(b) Running – tight shoulders and a high arm position can cause pain.

## Comment

I once cured a golfer's pain and reduced his handicap by four strokes, just by altering the 'hunched' shoulder position. Subscapular crepitus is a common finding, but not a common cause of clinical problems.

# Stress fracture of the humerus

## Cause

Rare. Sometimes occurs in throwing events and can occur at the epiphysis in children [10]. MRI changes near the elbow and in the medulla have been reported in tennis players.

# Coracoid tenderness

## Findings

May have pain on full shoulder internal and external rotation, plus circumduction, with the site of the pain lying over the coracoid process. Resisted rotator cuff testing is usually pain-free, whereas resisted adduction from the fully externally rotated and circumducted arm is painful. There is local point tenderness over the coracoid, conoid and trapezoid ligaments.

## Cause

The causes may be variable, possibly impingement of the clavicle onto the coracoid process, strain of the conoid or trapezoid ligaments, strain of the short head of biceps and coracobrachialis insertion. It is produced by forced or excessive external rotation in abduction, or muscle power being produced from this externally rotated and abducted position without upper body rotation (see Traumatic capsulitis of the shoulder).

## Investigations

None are clinically required but MRI may help with diagnosis.

## Treatment

Avoid an excessive externally rotated shoulder position. The tenderness may respond to local ultrasound or laser and is responsive to local corticosteroid, followed by controlled isometrics of adduction in external rotation and 90° circumduction.

## Sports

(a) Uncontrolled pectoralis deck machine exercises, when the elbow height is worked too high and no block is put onto the machine to prevent excess external rotation when the muscles fatigue.
(b) Throwing and bowling with a 'wide open' chest in a front-on position.
(c) Swimming freestyle, when the catch phase is applied with power and followed by an immediate pull phase, with no intervening glide phase. Excessive shoulder mobilizing exercises in swimming may contribute.

## Comment

This element always responds well to a local injection of cortisone over the coracoid and then appropriate rehabilitation of the adductors, plus correction of the technical fault. However, it is often part of a pectoral girdle instability where all the elements – anterior capsule, acromioclavicular joint and sternoclavicular joint – are involved and all must be treated. I have not seen shoulder mobilizing exercises produce this problem in gymnasts, possibly because they are naturally 'more supple' than the swimmers.

## Triceps origin strain or tear

### Findings

Pain and tenderness on the posterior aspect of the humerus, at the triceps origin. Resisted triceps, in the triceps curl position, are painful.

### Cause

An uncommon injury produced by supine lying, triceps curls with too heavy a weight, or whilst lying at the end of a bench so that the eccentric phase of contraction leaves the weight unsupported at the end of the movement.

### Investigations

None are clinically required, although diagnostic ultrasound can aid monitoring the injury and MRI may show muscle oedema.

### Treatment

(a) RICE (see Glossary).
(b) Electrotherapeutic modalities to settle inflammation, such as ultrasound and laser.
(c) Controlled triceps rehabilitation following the general muscle ladder principles (see Chapter 20).

### Sports

Weight training – beware anabolic steroid abuse.

### Comment

Very rare. I have seen only one in 35 years. Intramuscular ruptures are also very rare but have been reported [11]. They seem to be traumatic.

## Sternoclavicular joint strain

Pain, tenderness and, possibly, swelling over the sternoclavicular joint (see Chapter 6).

## References

1 Tibone J, Sellers R, Tonino P. Strength testing after third degree acromio clavicular dislocations. Am J Sports Med 1992;20:328–331

2 Krueger-Frank M, Siebert CH, Rosemeyer B. Surgical treatment of dislocations of the acromio clavicular joint in the athlete. Br J Sports Med 1993;27:121–124

3 Webb J, Bannister G. Acromio clavicular disruption in first class rugby players. Br J Sports Med 1992;26:245–247

4 Ellis R. Clinical examination. In: Hutson M, Ellis R (eds) Textbook of musculoskeletal medicine. Oxford: Oxford University Press; 2006. pp 133–134

5 Ferretti A, De Carli A, Fontana M. Injury of the suprascapular nerve at the spinoglenoid notch. The natural history of infraspinatus atrophy in volleyball players. Am J Sports Med 1998;26:759–763

6 O'Brien SJ, Pagnani M, Fealy S, McGlynn SR, Wilson JB. The active compression test: a new and effective test for diagnosing labral tears and acromioclavicular joint abnormality. Am J Sports Med 1998;26:610–613

7 Ellis RM, Remvig L. Frozen shoulder: a review of causation, progress and treatment. For the scientific committee of FIMM. J Orthop Med 2003;25(2):82–87

8 Cyriax JH, Cyriax PJ (eds). Cyriax's illustrated manual of orthopaedic medicine, 2nd edn. Oxford: Butterworth-Heinemann; 1993

9 Gado I, Emery P. Intra articular injection for resistant shoulder pain: a preliminary double blind study of a novel approach. Ann Rheum Dis 1996;55:199–201

10 Boyd KT, Batt ME. Stress fracture of the proximal humeral epiphysis in an elite badminton player. Br J Sports Med 1997;31:252–253

11 Singh RK, Pooley J. Complete rupture of the triceps brachii muscle. Br J Sports Med 2002;36:467–469

### Further reading

Bruckner P, Khan K. Clinical Sports Medicine, 3rd edn. New York: McGraw-Hill; 2006

Hutson MA (ed.). Sports injuries: recognition and management, 2nd edn. Oxford: Oxford Medical Publications; 1996

Hutson M, Ellis R (eds). Textbook of musculoskeletal medicine. Oxford: Oxford University Press; 2006

Reid D. Sports injury assessment and rehabilitation. Edinburgh: Churchill Livingstone; 1992

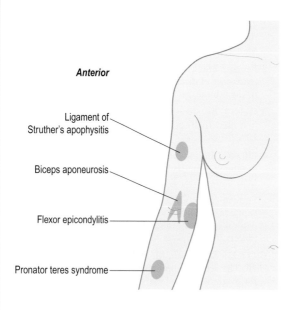

*Anterior*

Ligament of
Struther's apophysitis

Biceps aponeurosis

Flexor epicondylitis

Pronator teres syndrome

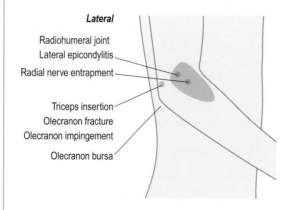

*Lateral*

Radiohumeral joint
Lateral epicondylitis
Radial nerve entrapment

Triceps insertion
Olecranon fracture
Olecranon impingement

Olecranon bursa

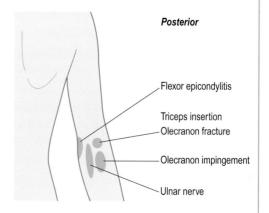

*Posterior*

Flexor epicondylitis

Triceps insertion
Olecranon fracture

Olecranon impingement

Ulnar nerve

# Chapter Eighteen

## 18

# Elbow

## CHAPTER CONTENTS

## Referred pain from the neck

Referred pain from the C5/6 roots commonly affects this area and must be excluded (see Chapter 3).

## Referred pain from the shoulder

The subacromial space, particularly, and occasionally the rotator cuff, can refer pain to the elbow, when elbow pain may be the only presenting symptom. Always check the shoulder first; if in doubt, inject the subacromial space with local anaesthetic and review the signs afterwards (see Chapter 17: Subacromial bursitis/inflammation).

## Lateral epicondylitis (tennis elbow/pitcher's elbow)

### Findings

Gradual or acute onset of pain over the lateral epicondyle or wrist extensor muscles, which is worse when gripping, hitting, digging, hammering, using a screwdriver or carrying a heavy briefcase with the palm down. The pinch grip to take down books or files off a shelf is a common cause. The pain is worse on making a fist, lifting a cup or kettle, or sometimes writing. Resisted wrist and finger extension are painful. Classically, resisted testing of the third and fourth finger cause pain, but if the index (second) finger and thumb are painful then the sports technique is possibly wrong (Figs 18.1 and 18.2). Tenderness to palpation will differentiate between:

Type 1   Tenoperiosteal
Type 2   Musculotendinous
Type 3   Muscular
Type 4   Posterior annular

## Cause

There is a tear or sprain of the extensor origin, particularly the extensor carpi radialis, and there may also be impingement of the extracapsular synovium from the radiohumeral joint.

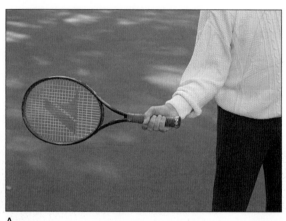

A

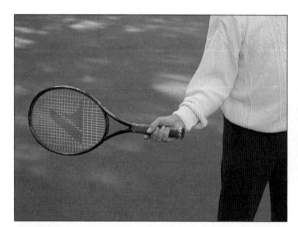

A

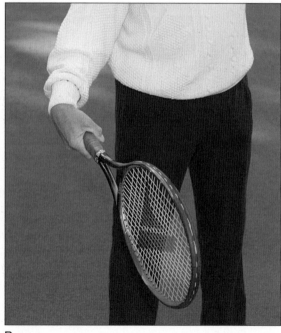

B

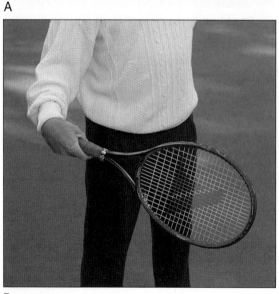

B

**Figure 18.1** • (**A** and **B**) The range of wrist movement when the thumb and index finger are relaxed.

**Figure 18.2** • (**A** and **B**) The reduced range when the thumb and index finger grip is tight.

## Investigations

None are clinically required, but if getting worse over the first 5 days of an acute injury then X-ray for myositis ossificans (Fig. 18.3), otherwise, to exclude a calcified ligament or radiohumeral arthrosis. Diagnostic ultrasound can also display the lesions, apart from radiohumeral arthrosis.

### Caveat

**Pain referred from cervical root C6, subacromial space or rotator cuff, radial nerve entrapment, forearm compartment syndrome.**

## Treatment

(a) RICE (see Glossary).

(b) NSAIDs, gel or ointment, or iontophoresis during the acute phase.

(c) Electrotherapy to settle inflammation, such as ultrasound, laser and interferential.

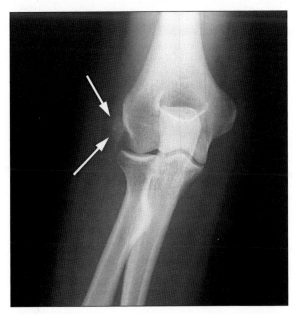

**Figure 18.3** • Myositis ossificans in the lateral epicondyle of a skier who had been performing rapid turns, with the ski poles 'picking' into the snow.

(d) Massage techniques to control scar tissue, such as frictions.

(e) Stretching of the muscle to stimulate the enthesis and prevent scar contraction.

(f) Isometrics of the extensors to organize scar tissue and strengthen the muscles.

(g) Dynamic exercises to increase muscle strength.

(h) Type 1 (tenoperiosteal) responds to physiotherapy and cortisone injections; type 2 (musculotendinous) responds to physiotherapy and cortisone injections; type 3 (muscular) responds to physiotherapy; type 4 (posterior annular) usually involves the extracapsular synovium of the radiohumeral joint and does not respond well to physiotherapy, requiring cortisone injection.

(i) Use the tennis elbow ladder (see Chapter 20).

(j) Chronic adhesions, with fixed flexion at the elbow but no radiohumeral arthrosis, responds to a Mills' manipulation (see Fig. 22.13) after injection of cortisone and local anaesthetic into enthesis (see Glossary: Mills' manipulation).

(k) Epicondylitis clasps help some people, but if applied too tightly they can compress the radial nerve/anterior interosseous nerve.

(l) Autologous blood injection into the origin for chronic resistant cases. Note that this is considered dope positive in sport [1].

(m) Failure to progress – rest for 1 year, work through the pain, or surgery.

### Caveat

**If the radiohumeral joint is involved, this must be treated before the epicondylitis. Myositis ossificans gives a history of getting much worse after about 5 days from the acute injury. Rest, sling, NSAIDs and analgesia, but an injection of cortisone may be curative.**

## Sports

### Golf – right-handed golfer (left hand)

(a) The left wrist is forced high so the extensors are overstretched.

(b) The left wrist at the address is in front of the hands, and take away is with flexion of the left

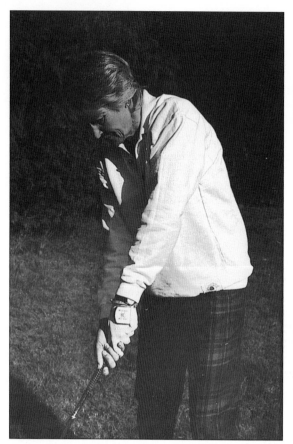

**Figure 18.4** • The left wrist is forced forwards, increasing the tension on the wrist extensors. If the club is blocked, for instance by thick grass, the wrist extensors, which are under tension, will be blocked and can tear at their origin, producing a tennis elbow.

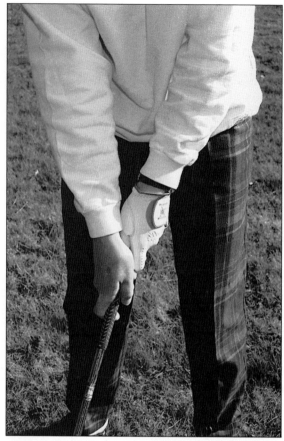

**Figure 18.5** • The right hand is closed and at the top of the back swing will not lie under the club but be forced into ulnar deviation. Unless the thumb and index finger are released, tension will develop in the extensor mechanism. Correction of technique is required.

wrist, not with shoulder rotation, so that, when hitting, the ground will acutely resist and block the extensors' movement into the shot (Fig. 18.4).

## Golf – right-handed golfer (right hand)

There is a closed grip with the right hand (Fig. 18.5).

## Tennis and squash

Pain occurs usually with backhands, serves or overhead shots.

(a) A grip that is too tight with the thumb and index finger prevents the full wrist flexion that the shot requires and stresses the restraining extensors. Treat by releasing the tension of the thumb and finger grip (Fig. 18.6); the patient needs to grip with the third, fourth and fifth fingers.

(b) Check other causes for gripping being too tight, such as a slippery handle, too thin a handle, too thick a handle, inappropriate tension of the racket strings, tension of the player, etc. (see Figs 18.5 and 18.6).

(c) Backhand problems, such as leading with the elbow and wrist into the shot (Fig 18.7), and dropping the racket head below the wrist (Fig 18.8).

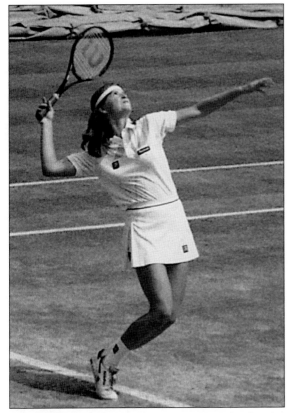

**Figure 18.6** • This professional tennis player (Hanna Mandlikova) clearly demonstrates release of the thumb and index finger.

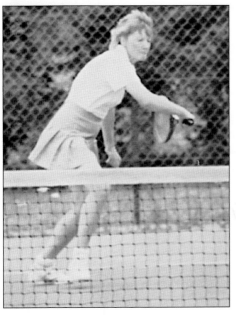

**Figure 18.7** • The elbow leads into the shot and the wrist is excessively cocked.

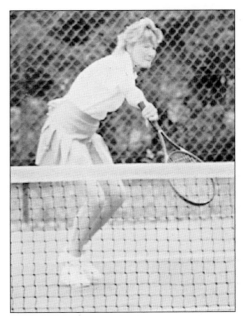

**Figure 18.8** • The racket head has now dropped below the wrist increasing tension on the wrist extensors.

(d) The top spun, single-handed, backhand may overload the extensors if the shot is over-practised without developing appropriate forearm strength.

## Badminton

(a) See tennis and squash above.

(b) The net player tends to intercept the shuttle and hit it acutely towards the floor, when a tight grip with thumb and second finger transfers the forces to the elbow, especially the radiohumeral joint, as well as the extensor complex.

## Water skiing

Beginners often hang on for dear life, with the tow bar held horizontally. This produces a tennis elbow that can be relieved by holding the tow bar vertically, as this uses the flexors and rests the extensors.

## Snow skiing

Can occur as an acute overload in good skiers, when the poles are used at speed on repeated rapid turns. 'Drag lifts' are being removed from the ski slopes, but if one has to use them then hold on to the tow bar with palms up.

## Fly fishing

Too much wrist, and not enough elbow and shoulder, in the casting technique. Extending the index finger along the top of the rod will help to prevent 'wrist break'.

## Office

(a) Writing – thicken the grip or hold the pen between the second and third fingers.

(b) Files – lift them out from a shelf with a palm-up grip, or use both hands.

(c) Computer mouse – work with a bent elbow and relax the grip to move the mouse, but it is important to select a size of mouse that allows a relaxed grip. Alter the left click 'pressing finger'.

(d) Brief case – carry with a palm-up grip and carry two light cases rather than one heavy one, or use a rucksack style case. Do not throw the case into the car.

## DIY and garden

Carry, weed, and dig palm up. Use a long-handled or power screwdriver to reduce the force onto the epicondyles at the elbows. Avoid hammering, or use a thicker grip, and release the second finger and thumb grip pressure. Use hand-held, not finger-held, secateurs.

## Comment

Most cases that have failed physiotherapy are posterior annular. These have often been treated for months before being referred on. One posterior annular injection that includes the radiohumeral joint often relieves the pain, and then rehabilitation of the extensors can be started as soon as the pain level permits. There seem to be three groups: those that settle after one episode, those that settle, but return whilst the technique or the strength is improved, and those who seem to improve but are never entirely cured, with the problem constantly returning. This is the group who often end up having surgery to the extensor origin, or they rest from activities and await healing to occur, which may be over a year. I cannot emphasize enough how many presentations of elbow pain are produced by referred pain from the neck or shoulder. All examinations of the elbow must include the neck and shoulder, and, if in doubt, inject the shoulder, usually the subacromial space, with 2% local anaesthetic to see if this relieves the elbow pain.

## Radiohumeral joint

### Findings

The findings are similar to a tennis elbow, with which it is often associated, so there is pain on making a fist and gripping with the palm down, as described in tennis elbow (see Lateral epicondylitis). There may also be night pain and pain on active or passive straightening of the elbow. Passive flexion, extension and, sometimes, pronation and supination are painful at the end of the range.

### Cause

Traumatic arthrosis of the joint, plus the extracapsular synovium may be impinged, and sometimes becomes atrophied and necrotic.

**Caveat**

**Gout, degenerative or inflammatory arthritis, and fracture of the proximal radial head if a history of trauma exists.**

### Investigations

None are clinically required, but X-ray for degenerative changes and a radial head fracture if the injury is failing to settle or there is a history of trauma. Ultrasound will display any lateral epicondylar or tendon damage.

### Treatment

(a) Treat the radiohumeral joint before any accompanying lateral epicondylitis.

(b) NSAIDs.

(c) Electrotherapeutic modalities to settle inflammation, such as interferential, pulsed shortwave diathermy and ultrasound.

(d) Injection of cortisone into the joint.

### Sports

**Tennis**

(a) Backhand grip for serve, and hitting the 'top spin' serve with pronation. In the early stages of learning to use a top spun service, the service shot snaps the radiohumeral joint into pronation and extension.

(b) Snatching the wrist movements to get on top of the serve when trying to induce top spin.

## Badminton

Usually, if the net player gets tense, they have too tight a grip between the thumb and second finger, so that the wrist will not release as easily into flexion when intercepting at the net. This restricted wrist range snaps the force into the radiohumeral joint. The correct shot should be a 'karate chop' with an angled racket, not a forced flexion of the wrist to drive the shuttlecock to the floor, but most net players want to kill the shot!

## Golf

The problem comes from gripping the club tightly and forcing extension of the elbows, particularly the left, whilst at the address position. Try a thicker grip on the clubs as this releases the grip pressure and relaxes the elbows, which may prove easier to achieve than by trying to 'relax' when tense.

## Comment

Tennis elbow does not hurt on passive flexion or pronation/supination. A 'soft block' to extension, short of the full range, is suggestive of joint involvement. If the faulty techniques are not corrected, the injury will return. Treating the epicondylitis before the radiohumeral joint does not seem to work – treat the radiohumeral joint first.

## Radial nerve entrapment

### Findings

(a) There is a clinical impression of a persistent tennis elbow, but with a description of intense pain that often wakes the patient at night. The pain is worse stretching out for something, and is easier in the fetal, flexed arm position. The pain can radiate to the back of the hand or up the arm.

(b) The signs at the elbow may be confusing, with no definite tennis elbow pattern (see Lateral epicondylitis). The extensor muscle group is tender, locally, to light palpation over the radial nerve.

(c) Brachial nerve tensioning tests may be positive, but neck movements do not seem to make it worse (see Glossary: Brachial nerve tensioning tests).

## Cause

The posterior interosseus branch of the radial nerve is caught under the ligament of Frohse, which forms a band between the two heads of the supinator muscle.

### Caveat

**C6/7 referral, referred shoulder pain.**

## Investigations

An EMG may or may not show nerve conduction deficit.

## Treatment

Surgical release of the ligament of Frohse to release the radial nerve.

## Sports

Sports are probably not causative, but implemental sports may make it worse.

## Comment

The clues seem to be night pain, with an intensity of pain description that is 'too strong' for a tennis elbow. The patient prefers the fetal arm position and there are unclear epicondylar signs. The surgical scar is much longer than the patient expects.

## Flexor epicondylitis (golfer's elbow)

### Findings

(a) Pain on pulling (weeds up), carrying boxes palms up, or scratching one's back using pulp pressure from the finger tips, as in cleaning or polishing a small object. There is no history of the 'pins and needles' or night pain that would suggest ulnar nerve involvement.

(b) The joint has a pain-free range.

(c) The ulnar nerve is not pathologically tender to palpation.

(d) The pain is always worse on resisted pronation, though resisted fingertip curl (flexor digitorum profundus) and resisted middle phalanx curl (flexor digitorum superficialis), especially of the third (mid) and fourth (ring) fingers, are usually, though not invariably, painful.

## Cause

An enthesopathy develops at the flexor origin from overload of the pronator and flexors of the wrist and fingers. There may be a musculotendinous disruption.

### Caveat

Neck C8, T1, ulnar nerve entrapment at the elbow, and avulsion of the medial humeral epicondyle (Little League elbow – apophysitis in children). Ulnar collateral ligament.

## Treatment

(a) RICE, but beware of ice irritating the ulnar nerve. Use 'wet ice'.

(b) Electrotherapeutic modalities to settle inflammation, such as laser and ultrasound.

(c) Cortisone to the locally tender area.

(d) Massage techniques to control scar tissue orientation.

(e) Stretch the fingers and wrist into extension to prevent scar contraction and orientate scar tissue.

(f) Isometric, resisted exercises against pronation, scratch one's back with finger pulp pressure, and squeeze objects with a finger tip grip. These activities will place a controlled load on the enthesis and scar tissue, and also maintain muscle strength.

(g) Gradually introduce larger loads (see Chapter 20).

(h) This injury takes time to heal, usually because rehabilitation is taken too fast and thus the injury has episodes when it reflares.

(i) Autologous blood injection [1].

(j) Failed conservative treatment requires a surgical release of the flexor complex at the enthesis, or a long period of rest and rehabilitation.

## Investigations

None are clinically required, unless the patient is failing to improve or following an acute severe episode, in which cases an X-ray or ultrasound to exclude avulsion and apophysitis is required (Fig. 18.9). Ultrasound may show musculotendinous damage and guide the placement of an injection. MRI can display the injury but probably does not alter the management.

## Sports

(a) Throwing or hitting with strong finger and wrist flexion to increase acceleration, such as throwing the javelin and, in baseball, the fast ball and curve ball.

(b) Rotational shot putt – if the shot slides off the tip of the fingers and thumb.

(c) Golf – strong right arm pull through the swing, especially with the right-hand grip being too open.

(d) Tennis – semi-Western forehand – top spun shots.

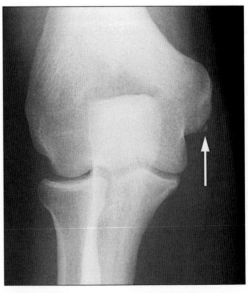

**Figure 18.9 •** A small avulsion fragment from the medial epicondyle (arrow).

(e) Sailing – winching the sails.

(f) Pulling, weeding and polishing, with a tight finger grip.

## Comment

This is not as common as tennis elbow, but it is fairly resistant to treatment. Cortisone removes the pain, but rehabilitation, which then must follow, will take several months. Do not take the patient up the rehabilitation ladder too fast. Proportionally, more of my patients with flexor epicondylitis have come to surgery than my patients with extensor epicondylitis, and it remains to be seen whether autologous blood injections will alter this.

## Ulnar neuritis

### Findings

(a) Pain at the elbow, which may refer upwards or down to the wrist and may wake the patient at night.

(b) 'Pins and needles', and possibly numbness at the fourth and fifth fingers and the ulnar half of the third finger.

(c) Tenderness to palpation of the ulnar nerve in the condylar groove, or just distal to the groove, which refers pain and 'pins and needles' to the fingers.

(d) Adverse neural tensioning tests, if positive, are not worse with neck movements.

(e) Muscle weakness of the interossei and hypothenar eminence wasting. If the damage is severe there may be clawing of the third and fourth finger, and Pope's sign and Froment's sign can be positive (see Glossary: Pope's sign and Froment's sign).

### Cause

Irritation or entrapment of the ulnar nerve in the condylar groove is often caused by external local pressure, such as leaning the elbow on the edge of the desk or window of the car when driving. Occasionally, after trauma to the elbow, the nerve is bound into the scar tissue.

### Investigation

EMG.

### Treatment

Avoid local pressure to the nerve, but, with night pain, a trial of perineural cortisone × 1 at the elbow may be successful. Surgical release and transposition of the nerve is required if the pain is not settling with conservative means.

### Sports

No sport is particularly relevant (see Chapter 19: Ulnar neuritis).

### Comment

Referral to the ulnar two fingers can be from carpal tunnel entrapment, as the ulnar and median nerves may link higher in the forearm. Damage to the superficial branch of the ulnar at the pisiform (Guyon's canal) produces no muscle weakness as this superficial branch is sensory. Avoidance of local pressure settles most of the problems and perineural steroids can reduce a flare, but chronic problems require transposition of the ulnar nerve.

## Ulnar collateral ligament

### Findings

There is pain on the medial aspect of the elbow, which is particularly noted in overarm, throwing sports athletes. A pop may be experienced in an acute episode, and further throwing becomes impossible. Forced valgus at the elbow becomes painful and lax, with increased elbow flexion [2]. Local tenderness is not diagnostic as the medial epicondyle and ulnar nerve are adjacent. Chronic cases may also show olecranon impingement (see below).

### Cause

Acute and chronic stress or partial rupture of the midsubstance anterior fibre of the ulnar collateral ligament, from trauma or repeated throwing, with a valgus strain.

### Investigations

Ultrasound and MRI may not be diagnostic. Stress X-ray, to gap the joint, will also show avulsion of the medial epicondyle, and olecranon osteophytes if they are present. Diagnostic arthroscopy may be required.

## Treatment

Care must be taken with the ulnar nerve, but rest and physiotherapy, and anti-inflammatories, such as NSAIDs and cortisone, will reduce the pain whilst rehabilitation back into throwing takes place. An unstable joint requires surgical repair of the ligament.

## Sports

(a) Those practising martial arts, and arm wrestlers, are prone to trauma.

(b) Baseball pitchers, tennis, javelin, quarter backs in American football.

## Comment

This injury can be difficult to diagnose. In overarm sports, a failure to diagnose other causes, such as medial epicondylitis or ulnar nerve irritation, should raise the index of suspicion.

## Triceps insertion

### Findings

Acute or chronic onset of pain at the insertion into the olecranon, which is worse with extending the elbow actively or on resisted extension. Passive elbow extension is pain-free and there is local tenderness to palpation over the enthesis.

### Cause

There has been a strain of the triceps insertion into the olecranon, usually in sports that accelerate extension at the elbow.

> ### Caveat
>
> Cervical spine C6/7. Ruptures at the triceps insertion have been reported [3]. Avulsion of the olecranon enthesis, olecranon fractures.

### Investigations

X-ray, as there are well-recorded incidences of olecranon stress fractures and avulsion of the apophysis. MRI will show both the soft tissue damage and the avulsion, but a small piece of cortical bone is better seen on X-ray and CT scan.

## Treatment

(a) RICE and NSAIDs.

(b) Electrotherapeutic modalities to settle inflammation, such as ultrasound and laser.

(c) Massage techniques to control scar tissue, such as frictions.

(d) Injection of cortisone to the enthesis to settle the inflammation and allow rehabilitation.

(e) Stretching, by passive flexion of the elbow and flexion of the shoulder, to prevent scar tissue contraction and to load the enthesis.

(f) Graded resisted isometrics to stress the enthesis and prevent scar tissue contraction.

(g) Increment the size of loads (see Chapter 20), but particularly through triceps curls, shoulder presses, dips and throwing.

(h) If avulsion has occurred then surgical fixation is required.

## Sports [4–7]

(a) Weightlifting – driving the arm into extension, when pressing weights, and triceps dips.

(b) Tennis – where there is a tendency to an arm-only serve that tries to hit the top spin serve.

(c) Baseball pitchers and javelin throwers.

(d) Martial arts, when the elbow is snapped into extension.

(e) Gymnasts.

## Comment

Like all enthesial problems, the inflammation responds well to anti-inflammatories, such as cortisone, but rehabilitation of the teno-osseous junction is vital for full recovery.

## Olecranon impingement

### Findings

Acute or chronic onset of pain at the posterior aspect of the elbow, which is worse on passive or active elbow extension, but not with resisted isometric testing of the triceps. It is locally tender in the groove between the lateral olecranon and the humerus. The area is usually not swollen. Check the Beighton–Horan score for hypermobility (see Glossary) as these patients often have increased elbow extension.

## Cause

Synovial or fat pad entrapment, between the olecranon and olecranon fossa of the humerus; usually because the elbow is whipped into extension or because the elbow hyperextends as a result of increased ligamentous laxity. Osteophytes may form, secondary to ulnar collateral ligament laxity.

 **Caveat**

C6/7 referral from the neck, triceps strain, stress fracture of the olecranon, avulsion from the olecranon, and gout.

## Treatment

(a) Avoid the causative mechanisms. See a coach.

(b) Electrotherapeutic modalities to settle inflammation, such as interferential and ultrasound.

(c) Inject cortisone to the tender area within the olecranon fossa, using a lateral rather than medial approach in order to avoid risk to the ulnar nerve. The needle should be placed into the olecranon condylar groove, and occasionally inject the fossa behind the triceps tendon.

## Sports

(a) Weightlifting – locking out 'presses' may cause impingement in the hypermobile elbows, and too heavy a weight in biceps curls can snap the elbow out into extension, in the eccentric phase.

(b) Baseball pitchers – particularly throwing the 'change up', which snaps the elbow into extension.

(c) Martial arts – snapping the elbow into extension.

(d) Gymnastics – sway back elbows. Gymnasts who possess a high Beighton–Horan score and who have a sway back elbow are unlikely to survive four-piece gymnastics. Rhythmic gymnastics may be preferable for them (see Glossary).

(e) Squash – the backhand shot, played too close to the body and with a straight elbow, and, especially, a little angled shot from the backhand corner to the forehand front wall, can lock out the elbow into extension (Fig. 18.10).

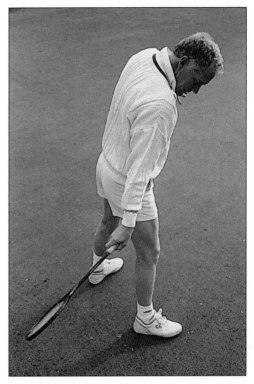

**Figure 18.10 •** A backhand shot at squash played with an extended elbow, racket below the wrist that jams the olecranon into its fossa.

## Comment

The injury does not respond well to physiotherapy. Cortisone and alteration in technique are the treatments of choice.

## Olecranon bursa

### Findings

Pain-free, palpable, fluctuant swelling, or swelling that occurs after localized trauma. There is stiffness of the elbow, but the joint movement is pain-free. Inflammatory, infective or systemic disease produce a red, warm and painful swelling, as may a traumatic haembursitis.

### Cause

(a) Frictional – from leaning on the elbow, or repetitive full flexion at the elbow, as reported by darts throwers.

(b) Traumatic – haembursitis of the olecranon bursa.

(c) Systemic – such as gout and the inflammatory arthritides.

## Treatment

(a) Avoid causative factors, such as leaning on the elbow.

(b) Aspirate and check for crystals, or culture.

(c) Hydrocortisone if required, for comfort.

(d) Rarely, surgical ablation.

## Investigations

X-ray for osteoarthritis, osteophytes or synovial chondromatosis (Fig. 18.11, and see Fig. 11.8) and send aspirate for polarized light microscopy (gout or pseudogout). Culture if infection is suspected.

## Sports

Said to occur in darts throwers during early training.

## Comment

Unless painful, most patients will accept the bursa. Try aspiration and cortisone, but if this does not settle after two treatments then leave well alone. Surgery may be required if synovial chondromatosis or osteophytes are troublesome.

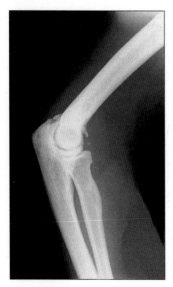

**Figure 18.11** • Degenerative changes in the elbow.

## Olecranon fracture

Apart from local trauma to the elbow, the olecranon can suffer a stress fracture or, in children, avulsion of the apophysis. The problems are those of a triceps insertion, but the bony damage requires longer to heal and a loose fragment may require surgical screwing (Fig. 18.12) (see Triceps insertion).

## Osteoarthritis of the elbow

### Findings

(a) There may be a history of previous trauma, followed much later by a gradual increase in pain and a decrease in range. The first sign is limitation of extension.

(b) Swelling, plus or minus limitation in passive flexion and extension, with pain at the limit of movement and a hard end feel.

(c) Pronation and supination are not limited unless the radiohumeral joint has been involved.

(d) Occasionally, osteophytes may irritate the ulnar nerve and produce symptoms in the hand.

### Cause

Degenerative changes, which are mainly post-traumatic are found.

### Investigations

X-ray for osteophytic lipping (see Fig. 18.11).

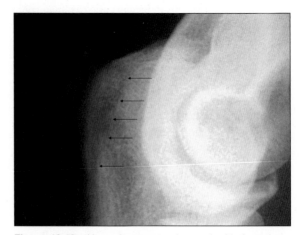

**Figure 18.12** • X-ray shows an early apophysitis from the olecranon at the triceps insertion.

## Treatment

(a) NSAIDs.

(b) Electrotherapeutic modalities to settle inflammation, such as shortwave diathermy and interferential.

(c) Allow movement in the pain-free range.

(d) Surgery.

### Caveat

**Systemic arthritis, gout or synovial chondromatosis.**

## Sports

Most problems occur with hitting sports, as in golf or racket shots, where the elbow straightens rapidly, extending the joint into the painful range. This is a difficult problem to get around. Attempting to lock out the elbow into extension, or a weight being heavy enough to passively force extension of the flexed elbow, can be very painful.

## Comment

Fortunately, osteoarthritis of the elbow is not that common, but really is quite limiting for implemental sporting activities when it does occur.

## Loose bodies

### Findings

There is a history of intermittent or persistent restriction or locking of the elbow, with swelling of the elbow joint, which may have followed trauma. There is a painful, restricted range of flexion and extension, which, with a radiohumeral loose body, will make pronation and supination restricted and painful as well.

### Cause

An osteochondral fragment, or a traumatic fragment, is trapped in the ulnar–humeral or radiohumeral joint.

### Investigations

X-ray is usually sufficient, and the best investigation to show a loose body or osteochondral defect on the humeral condyle (Fig. 18.13), but a cartilaginous loose body may not show. CT or MRI may be required, but these are also not good for visualizing a cartilaginous loose body.

## Treatment

Surgical removal of the loose body is required.

## Sports

(a) Gymnastics – the injury may signal the end of participation in four-piece gymnastics because the loose body is the end result of an avulsion of an osteochondral defect, but with careful monitoring the gymnast may be able to try the asymmetric bars, balance beam, and build into walkovers, and only later add flicks, somersaults and vaults.

(b) Loose bodies are usually post-traumatic in other sports.

## Comment

The osteochondral defect may be a compression stress fracture. The elbow does seem to suffer a reduction in range after the injury, and whether this elbow is truly capable of withstanding further attrition from gymnastics is highly debatable. Fortunately, it is not a common injury.

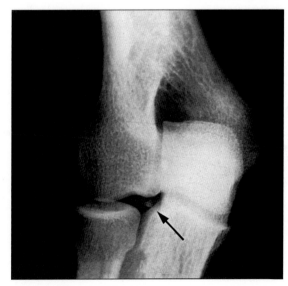

**Figure 18.13** • A loose body in the elbow.

## Osteochondral defect

A patient with a history of a loose body or of pain and swelling in an adolescent elbow should have an X-ray and, if normal, an MRI to look for osteochondral damage (see Loose bodies). Surgeons like to curette out the defect, but I wonder if rest from compression should not be the first line of treatment, especially if it is believed to be a compression stress fracture.

## Biceps aponeurosis/distal biceps tendon

### Findings

(a) Usually a gradual onset of pain, associated with elbow flexion under loads.

(b) There is pain on resisted supination and flexion, and Yergason's and Speed's tests may be positive (see Glossary).

(c) There is tenderness to palpation along the aponeurosis, to the radial insertion.

(d) Very rarely, the tendon may rupture at the distal end of the biceps [8], when bruising and weakness become apparent. If the aponeurosis, as well as the distal tendon, ruptures then the biceps will contract. If the aponeurosis is intact, the tendon length will be maintained.

### Cause

It is an uncommon consequence of strong biceps loading, usually with flexion and supination. Consider anabolic steroid abuse.

> ### Caveat
>
> C5/6 referral from neck, referral from the shoulder, or radial neck fracture.

### Investigations

None are clinically required if mild, but ultrasound or MRI may show a tendinosis and will show the rupture, if present (Fig. 18.14).

### Treatment

(a) The rupture requires surgery [8], but note that avulsion from the bone is particularly prone to complications, with or without surgery.

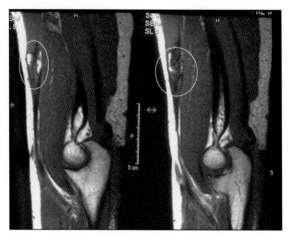

**Figure 18.14** • A distal biceps tear (circled) which should settle without complications.

(b) The tendinopathy is poor to respond and may take months to heal, so it is best to reduce loads and use controlled biceps exercises while the lesion heals over time.

(c) One can try local cortisone along the aponeurosis, but this has variable results.

### Sports

(a) Any requiring strong elbow flexion and supination can be at risk.

(b) Archery – the damage can be produced in beginners who draw the bow with elbow flexion rather than scapular retraction. Correct the fault, and use a lighter draw weight, until the injury has settled.

(c) Weightlifting and body building – avoid biceps curls and 'hand under' pull-ups. Check for anabolic steroid abuse.

(d) Cricket – a violent square cut by one of my patients produced this injury, as the right hand is whipped into supination during this shot.

### Comment

Fortunately, as it heals so slowly, the injury is rare. I now inform patients that treatment consists of time and controlled activities, as anything else does little to help. Tendon avulsions at the radius and ulna insertion have many complications and require specialist management.

## Pronator teres syndrome

### Findings

(a) A history of acute pain locally, over the mid-anterior forearm, and some anterior elbow pain that is locally tender to palpation.

(b) Gripping with the fingertips or middle phalanges, especially the third and fourth, give pain.

(c) Resisted flexor superficialis (middle phalanges) of the third and fourth fingers give pain in the forearm. Other authors have found that the profundus hurts (distal phalanges).

(d) Pain on forehand racket shots.

(e) If the nerve is involved then pins and needles in a median nerve distribution.

### Cause

Restriction of the median nerve as it passes through the pronator teres [9].

(a) Acute – a one-off retrieving shot (tennis or squash), when the ball is behind the player and the shot is played forehand with a straight arm and extreme flexion of wrist to achieve the correct direction of return.

(b) Chronic – if the acute mechanism (as above) is employed regularly, usually in squash.

(c) Perhaps these mechanisms, in fact, pull on the flexor muscle belly, and this is a muscle injury rather than a nerve entrapment. However, the findings are similar to that of the nerve entrapment reported as pronator teres syndrome [9].

### Investigations

None are clinically required, except if median nerve entrapment is envisaged, when the EMG may be positive.

### Treatment

For the acute type, local cortisone to the tender area may help. Correction of technique is required for the chronic problems. Rest from gripping, as in shot making in tennis and squash, for 12–18 months may be required. Surgery is required to release the tight pronator restriction band if nerve entrapment has occurred.

### Sports

(a) Tennis – may occur with a one-off shot (see Cause, above).

(b) Squash – instead of facing the back wall to hit the boast or drive out of the forehand back corner, the player faces the front to the side wall and tries to direct the shot straight to the front wall, with a straight arm and extreme wrist flexion.

### Comment

Fortunately, this is a rare condition. Although it is reported to do well with surgery to release the median nerve [9], my patients seem to have had an extreme resisted flexion injury, which should be a tear of superficialis, with scar tissue. The symptoms of the two descriptions seem to be similar, but they may be different conditions. Two of my patients did very well with steroid injections, two settled with altered technique, but one took a long time to rehabilitate. The technical fault was consistent with all four.

## Supinator strain

### Findings

Pain over the upper forearm that is worse with resisted supination. However, the passive elbow range is pain-free, passive supination is pain-free, resisted wrist and finger flexion are pain-free, and pure resisted elbow flexion is pain-free. The biceps aponeurosis is not tender to palpation.

### Cause

Rare. Biceps curls, which force the elbow into a full extension, with an oversupinated hand position. Sometimes this lift is called 'preacher curls'. When the weight is too heavy, a strain is produced at the supinator origin. There is acute pain, which appears to come with a number of different weight exercises, but careful analysis shows that the supinated position has been achieved during these exercises.

### Investigations

None are clinically required, but ultrasound and MRI may show the problem.

## Treatment

Difficult, but electrotherapeutic modalities, such as ultrasound, laser and interferential, plus reduced loading of the supinator, might help.

## Sports

Weight training, and in particular 'preacher curls'.

## Comment

I have seen only two cases, both of which took a long while to settle, but one player continued to play hockey, with pain, during the problem. Both had been performing preacher curls.

## Ligament of Struther's apophysitis

The ligament of Struther attaches to the humerus and may pull out a bony spur at its attachment. This can become vulnerable to direct trauma, as in boxing (Fig. 18.15).

## Compartment syndrome of the forearm

### Findings

A history of forearm flexor pain, worse after an increasing length of exercise. No evidence of referral from the neck or shoulder is found, and resisted flexors do not hurt unless seen acutely after the precipitating activity, when the forearm is tense and painful.

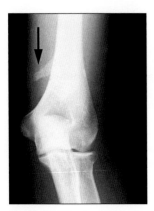

**Figure 18.15** • An ecchondroma or possibly the attachment of the ligament of Struther has been hit and fractured in this boxer.

## Cause

Possibly, a swelling of the flexor muscles within their fascial sheath. The sheath does not allow for this expansion and the increased pressure then reduces oxygen supply to the muscle.

### Caveat

**Carpal tunnel syndrome.**

## Investigation

Forearm, flexor compartment pressure studies.

## Treatment

(a) RICE.
(b) NSAIDs.
(c) Electrotherapeutic modalities to settle inflammation, such as ultrasound, laser and interferential.
(d) Surgical release of the tight fascia.

## Sports [10]

(a) Water ski racing – caused by the pure endurance of holding the tow bar, even though elbow and shoulder harnesses are used to relieve the problem.
(b) Motocross – as the rider stands most of the time, the clutch and brakes must be set at an angle about 45° to the horizontal. Sometimes they are set nearly horizontal for the sitting position, but when the rider stands the forearm flexors become continually stretched, and therefore work under continual tension whilst trying to control the bike.
(c) Rowing – occurs infrequently from the flexed fingers gripping around the oar.

## Comment

These are not common, but in the abovementioned sports an index of suspicion should be aroused.

## Stress fracture of the humerus

Tennis players have reported pain around the elbow and MRI has shown increased signal on STIR and T2 sequences, in the marrow of the humerus.

# References

1 Suresh SPS, Ali KE, Jones H, Connell DA. Medial epicondylitis: is ultra sound guided autologous blood injection an effective treatment? Br J Sports Med 2006;40(11):935–939

2 O'Driscol WM, Lawton RL, Smith AM. The moving valgus stress test for medial collateral ligament tears of the elbow. Am J Sports Med 2005;33(2):231–239

3 Stannard JP, Bucknell AL. Rupture of the triceps tendon associated with steroid injections. Am J Sports Med 1993;21:482–485

4 Rao PS, Rao SK, Navadgi BC. Olecranon stress fracture in a weight lifter. Br J Sports Med 2001;35:72–73

5 Gordon WN, Michael TD. Olecranon stress fractures in throwers: a case report of two cases and a review of the literature. Clin Orthop 278:58–61

6 Hulko A, Orava S, Nikula P. Stress fractures of the olecranon in javelin throwers. Int J Sports Med 1986;7:210–212

7 Chan D, Aldridge MJ, Maffulli N, Davies AM. Chronic stress injuries of the elbow in young gymnasts. Br J Radiol 1991;64(768):1113–1118

8 D'Alessandro DF, Shields CL, Tibone JE, Chandler RW. Repair of distal biceps tendon ruptures in athletes. Am J Sports Med 1993;21:114–119

9 Hartz CR, Linsheid RG, Gramse RR. The pronator teres syndrome. Compression neuropathy of the median nerve. J Bone Joint Surg 1981;63(6):885–890

10 Wasilewski SA, Asdourian PL. Bilateral chronic exertional compartment syndromes of forearm in an adolescent athlete: case report and review of literature. Am J Sports Med 1991;19:665–667

## Further reading

Altchek D, Andrews J (eds). The athlete's elbow. Baltimore: Lippincott, Williams and Wilkins; 2001

Bruckner P, Khan K. Clinical sports medicine, 3rd edn. New York: McGraw-Hill; 2006

Hutson MA (ed.). Sports injuries: recognition and management, 2nd edn. Oxford: Oxford Medical Publications; 1996

Hutson M, Ellis R (eds). Textbook of musculoskeletal medicine. Oxford: Oxford University Press; 2006

Reid D. Sports injury assessment and rehabilitation. Edinburgh: Churchill Livingstone; 1992

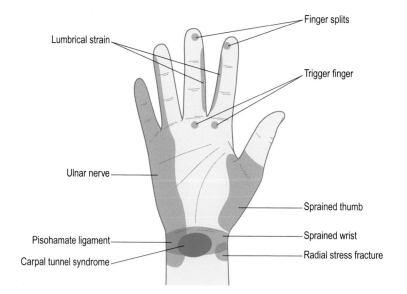

Finger splits

Lumbrical strain

Trigger finger

Ulnar nerve

Sprained thumb

Pisohamate ligament

Sprained wrist

Carpal tunnel syndrome

Radial stress fracture

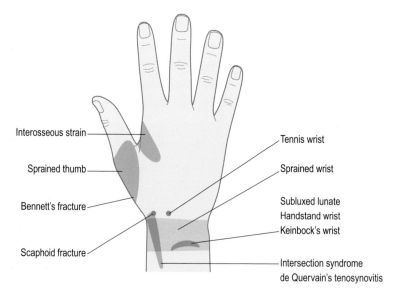

Interosseous strain

Tennis wrist

Sprained thumb

Sprained wrist

Bennett's fracture

Subluxed lunate
Handstand wrist
Keinbock's wrist

Scaphoid fracture

Intersection syndrome
de Quervain's tenosynovitis

# Wrist and hand

## Acute traumatic injuries

Falls, implemental trauma or karate-like blows may produce fractures and internal ligament derangement. X-rays should be taken. The Terry Thomas sign and Watson test suggest scapholunate dissociation, which can cause on-going problems (see Glossary). Particular care, and a high index of suspicion, are required to diagnose scaphoid and hamate fractures. Internal ligamentous damage is difficult to diagnose and often requires an MRI arthrogram. Their general management is for experts in hand and wrist problems. A patient whose wrist pain continues to get worse with activities should be investigated further for lunate and perilunate dislocation, as intracarpal instability can be helped by early surgery before permanent destruction occurs. Finger fractures, avulsions and ligament sprains are common, and, although the adjacent fingers may act as splints, mallet and boutonnière deformities and spiral fractures do require specific management by a hand specialist. The attitude of the open hand and clenched fist will give clues to metacarpal and phalangeal stress fractures. A spiral fracture will distort the alignment. The distal end of the fourth and fifth metacarpals are classically broken by a punch, but a subluxation of the fifth metacarpal and of the proximal end of the second metacarpal also occurs in boxers. Triangular fibrocartilage tears can be caused by impingement, with excessive ulnar deviation, but they are usually traumatic. Imaging the triangular fibrocartilage is difficult, but MRI may show the damage, and an MRI arthrogram may be more definitive, before arthroscopy and repair is undertaken.

# Mallet finger

A rupture of the terminal insertion of the extensor tendon into the distal phalanx is usually caused by a fall, or an implement, such as a ball, striking the digit and forcing the distal interphalangeal joint into flexion. The joint should be splinted into extension and held in a splint for 6 weeks, day and night, followed by night splints for a further 4–6 weeks. If a fracture is present then surgical repair and reattachment of the tendon is required. Some extensor lag is common but gradually reduces.

# Flexor injuries of the fingers

The forces applied by climbers to their flexor tendons are sufficient for the fibrous flexor sheath to be pulled away from the bone, producing a bowstring injury to the A2 pulley, usually of the fourth finger. Small tendon nodules, suggesting old tears, are present and collateral ligament sprains are chronic in climbers [1]. The forces required for climbing will overcome any surgical repair, so this injury is best left alone unless there has been a volar plate rupture, when splinting in 20° of flexion for 1 week and then active range of movement with a 'neighbour' strap is required, but contractions can occur.

## a) Boutonnière deformity

The dorsal fibrous sheath over the proximal interphalangeal joint splits into its lateral bands, a central slip rupture, and allows the joint to flex through the defect. Though this can be caused by systemic problems and respond to surgery, when trauma has been the cause then surgical repair is not strong enough to withstand a return to sport.

## b) Jersey finger

This injury occurs in sports that utilize a grip on the opponent's clothes: martial arts, rugby, illegally in soccer, etc. The opponent breaks clear of the grip by avulsing the tendon from the bone. Commonly, the fourth finger (ring) profundus tendon is avulsed from the distal phalanx and the joint lies in extension. The tendon should be reattached if possible and, if not, then fusion of the joint in neutral to slight flexion is preferred.

## c) Trigger finger

### Findings

There is a history of triggering of the finger, which can sometimes be painful when holding a racket. There may be obvious triggering, with a tender, mobile nodule, palpable on the palmar surface above the metacarpophalangeal joint.

### Cause

A nodule on the flexor tendon of the finger catches as it moves though a stenosis in the flexor sheath, usually over the metacarpophalangeal joint at the entrance to the A1 pulley.

**Caveat**

**Dupuytren's contracture.**

### Investigations

None are clinically required but ultrasound can localize the nodule and guide an injection.

### Treatment

- **(a)** Injection of the tendon sheath stenosis.
- **(b)** Surgery to release the stenosis, by either needle or open surgery.

### Sports

The lesion is not commonly caused by sport, but too large a grip in racket games may effectively bow the flexor tendons, which then become irritated by the pressure of the grip. A reduction of handle size will treat the problem. However, once established, then too small a grip may promote a tight flexion that maintains and irritates the flexor nodule within the stenosis.

### Comment

Many cases of trigger finger are functionally 'cured' without surgery, so it is well worth trying cortisone in the early stages.

# Finger splits

## Findings

Common in implemental games, when a painful, persistent, open linear wound on the pulp of the finger is found. Rock climbers produce an abrasive erosion of the skin at the tips of the fingers [2].

## Cause

Frictional twisting of the finger on the handle splits the skin over the pulp of the finger.

## Investigations

None are clinically required.

## Treatment

(a) Tape the fingers, over the wound, for games and keep clean.
(b) Try using gloves.
(c) Try another handle cover, possibly a soft rubber application, as towelling needs replacing frequently, and dry, worn towelling is often to blame.
(d) Embucrylate, cyanoacrylate, or superglue to 'stick' the split edges together.

## Sports

(a) Implemental games, such as hockey and racket sports (e.g. tennis and badminton).
(b) Climbing.
(c) Some events, such as shot putting, may ban taping in certain forms – check.

## Comment

Finger splits are quite painful and usually occur at the start of the season. Replaceable rubber taping to the handle seems to prevent this injury.

# Lumbrical muscle strain (shot putter's finger)

## Findings

Pain, whilst shot putting, along the medial and lateral borders of the third and fourth fingers. Resisted flexion of the extended phalanges at the metacarpophalangeal joint is painful.

## Cause

A very rare cause of pain in the lumbricals, which are used to flex the fingers, whilst putting the shot.

## Investigations

None are clinically required.

## Treatment

Rest from shot putting. However, the inflammation may respond to local steroids. Taping may ease the injury during practice, but check the current rules as taping is severely limited for competition.

## Comment

Very rare. I have seen only one case. Anabolic steroids may have an influence on tendon strength.

# Interosseous muscle strain

## Findings

Usually occurs in racket players, such as squash players. Pain and tenderness is palpated over the first interosseous muscle, which is also sore on resisted adduction.

## Cause

The index finger is held, stretched, too far along the racket handle, and the index finger applies constant excessive force to the grip, which is opposed by a constant thumb force.

## Investigations

None are clinically required.

## Treatment

(a) Electrotherapeutic modalities to settle inflammation, such as ultrasound and laser.
(b) NSAIDs.
(c) Alter the grip by reducing the extension of the index finger along the racket.

## Sports

Racket games, particularly squash.

## Comment

Some coaching manuals encourage the index finger grip to be laid along the racket handle, but someone always overdoes this grip and applies great force between the thumb and index finger. A simple adjustment in technique improves their squash, and their injury.

# Metacarpal fracture

A fracture of the distal end of the fourth or fifth metacarpal caused, commonly, by punching. If there is rotation caused by a spiral fracture, or if the angle of deviation of the fracture is greater than 40°, then a K wire or plating is required. Discussion continues as to whether boxers should return to their sport with the plates still in situ. Certainly the K wire must be removed. Active range of movement should be obtained as soon as possible. Light 'weights' can be lifted at about 6 weeks, and light impact at 3 months. Full impact on a punch bag may be utilized at 6 months, if there is a good callus and/or sound surgical plating.

# Impingement injuries

The wrist has a rotatory movement between the radius and the ulnar that permits supination and pronation. The major movements are ulnar and radial deviation (and some flexion and extension) between the radius and ulna, on one side, and the proximal carpal bones – scaphoid, hamate and triquetral – on the other. A hinge joint is formed between this proximal row and the distal row of hamate, capitate, trapezoid and trapezium. The hinge movement is especially prone to impingement in extension and distraction of intracarpal ligaments in flexion:

(a) Tennis wrist is caused by impingement of the carpals and metacarpals at the base of the second and third metacarpals, when playing with a full Western grip (Figs 19.1–19.3). Here, the very open hand-grip allows full extension and takes all the impact of the forehand tennis shots over this area. The grip must be weakened to a semi-Western style.

(b) Handstand wrist is an impingement in extension whilst doing a handstand or press-up. Turning the hand out into ulnar deviation will relieve

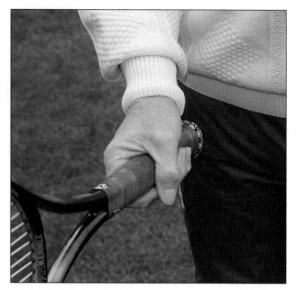

**Figure 19.1** • Standard grip.

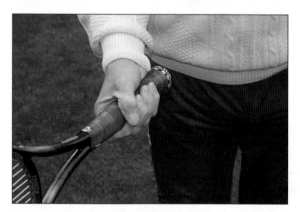

**Figure 19.2** • Semi-Western grip.

this. A half-glove filled with padding over the butt of the hand, or performing press-ups on a pile of books or a bench, so that the wrist is held in a neutral position, aids training.

# Subluxed lunate

The lunate may sublux with wrist flexion. Manipulation and splinting in a cock-up splint may help.

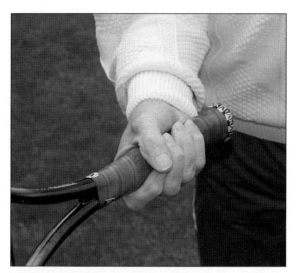

**Figure 19.3** • Western grip.

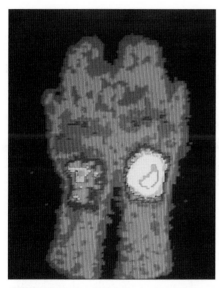

**Figure 19.4** • A positive scan of Keinbock's avascular necrosis of the lunate.

## Keinbock's avascular necrosis of lunate

Rest in a cast brace or cock-up splint may help. Pami-dronate may have a place. Surgery may be required in chronic cases (Fig. 19.4).

## Collateral ligament injuries

### a) Little or fifth finger

In right-handed golfers the little finger may be over-lapped, as opposed to interlocked, with the index finger of the left hand. This can produce a strain of the radial collateral ligament of the metacarpophalangeal joint, or the proximal interphalangeal joint, of the right little finger.

### b) Fourth finger

Nine- or tenpin bowlers usually insert their thumb, index, and fourth finger into the carrying holes drilled into the ball. Many amateurs who use a ball provided by the bowling lanes may find the holes wider apart than they should be using. When some spin is generated on the ball by a pronatory movement, the fourth finger may be strained across the radial collateral ligaments.

### c) Sprained thumb, metacarpophalangeal joint

#### Findings

There is a history of an acute injury, with swelling and bruising of the thenar eminence. Pain is centred in the metacarpophalangeal joint capsule. Passive abduction of the first metacarpophalangeal joint is painful, unless complete rupture has occurred, and the range of move-ment may be increased. However, this range must be checked against the contralateral thumb to establish the normal range of movements, which may be extreme. The patient may not be able to lift a bottle or a glass in a one-hand grip.

#### Cause

Forced abduction of the thumb, such as when the thumb is caught in clothing during a tackle, or forced abduction from a ball or implement, when the ulnar collateral ligament and capsule, and occasionally radial collateral ligament, are damaged.

#### Investigations

X-ray for a flake fracture of the ulnar collateral ligament.

## Treatment

(a) RICE.

(b) NSAIDs.

(c) Strapping of the joint to limit abduction, but encourage flexion and extension.

(d) Electrotherapeutic modalities to settle inflammation, such as ultrasound and laser.

(e) If the joint range is increased, the ligament is torn, and it will require surgery to the ulnar collateral ligament.

## Sports

(a) Strap for activities in sports that permit this form of strapping, strap between the thumb and base of the index finger, to form a web between the fingers.

(b) Skiing – caused by the thumb catching in the diamond of a dry ski slope. A pair of socks worn over the gloves or taping the first metacarpophalangeal joint may help prevent this problem. Safety straps, for ski poles, pull on the thumb when the skier falls. Use release handles on ski poles, or allow the strap to hang over the wrist, so that the straps are not held down by the hand-grip. Thermoplastic thumb splints are appropriate.

## Comment

This is a very common lesion. The major problem occurs in deciding how to strap the thumb in sports that need to hold an implement. Probably it is best to tape during activities, and use an elasticated bandage for normal use. Unfortunately the unstable ulnar collateral ligament is often overlooked.

## Metacarpotrapezial joint

### a) Sprained

### Findings

Either an acute injury or (more usually) one with a gradual onset, and pain at rest, in the metacarpotrapezial joint. The pain is worse with writing, gripping, polishing or picking up a glass. There is pain on extension, circumduction and opponation of this carpophalangeal joint. There is tenderness to palpation over both the dorsal and volar aspect of the joint.

## Cause

Strain of the joint capsule, usually from hyperextension (see Osteoarthritis of the metacarpotrapezial joint and Bennett's avulsion fracture).

## Investigations

If the sprain is failing to progress, then X-ray or CT scan for degenerative changes. Blood test for rheumatoid factors and autoimmune profile should be taken if systemic disease suspected.

### Caveat

**Rheumatoid arthritis.**

## Treatment

(a) NSAIDs.

(b) Injection of cortisone into the first carpometacarpal joint.

(c) Electrotherapeutic modalities that settle inflammation, such as shortwave diathermy and interferential.

(d) Strapping, or a thermoplastic splint, for sport.

## Sports

(a) Fishing – may have to relax thumb pressure on the grip or use the index finger on the top of the rod, as opposed to the thumb, when casting.

(b) Golf – may have to relax thumb pressure on the golf club or thicken the grip. This problem can occur in the left thumb, with a split grip, in either the take away or the follow through with a drawn shot, when the top of the back swing or follow through extends the thumb further. A power fade seems to relieve the pressure on the thumb.

## Comment

An acute flare is a capsulitis, which responds very well in 48 hours to an intra-articular injection of cortisone, but the chronic stresses seem to return with minor loads, and osteoarthritis is often insipient.

## b) Osteoarthritis of the metacarpotrapezial joint (first CMC joint)

Degenerative change is very common in this joint and it responds to conservative measures that are required for a sprained joint (see above). Intra-articular sodium hyaluronate injections can be helpful. A splint or support during activities is essential. Surgical excision of the trapezium or replacement of the trapezium may be required, though both have complications. The grip size may have to be narrowed.

## Bennett's avulsion fracture

### Findings

There is a history of an acute axial injury to the top of the thumb, with swelling and bruising around the thenar eminence. There is a painful, increased range at the first metacarpotrapezial joint in abduction, and the patient cannot hold a wide grip, such as is needed to hold a bottle or glass. Although the range of movement is increased, the painful side must be compared with the normal side on account of the great variation in the normal range that can exist.

### Cause

Abduction, impaction injury, with a transarticular fracture dislocation of the first metacarpal at the metacarpotrapezial joint, in which a small fragment remains held in situ by the strong volar ligament. This fracture may be further graded by the surgeons, into a Rolando Y- and Rolando T-shaped fracture.

### Investigations

X-ray of the thumb (Fig. 19.5).

### Treatment

Immediate cast bracing for comfort, but surgical repair is usually required for stability.

### Sports

Certainly after injury and repair of this joint, and perhaps prophylactically, a thermoplastic splint should be used. This is particularly so for skiing and, if permitted, in any other relevant sport.

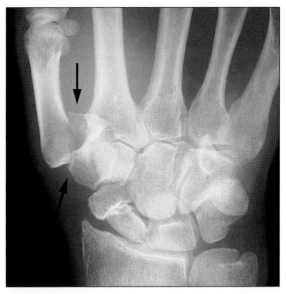

Figure 19.5 • A Bennett's fracture. (Mr John Challis)

Caveat

**A permanent, unstable, weak grip and osteoarthritis will occur if the thumb is not repaired successfully.**

### Comment

This injury is much more likely to end in accident and emergency, where the history of the mechanism of injury and the deformity should alert to the need for X-ray and surgical referral.

## de Quervain's tenosynovitis

### Findings

There is pain over the dorsal, radial aspect of the wrist, which may radiate up over the distal radial half of the forearm. It is worse with resisted or active movement of the abductor pollicis. Finklestein's test is positive (see Glossary).

Type 1   The tendon is tender to palpation and may be swollen as it passes over the radial styloid.

Type 2   The junction where the abductor pollicis tendon is crossed by the extensor communis is tender to palpation, and there may be crepitus in the early stages.

Type 3    Resisted abduction of the thumb is painful over the muscle, due to a tight fascial band or tendon sheath causing stenosis.

## Cause

Tenosynovitis of the abductor pollicis longus and extensor pollicis brevis from overuse, usually with a wide spread grip. The thumb is spread into abduction, such as the feathering hand in rowing, opening jam jars and polishing.

### Caveat

Referral from neck C6/7, arthrosis of the trapezium first metacarpal joint, scaphoid fracture.

## Investigations

None are clinically required, but ultrasound may be of value. MRI can show muscle oedema.

## Treatment

Type 1    Injection of cortisone around the tendon at the radial styloid. If this does not settle after two injections then surgery over the radial styloid to free the tendon sheath will be required.

Type 2    NSAIDs, laser, ultrasound, frictional massage, an injection of cortisone; surgery to free the sheath if progress is not being maintained. It can recur.

Type 3    As for type 2.

## Sports

(a)   Rowing – usually in the feathering wrist, when a smaller oar grip may be tried. The 'gate' for the oar must not be so tight that it resists rotation of the oar. Rough water does not always let the oar clear the water and can produce a resistance to feathering.

(b)   Tenpin bowling – when the 'thumb hole' in the ball is too far away from the finger holes.

(c)   Golf – overforcing the (mainly right) thumb down the handle, with a high wrist – relax the wrist and thumb, or thicken the grip, or place a pad under the thumb, which is equivalent to thickening the grip in this specific area.

(d)   Kayaking – several adaptations of paddle shape are available that may help the grip to reduce the functional spread of the thumb.

(e)   Shooting – the normal stock of the gun can encourage an ulnar-flexed wrist, with a wide abducted thumb. Switching to a pistol style stock will overcome this problem.

(f)   Tennis – too thick a Western-style grip encourages increased abduction of the thumb.

(g)   General – avoid wide abduction of the thumb with daily activities. Many mothers who breast feed support their baby's head in their hand, with the thumb held in a wide abducted position that produces de Quervain's.

## Comment

Rowers often get the 'intersection' de Quervain's, type 2, and some surgeons release the sheath on the first occasion. The radial styloid de Quervain's almost never responds to physiotherapy, so early cortisone and correction of the technical problem is the treatment of choice.

## Intersection syndrome

Pain and swelling over the distal radial forearm, which may have crepitus and be tender to palpation, and is worse with resisted abduction or extension of the thumb (see de Quervain's tenosynovitis, type 2).

## Carpal tunnel syndrome

### Findings

The patient has pain in the wrist and forearm, which may spread more proximally and often wakes the patient at night, when it may be eased with elevation of the hand. There is, classically, numbness and 'pins and needles' of the thumb, index finger and radial side of the middle finger. Because of an anatomical, proximal anastomosis in the forearm that can occur between the ulna and median nerve up to 30% of patients may have referral into the ulnar two fingers. Phalen's test and Tinel's sign may be positive (see Glossary). Kuschner et al [3] suggested that Phalen's test is much more sensitive than the Tinel sign. Wasting of the thenar eminence will be apparent when chronic or severe damage has occurred.

## Cause

Compression of the median nerve as it passes through the carpal tunnel.

## Investigations

Clinically are not required, but when the diagnosis is in doubt:

(a) a trial of local injection therapy into the carpal tunnel

(b) EMG if doubt about the forearm pain exists, but thenar wasting is almost pathognomonic

(c) thyroid function tests should be taken for hypothyroidism, and investigation of causes of systemic or local fluid retention.

## Treatment

(a) Treat the systemic causes long term, and acutely with diuretics, as the reduced swelling may ease the pain.

(b) Injection of cortisone into the carpal tunnel under ultrasound guidance, although this can be performed safely without ultrasound if care is taken to avoid the median nerve.

(c) Surgical release of the retinaculum, especially if muscle wasting is present. Prolonged cases of nerve entrapment may not respond.

**Caveat**

Diuretics may be banned in some sports.

## Sports

Occurs in cycling and motor cycling if the brake or gear levers force the wrist into extension. Tribars may also produce the same problem [4]. Treat by moving the gears downwards, out of the horizontal plane, to lessen wrist extension. Reduce the angle of extension at the wrist when holding tribars.

## Comment

The pain settles well with a cortisone injection and correction of the technical problem, but muscle wasting and failure to respond long term should be treated by surgical release. This is a problem seen in typists and IT workers, owing to their extended wrist position during keyboard use.

# Ulnar neuritis

## Findings

Pain, 'pins and needles' and numbness in the hypothenar eminence and ulnar two fingers (fourth and fifth), but this is not accompanied by weakness, as the motor and sensory nerves divide at the wrist, proximal to Guyon's canal, and only damage more proximal will cause motor weakness as well. There may be a definable sensory disturbance. Pope's and Froment's signs are negative as there are no motor problems (see Glossary; Chapter 18: Ulnar neuritis).

## Cause

Pressure on the ulnar nerve, around the pisiform at Guyon's canal.

**Caveat**

Pisohamate ligament strain, ulnar nerve damage proximal to Guyon's canal, C8/T1 lesion, carpal tunnel and ulnar artery occlusion [5].

## Investigations

An EMG is probably unhelpful, but, if trauma is suspected, an X-ray to exclude a hook of hamate fracture is advisable.

## Treatment

Remove the cause of pressure. Surgery if a hamate fracture or gross pisiform instability is present.

## Sports

(a) Reported in cyclists holding the curve of the handlebars so that the ulnar border is compressed. Pad the handlebars, avoid this grip, and use tribars if permitted, but note that tribars can produce a carpal tunnel syndrome (see above).

(b) Tennis players or golfers may hold the handle at the end of the grip, which digs into the ulnar nerve during the shot. The handle must be held shorter, allowing the end to project beyond the pisiform. This is particularly so with the semi-Western grip and top spun forehand (Figs 19.6 and 19.7).

## Comment

Not a common lesion, it is rarely reported in any other than cyclists (occasionally in golf and racket games) unless accompanied by trauma. Correction of the grip may be curative, and surgery should not be considered until this has been corrected.

## Pisohamate ligament strain

### Findings

Localized pain over the pisiform when using a racket or club. Gliding the pisiform on the hamate to strain the pisohamate ligament reproduces this pain (see Figs 19.6 and 19.7).

### Cause

Pressure on the pisohamate ligaments from implements such as a tennis racket or golf club handle.

### Caveat

**Ulnar nerve compression through Guyon's canal (see Ulnar neuritis).**

## Investigations

None are clinically required, although possibly a hook of hamate view on X-ray for a fracture if there is a history of trauma.

## Treatment

(a) Electrotherapeutic modalities to settle inflammation, such as ultrasound and laser; but beware of the nerve.

(b) Injection of pisohamate ligaments with cortisone.

(c) Correct the cause.

(d) Surgery.

## Sports

(a) Mainly tennis, especially with the semi-Western grip on the forehand shot, with the racket held too near the end of the handle, which therefore digs into the pisiform when rolling the top spun shot. Hold the handle shorter (see Figs 19.6 and 19.7).

(b) Golf – same cause in the left hand as in tennis above, but usually forcing the handle into the pisiform and then being acutely traumatized because the club is blocked, e.g. by a tuft of grass or tree root.

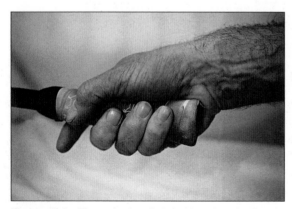

**Figure 19.6** • The racket handle is held too long so that the handle end levers across the pisohamate ligament and Guyon's canal.

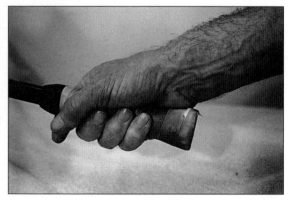

**Figure 19.7** • A correct grip to avoid the problems of Fig. 19.6.

## Comment

Physiotherapy does little and, although an injection helps, avoidance of the cause is most important, and may involve a lay off to allow the ligaments to settle, certainly before surgery is considered.

## Extensor and flexor carpi, ulnaris and radialis insertional strain

Pain at the wrist that is worse with extension and radial deviation (extensor carpi radialis), ulnar deviation (extensor carpi ulnaris), flexion and radial deviation (flexor carpi radialis) and flexion with ulnar deviation (flexor carpi ulnaris) are usually part of a traumatic sprain of the wrist, rather than being produced by a poor technique. They will require standard management of a tendon injury:

(a) RICE, but care must be taken with ice in view of the nearby nerves.

(b) NSAIDs.

(c) Local cortisone to settle inflammation.

(d) Electrotherapeutic modalities to settle inflammation, such as ultrasound and laser.

(e) Massage techniques to prevent scar tissue adhesions, such as frictions.

(f) Isometric loads to organize and lengthen scar tissue, plus maintain muscle strength.

(g) Isotonic and skill-orientated loads using the principle of the general muscle ladder (see Chapter 20).

(h) Surgery may be particularly required for flexor carpi ulnaris tears, as the tendon will often keep subluxing.

## Radial stress fracture and ulnar congruency

### Findings

The adolescent gymnast presents with a gradual onset of pain in the wrist, particularly on the radial volar aspect, which might be associated with a particular gymnastic movement. The lesion is often unilateral in girls and bilateral in boys. The wrist movement is often pain free, but tenderness is palpated over the volar and dorsal surface of distal radius. Volar pain over the distal radius should raise a high index of suspicion of a radial stress fracture.

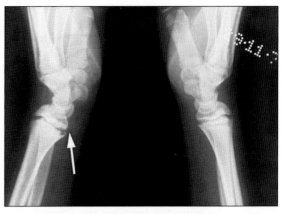

**Figure 19.8** • Lateral X-ray showing a hooked appearance of the radial metaphyseal stress fracure (*arrow*).

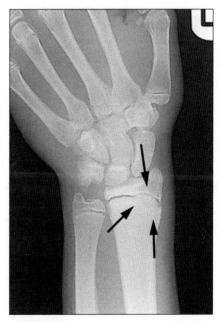

**Figure 19.9** • The more frequently seen 'moth-eaten' early changes in the radial epiphysis (*arrow*).

### Cause

A stress lesion of the radial epiphysis/metaphysis, from repetitive weight-bearing movements of compression and rotation across the wrist. Almost always confined to adolescent gymnasts and tumblers.

### Investigations

(a) X-ray, anteroposterior and lateral (Figs 19.8 and 19.9).

(b) MRI scan.

## Treatment

Rest from compressive exercises, or all arm exercises, for 7–12 weeks. Some gymnasts have been successfully treated by permitting traction exercises, such as training on the asymmetrical bars, balancing on the beam, etc., but stopping compression exercises, such as training on the floor and vault, until healing has occurred [6].

## Sports

Particularly seen in adolescent gymnasts during vaults and floor work, perhaps twisting vaults such as the Tsukahara for girls, and for boys, the Diamadov on parallel bars and pommel horse are causative.

> ### Caveat
>
> Injury may produce premature fusion of the radial epiphysis and a long ulna (ulna congruence, ulnar variance) – effectively a short radius [7,8] (Fig. 19.10).

## Comment

Palpable pain over the volar radial surface must be investigated as a possible stress fracture in adolescent gymnasts or tumblers. The fuzzy, moth-eaten appearance of the metaphysis is diagnostic (see Fig. 19.9). All my cases have healed by just avoiding competitive and causative compression exercises until pain-free.

## Ulnar stress fracture

An unusual stress fracture in the non-dominant arm with a double-handed backhand, with only localized tenderness over the middle third of the ulnar to palpation, and pain on resisted pronation. X-rays were negative and the bone scan positive. Tennis players using a double-handed backhand with these symptoms must be considered as possible stress fractures [9]. It has also been reported in tenpin bowling [10], weightlifting and volleyball players, and is seen in the tennis serve, whilst cutting the serve [11].

## Ulnar digital neuritis of the thumb

Reported in tenpin bowling as a neuropraxic injury to the ulnar digital nerve, with pain, hypersensitivity and

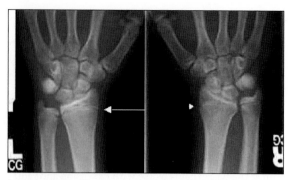

**Figure 19.10 •** Damage to the right radial epiphysis has caused premature fusion of the radius, but the ulnar continues to grow, producing a long ulnar and radial deviation of the wrist. Ulnar congruence.

a thickened palpable nerve, caused by rubbing of the thumb in its thumb hole, which produced fibrosis around the nerve [12].

## References

1 Bollen SR, Gunson CK. Hand injuries in competition climbers. Br J Sports Med 1990;24:16–18

2 Cole AT. Fingertip injuries in rock climbers. Br J Sports Med 1990;24:14

3 Kuschner SH, Ebramzadeh E, Johnson D, Brien WW, Sherman R. Tinel's sign and Phalen's test in carpal tunnel syndrome. J Orthop Med 1996;18(1):24–27

4 Braithwaite IJ. Bilateral median nerve palsy in a cyclist. Br J Sports Med 1992;26:27–28

5 Koga Y, Seki T, Car LD. Hypothenar hammer syndrome in a young female badminton player. A case report. Am J Sports Med 1993;21:890–892

6 Read MTF. Stress fractures of the distal radius in adolescent gymnasts. Br J Sports Med 1981;15:272–276

7 DiFiori JP, Puffer JC, Mandelbaum BR, Dorey F. Distal radial growth plate injury and positive ulnar variance in non elite gymnasts. Am J Sports Med 1997;25:763–768

8 De Smet L, Claessens A, Lefevre J, Beunen G. Gymnast's wrist: an epidemiological survey of ulnar variance and stress changes of the radial physis in elite female gymnasts. Am J Sports Med 1994;22:846–850

9 Bollen SR, Robinson DG, Crichton KJ, Cross MJ. Stress fractures of the ulna in tennis players using a double handed backhand stroke. Am J Sports Med 1993;21:751–752

10 Escher SA. Ulnar diaphyseal stress fracture in a bowler. Am J Sports Med 1997;25:412–413

11 Bell P. Personal discussion after incident at Wimbledon tennis tournament; 2005

12 Dobyns JH, O'Brien ET, Linscheid RL, Farrow GM. Bowler's thumb: diagnosis and treatment. A review of seventeen cases. Am J Bone Joint Surg. 1989;14:241–243

## Further reading

Bruckner P, Khan K. Clinical sports medicine, 3rd edn. New York: McGraw-Hill; 2006

Hutson M, Ellis R (eds). Textbook of musculoskeletal medicine. Oxford: Oxford University Press; 2006

Reid D. Sports injury assessment and rehabilitation. Edinburgh: Churchill Livingstone; 1992

# Chapter **Twenty**

# 20

## Rehabilitation and training with an injury

## General principles of rehabilitation

(a) Rehabilitation needs to be performed little and often, at least three to five times a day. Thirty minutes, three times a week is not sufficient.

(b) Exercises should be developed to train the uninjured parts of the body and maintain cardiovascular fitness, but rest the injured part until the injury can withstand controlled incremental loads.

(c) Athletes are target achievers and will use any method to achieve the goals that are set for them. This will include 'cheating' by developing new skills with which to achieve their current target. This new skill may not be the best skill for the highest levels of performance. For example an injured athlete at point A has to recover to a skill level C. It is better to move slowly along the path to C than rush to skill level point B and then discover that no path links point B to point C. A prime example would be retraining quadriceps, only to find that the fast progress made to achieve a straight leg raise has been made by rotating the tibia externally so that the knee joint is held straight by the articular surfaces locking across the joint, rather than by the quadriceps strength. This athlete is then unable to support a step down, which loads the joint through the knee as opposed to locking the articular surfaces. Later, this athlete will have to stop rehabilitation and return to basics to reprogramme the correct skill.

(d) Rehabilitation of a skill that produces the best performance must not be sacrificed for a skill that enables a return to match play faster but which has a less effective performance.

(e) Target setting should always be positive: 'do this' rather than 'don't do that'.

(f) 'Overload' injuries should not occur in training.

(g) Training must not delay or retard healing.

(h) Skill function and pain should control rehabilitation, not an arbitrary time scale.

(i) It is better to delay a week or two to play at 100% than return and play all season at 90%.

(j) Stretch injured muscles before and after training.

(k) Left to themselves, athletes will tend to train what they are good at; therefore, rehabilitation is the time to work on their weaknesses.

## How much training per session?

There is no perfect answer but, for instance, when training to run, the rhythm between both legs should be balanced, and the injured side should be sharing the load equally with the uninjured side. If the required skill or rhythm breaks down, the speed or loading should not be increased until the rhythm is corrected. Work up to the commencement of pain only, because rolling eyeballs and gritted teeth are for training, not rehabilitation. Within reason, 'wimping out' is permitted.

Pain may occur during rehabilitation or after the session is over, in which case:

(a) If the pain stops immediately on cessation of the activity – continue at this level.

(b) If the pain continues for 20–30 seconds – stop the session! Start the exercise again from the lowest loads at the next training session, or the next day.

(c) If the injury does not hurt at the time but hurts later – use NSAIDs.

(d) If the pain has settled by the following morning – training is within injury tolerance but should not be increased.

(e) If the pain is worse the following morning but settles by midday – training is at the maximum so reduce the load by 10%.

(f) If the pain is worse for the following 24–48 hours – training has been well over the maximum recommended. Rest until the pain has settled. Start again with a considerable reduction in load, about 50%, even if there is no pain at that stage.

(g) Isokinetic training (see Glossary) has the advantage of providing a fast angle of rotation, which has a low resistance, or a slow angle of rotation with a high resistance, and the advantage that the machines will 'quit' when the patient 'quits', thus preventing muscle damage [1].

Always stretch the injured part properly before and after exercising (see Stretching).

## Psychological help

Sometimes, athletes who seem to have all the motivation possible to drive through rehabilitation appear to progress very slowly. Either the clinician or a psychologist should explore the athlete's picture of the internal damage that they have suffered. Invariably this picture is at total odds with the actual healing process. However, athletes envisage their own picture of the problem and often feel that the rehabilitation they are being asked to undertake is going to make them worse. Once they understand the true injury pattern and the nature of healing, and their inbuilt picture has been disabused, they will again make progress.

## Open chain and closed chain exercises

### Open chain exercises

Open chain exercises are those that fix the body, load the distal part, and then move the distal part. Thus leg extension exercises require the athlete to sit, place a weight or resistance over the foot and then extend the knee. This exercise will strengthen the quadriceps but will also produce forces that can translate across the knee joint as well as through the articular surfaces. This can cause problems for the cruciate-deficient knee [2]. These exercises do not train coordination and balance at the same time. Thus, for joint problems closed chain exercise are better, but for muscles either can be used.

### Closed chain exercises

Closed chain exercises, in principle, fix the periphery and work the proximal joints and muscles. Thus, leg presses and press ups are closed chain and the forces travel through the joint, not across it. Coordination can be developed at the same time by performing exercises such as balancing on one leg, squats, hopping and jumping. These have the advantage of training the mechanoreceptors in the joints and the proprioceptive coordination required to balance and move properly, at the same time as building strength.

## How to increment loads

### Non-committal loads

These are exercises that can be aborted at any stage without further damage or harm to the injury, and they may be performed as isometrics, closed chain exercises, counter-balanced weights or resistance elastic bands.

### The 'rule of 7'

This can be used for the above exercises when inviting patients to build them into their normal day, but the timing can be pushed to a 'rule of 10' for full training sessions.

The 'rule of 7' is: 7 seconds work, 7 seconds rest, repeat seven times, preferably seven times a day, but three to five will do and is more achievable for the amateur than a 10 second rule.

### Committal loads

These are movements that once initiated cannot be stopped, or cannot be stopped without damage, such as running, jumping, throwing, hitting and using free weights.

## Early stages of rehabilitation

Should utilize non-committal loads and non-committal exercises. Isometrics should be used in the inner range (with the muscle short), progressing to mid-length, and then the outer range.

## Middle stages of rehabilitation

Committal loads should be added – at low speed and slow acceleration.

## Later stages of rehabilitation

The endurance of the committal movement is built up, and then speed and acceleration is incremented.

(a) Weights – use body weight and build up repetitions until the patient can handle 25–30 repetitions, and then increase the weight by, for instance 2 kg, until the patient can manage 25–

30 repetitions, and then continue in the same way until the desired weight is reached.

(b) Running – run 1500 metres at 10 min/km pace. If there is no flare of the injury to this, increase the speed in stages, such as 9, 8 and 7 : 30 min/ km running pace, until the desired running pace is reached. Run each speed on two occasions, without problems, before increasing the speed. When the desired running speed is reached then increase the distance, but drop the speed down to 10 min/km pace and repeat, as above, until the desired speed and distance are again reached. The distance should be incremented more slowly, probably in 1500 metre steps after the first 3 km.

(c) Hitting, throwing and kicking – these should be performed at slow speed, over short distance, until 25–30 repetitions produce no reaction, and then increase the distance of the throw, kick, or hit, still at a slow speed, until the limit of easy movement is reached, and then reduce distance and increase the speed or force, gradually moving out the distance. Finally return to a short distance in order to increase speed and force up to the desired power.

## Final stages of rehabilitation

Add pliometrics, such as bounding and depth jumping, and use the rehabilitation ladders (see the end of this chapter).

## Principles of the training ladders

The training ladders are designed not only to increment loads on the target muscles but also to give time for the correct skills to be redeveloped. A trick movement may have been incorporated previously to get round the problem (e.g. turning the foot out to run off the posterior tibialis rather than the injured Achilles), but this movement is not the most efficient to achieve the end point skill, so it must be eliminated and the correct movement skill reintroduced (see General principles of rehabilitation (c)). The stop points for moving up the ladder are pain lasting 20–30 seconds (see How much training?) or failure to put together the correct rhythm. Rhythm, which is a way of checking movement skill and, in running, that one leg is working as hard as the other, is a vital ingredient of rehabilitation. Some people may find counting can impose a flow of rhythm to the body. This counting should be to an odd number, not lower than 9. The patient feels, say, the right leg movement on counts 1, 3, 5, 7, and 9, and matches the left leg on 2, 4, 6, and 8. However, the next cycle will count the left leg as 1, thus switching the odd numbers to the left leg. Patients automatically switch their concentration between both legs, so that a flow of rhythm is maintained. Do not let patients be logical, but just make them pick up the rhythm from the good leg, and try to match it on the bad leg. If they cannot put together the skills to maintain rhythm at the lower stages of the ladder, they certainly will not be able to put these skills together at the top end, and, although they return to the sporting field, their ultimate skills will remain severely compromised. Each new training session should be started at the bottom of the ladder, but once the higher stages are reached then the first stages can be reduced to warm up, i.e. only one or two repetitions. The ladders must be looked upon as skill training (running is a skill), and not fitness training, although they will take on both roles at the later stages.

## Cross-training

Aerobic fitness, and to a certain extent anaerobic fitness, may be maintained by removing impact or by changing a technique so that the injury is rested but the heart and lungs are exercised. This is known as cross-training. For instance, 'pattering' is low-load impact cross-training and 'cycling' is non-impact cross-training.

### Patter routine

This simple exercise is effective in raising the pulse rate and building fitness without straining the knees or hips. It also takes up very little time. Quality, not quantity, is vital in fitness training. The secret to pattering is not to lift the feet far off the ground. A slow patter is more like a fast jog on the spot, with the knees kept low. The feet must be lifted only 2.5–5 cm off the floor. A fast patter has the same low knee and foot lift, but pattering is done as fast as possible. It is testing, but simple.

#### Routine for an unfit athlete (3 minutes)

| | |
|---|---|
| 1 min | slow patter |
| 5 s | fast patter |
| 50 s | slow patter |
| 5 s | fast patter |
| 50 s | slow patter |
| 10 s | fast patter |

Rest for 3 minutes, whilst doing stretching exercises. Repeat the above routine at least twice, preferably four times.

#### Routine for a fairly fit athlete (5 minutes)

| | |
|---|---|
| 50 s | slow patter |
| 10 s | fast patter |
| 40 s | slow patter |
| 20 s | fast patter |
| 50 s | slow patter |
| 10 s | fast patter |
| 30 s | slow patter |
| 10 s | fast patter |
| 50 s | slow patter |
| 30 s | fast patter |

Then rest for 3 minutes, whilst doing stretching exercises. Repeat the above training routine at least once, preferably three times.

#### Routine for a fit athlete (16 minutes)

Perform the routine as for the unfit athlete once, followed immediately by the routine for the fairly fit athlete, repeat.

### Skipping routine

If the patient is good at skipping, use the same timing as for the patter routines. This gives the calf muscles a particularly good workout.

### Swimming routine

Swimming is an excellent way to keep the muscles toned up, especially when the patient cannot 'run through' an injury. The water supports the body's weight but does not offer great resistance. Although less muscle power is required, the pulse rate is still raised by swimming. Running in water whilst using a flotation jacket for stability may be used instead of actual swimming. The patient should not just run with a high knee lift but take large strides, really pulling with the hamstrings, trying to mimic their running style.

#### Routine for a poor swimmer/non-swimmer

The athlete should jump in, swim or flounder across the width of the pool, climb out using the good leg and stand up, turn around, and then repeat the routine for 3–5 minutes. After the exercise, the patient should rest for 3 minutes while doing stretching exercises. Repeat the above routine at least twice, preferably three times.

## Routine for a good swimmer

As above, but swim one length of the pool each time.

## Rowing routine

A rowing machine is required for this. It gives a thorough workout for legs, arms and abdominal muscles, and also builds up stamina. Untrained rowers will find this much harder work than expected. Lying back at the end of each stroke will exercise the stomach muscles. The hand grip can be varied, either over the top or underneath, if the arm muscles ache. Patients with knee problems should not drop the knees out to the side but try and keep them in line with the first and second toes as they move backwards and forwards. Drawing a mark over the midline of the knee caps will help to keep the knees in line. Make sure the athlete presses equally hard with both legs, trying to get both knees to travel at the same rate, especially when locking them straight. Patients with back problems should 'core stabilize' their back and should not reach too far forwards, or lay back at the end of the stroke.

## Routine for patients doing long-distance/ stamina events

The patient should be able to carry on a conversation, even if they are panting a bit, and exercise for at least 10 minutes, although more than 30 minutes is preferable.

## Routine for patients doing middle-distance events and running ball games

This should include aerobic and anaerobic training such as 2 minutes long distance, 1 minute sprint followed by a 3 minute rest. To be repeated as often as required.

## Routine for sprint events and martial arts

Exercise with at least 30 hard strokes per minute, for 1–2 minutes. Rest for 5 minutes. Repeat as often as required.

## Cycling routine

This removes impact from the ankles, knees and hips, and avoids jarring the back, whilst still allowing an excellent workout for heart and lungs. It may be done on a stationary exercise bike in a gym or on an ordinary pedal cycle out on the road. For stamina training athletes should use easy low gears, at a pace where they are able to talk whilst only slightly panting, but, for sprint training, harder, higher gears are used. Those with knee problems should keep the knees vertical over the first and second toes to avoid a varus or valgus action at the knee, and try to take up pedal pressure at the top of the pedal cycle, not half way down when it becomes easier. Count for rhythm.

## Routine for long-distance running

The time on the bike should be equal to the time normally spent training on foot, but over a much longer distance, preferably 2–2.5 times longer than they would usually run. Few of us have the skill to move a bike that fast, but it is the approximate physiological equivalent.

## Routine for middle-distance running and ball games (5 minutes)

4.5 min   stamina training
30 s      sprint training

Rest for 3 minutes, while doing stretching exercises. Repeat at least twice, preferably four times.

## Routine for sprint events, strength events, volleyball, basketball, etc. (5 minutes)

2 min    stamina training
30 s     sprint training
90 s     stamina training
1 min    sprint training

Rest for 4 minutes, while doing stretching exercises. Repeat at least twice, preferably four times.

## Change of direction training

(a) Cross-over steps. This is a sideways step sequence, crossing one foot in front and then behind the other. This works the hip adductors and the ligaments of the knees and ankles.

(b) Side to side steps. Step sideways, draw the other leg up to the first, and repeat with the first leg abducting sideways. This can be done at speed.

(c) Figure-of-eight runs particularly stress the ligaments of the knees and the ankles. The arc of the '8' can be reduced to increase the stresses on the ligaments.

(d) Side stepping. Run in a straight line and add in side steps.

(e) Shuttle or doggy runs. Sprint out to a mark, turn as fast as possible and sprint back.

(f) Kicking a ball against a wall. Kick the ball with the inside or outside of the foot. This stresses ankle and knee ligaments.

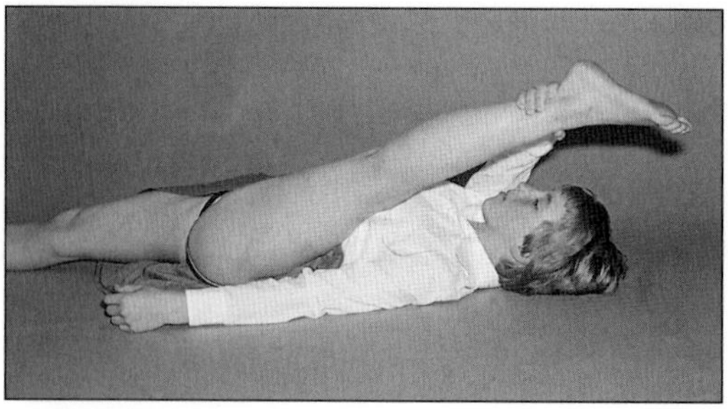

**Figure 20.1** • Passive stretching is limited only by joint range and soft tissue abutment!

## Stretching

(a) Increases the number of sarcomeres.

(b) Stresses the stretch elastic component of the muscle/tendon complex.

(c) Can reset the gamma efferents, which control muscle tension, allowing a fuller range of movement.

(d) Can prevent adhesions following injury.

(e) Provides a low load across the scar tissue, helping to orientate healing fibroblasts.

Static stretching does not prevent injuries.

## Methods of stretching

### General

Stretching is for the antagonist, which is the muscle that resists the direction of movement, and should be done with a relaxed, passive muscle, which is achieved by breathing out and relaxing to reduce muscle tension whilst the stretch is employed.

### Passive stretching

This type of stretching is limited by joint range and soft tissue abutment (Fig. 20.1).

### Proprioceptive neuromuscular facilitation

This is a method that tries to enhance the relaxation for passive stretching.

Method 1   Actively works the antagonist against the resistance of the therapist, and then relaxes this muscle while the agonist is passively stretched by the therapist.

Method 2   The antagonist should relax when the agonist is worked, so the therapist resists the agonist, the muscle that initiates the movement, gradually stretching the antagonist at the same time [3].

### Active stretching

This requires muscle work from the agonist and relaxation from the antagonist.

### Yoga stretching

This allows the gamma efferents, which control muscle tone, to be reset, producing long-term elongation, and does not habituate protective spasm from an injury.

### Bounce stretching

Habituates protective spasm from an injury and does not permanently lengthen the tendon muscle complex, but it does increase teno-osseous junction strength [4].

### Ballistic stretching

Actively kicking a straight leg raise into the air, with increasing rapidity, will train the hamstrings (which are decelerating this movement) to decelerate the movement over a longer arc. EMG shows that the hamstring actively decelerates the swing phase of running so that the leg is braced ready for impact, and this combination of agonist and antagonist contracting together is known as coactivation [5]. If the hamstring is stretched forcibly, it will encourage a contraction when the knee is nearly straight. Thus jumping into 'front back' splits and 'hurdle' stretches, if forced, may recruit active hamstring contraction at the very moment that relaxation is required, and therefore must be trained as a ballistic movement, or done slowly, with relaxation of the target muscle group at the end of range [5].

## Caveat

**I have seen several hamstring avulsions of the ischial tuberosity, from forced intentional stretching of the hamstring (see Fig. 9.1).**

## Stretching pre-exercise

(a) Gently warm up first.

(b) Active yoga stretch for muscle relaxation for 15–20 seconds.

(c) Passive stretch using gravity, or a partner for muscle relaxation, of both agonist and antagonist [6,7].

(d) Bounce stretch for teno-osseous strength [4].

(e) Ballistic stretch for muscle coactivation [5].

(f) Slow mimic of sport activities.

(g) Stretch on warm down.

## Stretching for injury

(a) Gently warm up.

(b) Active yoga stretch to stretch out scar tissue.

(c) Proprioceptive neuromuscular facilitation stretch, for scar tissue.

(d) Ballistic stretch, for scar tissue and muscle coactivation.

(e) Stretch on warm down.

(f) The warm up can slowly mimic activities required by the game, and this, therefore, encourages both active and ballistic stretching [4].

## Useful simple stretches

- Calf stretches (Figs 20.2 and 20.3).
- Hamstrings (Fig. 20.4).
- Quadriceps (Fig. 20.5).
- Adductors (Fig. 20.6).
- Spine (Figs 20.7 and 20.8).
- Shoulders (Fig. 20.9).
- Hamstring, quadriceps, and adductors (Fig. 20.10).

## Proprioception

Mechanoreceptors in the joints, and the position sense in space, are enhanced by balancing exercises. However, if the eyes can be removed from helping the patient to

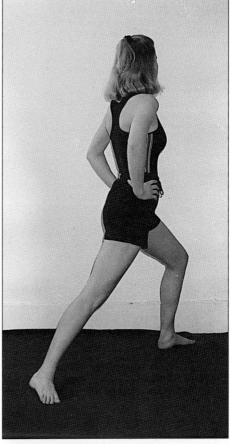

**Figure 20.2** • Gastrocnemius stretch of the back leg. The knee and foot must be kept straight. However, the turned out foot shown here increases the range of forward movement but achieves less stretch of the calf.

balance, then the mechanoreceptors must contribute more. So balances may be done with the eyes shut or, on a busy day, by balancing whilst brushing the hair, cleaning teeth or talking on the telephone, because doing something else stops the eyes and brain from helping the balance This makes the mechanoreceptors contribute more, which is of course more representative of normal life. Proprioception can also be enhanced by support strapping, which recruits the skin receptors into providing additional positional information [8].

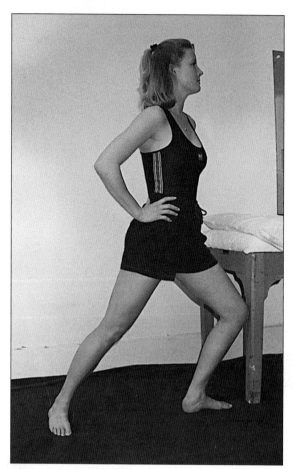

Figure 20.3 • Soleus stretch of the front leg with the knee bent.

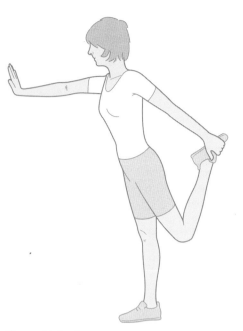

**Figure 20.5** • Quadriceps stretch. Stand on the right leg and hold the left foot in the left hand, and pull the left knee backwards, keeping the back straight. When the pull is felt in front of the thigh, breathe out, and hold for 20 seconds. Now stretch the knee away from the bottom. Keep the knee in line with the hips to stretch the quadriceps and the iliotibial band. Repeat exercise on the other side.

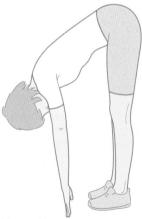

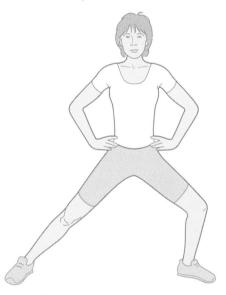

**Figure 20.4** • Hamstring stretch. Stand upright with feet wide apart and hands on hips. Push the bottom backwards, then pivot forwards from the hips with the back straight and the chest forward, and reach out towards the feet. Rolling the spine down from the shoulders does not achieve a full hamstring stretch.

**Figure 20.6** • Adductor stretch. Stand with the feet wide apart, bend the left knee but keep the weight over the straight leg and do not lean forwards. When a pull is felt in the groin of the straight leg, increase the stretch by leaning further over the straight leg, keep the bottom in, and breathe out. Repeat exercise to the other side.

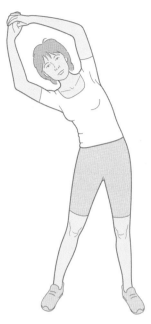

**Figure 20.7** • Stand comfortably and clasp the hands at full stretch above the head. Keep the trunk upright and lean sideways, not forwards, until a pull is felt down the opposite side. Breathe out. Repeat to the other side.

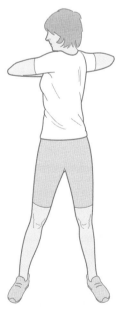

**Figure 20.8** • Stand comfortably with hands clasped in front of the chest and slowly rotate the body to the right. Breathe out. Repeat to the other side.

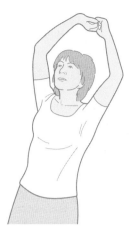

**Figure 20.9** • Clasp the hands behind and slightly above the head. Press the shoulders and arms backwards. Breathe out.

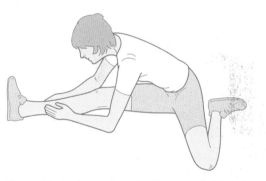

**Figure 20.10** • Hamstring, quadriceps and adductor stretch. Try to get the legs at right angles with the back leg bent, then keeping the back straight try to place the chest over the straight leg. When a pull is felt at the back of the knee, hold the stretch and breathe out. It is essential not to force this movement as this can damage the ischial hamstring attachment. Leaning backwards in line with the straight leg will stretch the adductors and quadriceps of the bent leg. Repeat on the other side.

## Prophylactic strapping

Evidence from American basketball teams suggests that this does help reduce the number of ankle sprains. However, no increased protection from knee injury has been shown. Fingers and wrists seem to benefit, and thermoplastic splints for skiers' thumbs are invaluable. Sometimes strapping a muscle may be of help, possibly by acting as an exoskeleton so that the muscle achieves purchase on the support, which reduces the loads being transferred to its tendons. A particular example may be the tennis elbow supports. Some prophylactic strapping requires 'underwrap' and metres of tape to be purchased, and these can be replaced by custom-made plastic, pneumatic, Velcro, or lace-up supports [8].

# Convenient home rehabilitation

Most sportspeople are amateurs, with jobs to hold down, and exercises should be built into their working day if possible. They may attend two physiotherapy sessions a week for 15 minutes, which is hardly sufficient, but as they improve or run out of money, this attendance will be rapidly abandoned. They will have to be given formal exercises at home, although some exercises can be designed for the journey or workplace.

## General proprioceptive exercises for ankle, knee, hip and back

Balance on one leg whilst cleaning the teeth, brushing the hair, putting on clothes, answering the telephone or waiting for the train, and indeed standing on the train.

## Quadriceps and proprioceptive exercises

Balance, and hold a half knee squat on one leg, whilst doing the general exercises above. Walk upstairs placing the whole foot flat on each tread, so that no additional thrust is obtained from the calf, and propulsion is obtained only from the quadriceps. Walk slowly down stairs or slopes, trying to hold the rhythm consistent between both legs.

## Calves

These should be trained one at a time by doing heel raises on one leg whilst, for example, waiting for a train, cleaning the teeth or answering the phone.

## Hamstrings

Very adequate eccentric and concentric work can be performed at home by lying supine on the floor and placing the heels on the seat of a chair. Then raise one's backside as high as possible off the ground and then lower it back to the floor again. This can be performed fast or slow, one legged or both legged, with the knees bent or nearly straight, and is referred to as 'chair raises' (see Glossary: Chair test).

# Isometrics using the 'rule of 7' (see The 'rule of 7')

(a) Peroneals. Cross the ankles, with plantar flexed feet, and force the outside of both feet against each other. Do not turn the foot so that the tibialis anterior is doing the work.

(b) Posterior tibialis. Push the big toe joint of the target foot against the inside heel of the other foot.

(c) Tibialis anterior and flexor hallucis. Pull the dorsum of the foot and great toe up into the sole of the other foot.

(d) Quadriceps and hamstrings. Sit on a desk, cross the ankles and push away with the hindmost foot to extend the knee and work the quadriceps of that leg, whilst pulling back with the front leg heel, into the ankle of the back foot, to work the hamstrings of the other. This can be done sitting on the train, if required.

(e) External hip rotators. Whilst standing, tighten the buttocks, drive the knees straight and externally rotate the knees (the movement comes from the hip, but the patient often understands this phrase better). This then may be done whilst standing on one leg, and then drop into a half squat balance on this leg. However, the knee must not be allowed to drift into valgus, the foot of the unsupported leg swing behind the other leg, nor the anterior superior iliac spine on the ipsilateral side swing forward. All of these unwanted movements are produced by the external rotators of the hip being weak (Figs 20.11 and 20.12).

(f) The rotator cuff of the shoulder may be exercised by isometrics against the resistance of the restraining other hand. External rotation for the infraspinatus, internal rotation for subscapularis, and elbow abduction, from a position tucked in to the side, for supraspinatus. The drop tests may be used for rehabilitation (see Glossary: Drop tests for the shoulder).

(g) Exercises for tennis elbow can incorporate: with the elbow held straight, resisted extension of the wrist, and then, as the pain settles, resist the extended fingers against the other hand.

(h) Exercise for golfer's elbow may include pressing the pulps of the fingers into the trapezius and trying to pronate the target hand against the resistance of the other hand.

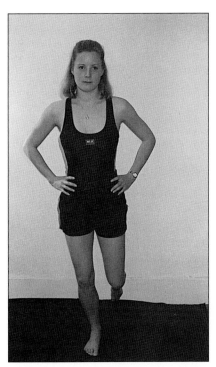

**Figure 20.11** • The half-knee squat. The pelvic stabilizers and external rotators of the hip have held the knee in line over the foot.

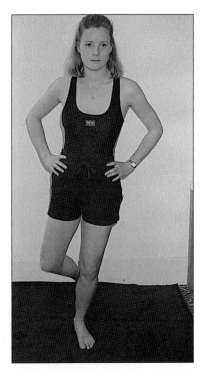

**Figure 20.12** • The dropping down of the left hand on the anterior superior iliac spine shows that the left pelvis has rotated forward, allowing the right leg to swing behind the left leg. The pelvic and hip stabilizers are not controlling stability and tracking problems will ensue.

(i) Biceps isometrics, such as pulling the forearm up to the shoulder, can be done against the resistance of the contralateral hand.

## Rehabilitation ladders

See the following 13 pages.

## General muscle ladder

At levels 7 or 8 of the general muscle ladder, use closed chain rather than open chain work for the legs.

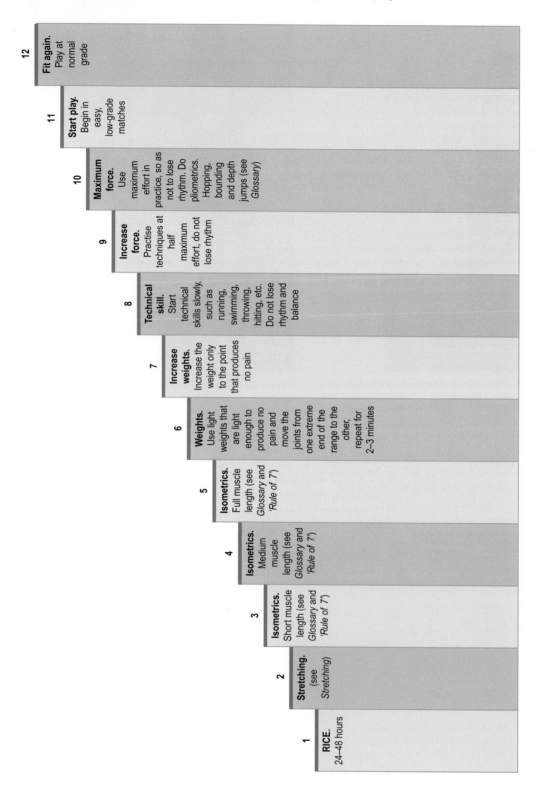

**12 Fit again.** Play at normal grade

**11 Start play.** Begin in easy, low-grade matches

**10 Maximum force.** Use maximum effort in practice, so as not to lose rhythm. Do pliometrics. Hopping, bounding and depth jumps (see *Glossary*)

**9 Increase force.** Practise techniques at half maximum effort, do not lose rhythm

**8 Technical skill.** Start technical skills slowly, such as running, swimming, throwing, hitting, etc. Do not lose rhythm and balance

**7 Increase weights.** Increase the weight only to the point that produces no pain

**6 Weights.** Use light weights that are light enough to produce no pain and move the joints from one extreme end of the range to the other, repeat for 2–3 minutes

**5 Isometrics.** Full muscle length (see *Glossary* and *Rule of 7*)

**4 Isometrics.** Medium muscle length (see *Glossary* and *Rule of 7*)

**3 Isometrics.** Short muscle length (see *Glossary* and *Rule of 7*)

**2 Stretching.** (see *Stretching*)

**1 RICE.** 24–48 hours

## Quadriceps ladder, strength

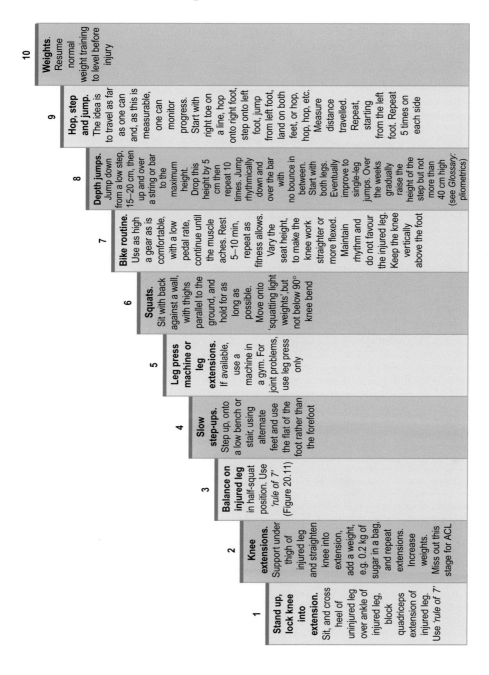

**1. Stand up, lock knee into extension.** Sit, and cross heel of uninjured leg over ankle of injured leg, block quadriceps extension of injured leg. Use *'rule of 7'*

**2. Knee extensions.** Support under thigh of injured leg and straighten knee into extension, add a weight, e.g. 0.2 kg of sugar in a bag, and repeat extensions. Increase weights. Miss out this stage for ACL

**3. Balance on injured leg** in half-squat position. Use *'rule of 7'* (Figure 20.11)

**4. Slow step-ups.** Step up, onto a low bench or stair, using alternate feet and use the flat of the foot rather than the forefoot

**5. Leg press machine or leg extensions.** If available, use a machine in a gym. For joint problems, use leg press only

**6. Squats.** Sit with back against a wall, with thighs parallel to the ground, and hold for as long as possible. Move onto 'squatting light weights', but not below 90° knee bend

**7. Bike routine.** Use as high a gear as is comfortable, with a low pedal rate, continue until the muscle aches. Rest 5–10 min, repeat as fitness allows. Vary the seat height, to make the knee work straighter or more flexed. Maintain rhythm and do not favour the injured leg. Keep the knee vertically above the foot

**8. Depth jumps.** Jump down from a low step, 15–20 cm, then up and over a string or bar to the maximum height. Drop this height by 5 cm then repeat 10 times. Jump rhythmically down and over the bar with no bounce in between. Start with both legs. Eventually improve to single-leg jumps. Over the weeks gradually raise the height of the step but not more than 40 cm high (see *Glossary:* pliometrics)

**9. Hop, step and jump.** The idea is to travel as far as one can and, as this is measurable, one can monitor progress. Start with right toe on a line, hop onto right foot, step onto left foot, jump from left foot, land on both feet, or hop, hop, hop, etc. Measure distance travelled. Repeat, starting from the left foot. Repeat 5 times on each side

**10. Weights.** Resume normal weight training to level before injury

## Quadriceps ladder, heart and lungs

The heart and lung ladder builds up stamina. To rebuild muscle strength, use the strength ladder. These two may be used in parallel. Competitors in power events should concentrate on strength, whilst speed and endurance competitors will find the heart and lungs ladder more appropriate. Competitors in most ball games will use both ladders.

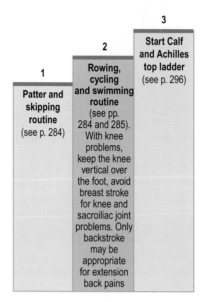

**3**

**Start Calf and Achilles top ladder** (see p. 296)

**2**

**Rowing, cycling and swimming routine** (see pp. 284 and 285). With knee problems, keep the knee vertical over the foot, avoid breast stroke for knee and sacroiliac joint problems. Only backstroke may be appropriate for extension back pains

**1**

**Patter and skipping routine** (see p. 284)

## Knee ladder

The knee should be strapped or braced for the first 6 weeks of match play. This ladder should be started only after level 7 of the Achilles or hamstring top ladder has been reached. Kicking can start at the same time. Using a soccer ball:

1 Standing 2 metres away from a wall, kick using the side foot and instep.

2 Move 6 metres from the wall and repeat kicking.

3 With a partner, gradually move further apart.

Using a football or rugby ball:

4 Kick from the hand (caressing the ball).

5 Hard punt.

6 Hard kick from the ground.

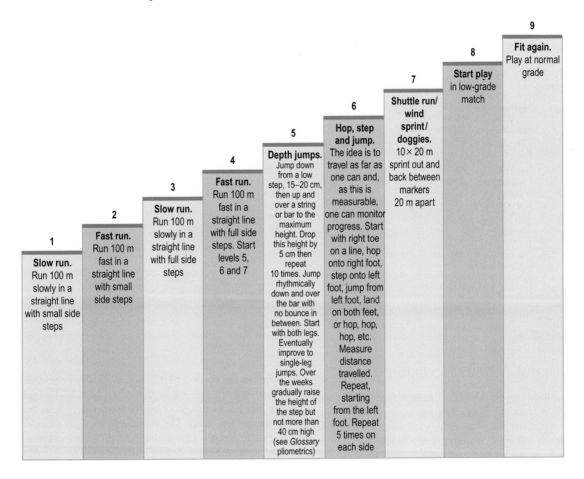

**1 Slow run.** Run 100 m slowly in a straight line with small side steps

**2 Fast run.** Run 100 m fast in a straight line with small side steps

**3 Slow run.** Run 100 m slowly in a straight line with full side steps

**4 Fast run.** Run 100 m fast in a straight line with full side steps. Start levels 5, 6 and 7

**5 Depth jumps.** Jump down from a low step, 15–20 cm, then up and over a string or bar to the maximum height. Drop this height by 5 cm then repeat 10 times. Jump rhythmically down and over the bar with no bounce in between. Start with both legs. Eventually improve to single-leg jumps. Over the weeks gradually raise the height of the step but not more than 40 cm high (see *Glossary* pliometrics)

**6 Hop, step and jump.** The idea is to travel as far as one can and, as this is measurable, one can monitor progress. Start with right toe on a line, hop onto right foot, step onto left foot, jump from left foot, land on both feet, or hop, hop, hop, etc. Measure distance travelled. Repeat, starting from the left foot. Repeat 5 times on each side

**7 Shuttle run/ wind sprint/ doggies.** 10 × 20 m sprint out and back between markers 20 m apart

**8 Start play** in low-grade match

**9 Fit again.** Play at normal grade

## Calf and Achilles bottom ladder

**1**

**RICE.**
24–48 hours. Elevate heels with a heel raise. If appropriate, wear high heels

**2**

**Encourage active plantarflexion**, followed by active dorsiflexion to pain. Start stages 3, 4, 5 and 6

**3**

**Stretching.**
See Figures 20.2 and 20.3

**4**

**Buttock strength.**
On all fours, bring the knee up to the chest, then swing the leg backwards and upwards, the heel swings towards the back of the head. Use gluteal exercise machine in the gym

**5**

**Non-impact cross-training** via swimming and rowing routines (see pp. 284 and 285). May have to place pedal under arch of foot and later move to ball of foot

**6**

**Heels.**
Do plantarflexed heel raises with both feet together to 20–25 repetitions. Do not work through pain. When successful, start one-legged heel raise to 20–25 repetitions

**7**

**Heel drops on staircase.**
Stand with balls of feet on staircase. Drop the heels as low as possible below the stair, and then rise to tiptoe, repeat. Start with both legs together. When 20–25 can be done pain-free, use one leg

**8**

**Hop test.**
When 50 pain-free hops can be completed on the injured leg, move to Calf and Achilles top ladder. This is a test, not a training session

## Calf and Achilles top ladder

Continue cross-training, for fitness. Start each training session from the bottom of the ladder. Perform six of stage 1, then six of stage 2, etc., until pain or loss of rhythm halts the training. Early ladder steps may be cut from six to two repetitions when working at the higher stages. Check that the leg rhythm is equal and do not gallop. One way to avoid favouring an injured leg is to count from 1 to 9 whilst running, which sets a rhythm for the legs to follow and allows concentration to move from one leg to the other. Match the feel of the bad leg to the good leg, counting 1, 2; 1, 2; tends to stress any limp. Do stretching exercises between each 100 metres. Check that heel pick up and knee lift are the same height. Stop if any pain lasts for more than 20–30 seconds, and do not progress up the ladders if there is loss of rhythm.

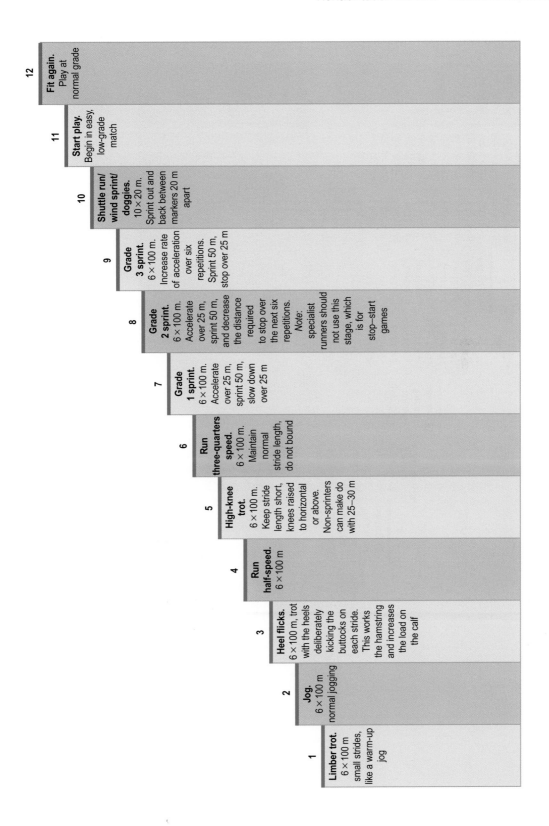

**1** Limber trot. 6 × 100 m small strides, like a warm-up jog

**2** Jog. 6 × 100 m normal jogging

**3** Heel flicks. 6 × 100 m, trot with the heels deliberately kicking the buttocks on each stride. This works the hamstring and increases the load on the calf

**4** Run half-speed. 6 × 100 m

**5** High-knee trot. 6 × 100 m. Keep stride length short, knees raised to horizontal or above. Non-sprinters can make do with 25–30 m

**6** Run three-quarters speed. 6 × 100 m. Maintain normal stride length, do not bound

**7** Grade 1 sprint. 6 × 100 m. Accelerate over 25 m, sprint 50 m, slow down over 25 m

**8** Grade 2 sprint. 6 × 100 m. Accelerate over 25 m, sprint 50 m, and decrease the distance required to stop over the next six repetitions. *Note:* specialist runners should not use this stage, which is for stop–start games

**9** Grade 3 sprint. 6 × 100 m. Increase rate of acceleration over six repetitions. Sprint 50 m, stop over 25 m

**10** Shuttle run/ wind sprint/ doggies. 10 × 20 m. Sprint out and back between markers 20 m apart

**11** Start play. Begin in easy, low-grade match

**12** Fit again. Play at normal grade

## Hamstring bottom ladder

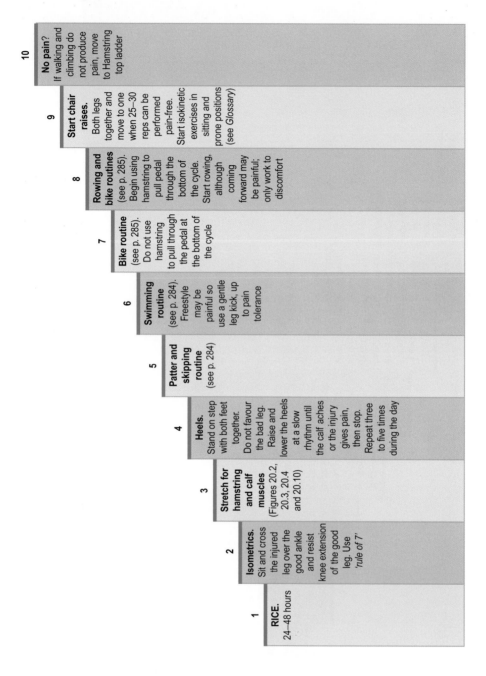

**1**
RICE. 24–48 hours

**2**
Isometrics. Sit and cross the injured leg over the good ankle and resist knee extension of the good leg. Use 'rule of 7'

**3**
Stretch for hamstring and calf muscles (Figures 20.2, 20.3, 20.4 and 20.10)

**4**
Heels. Stand on step with both feet together. Do not favour the bad leg. Raise and lower the heels at a slow rhythm until the calf aches or the injury gives pain, then stop. Repeat three to five times during the day

**5**
Patter and skipping routine (see p. 284)

**6**
Swimming routine (see p. 284). Freestyle may be painful so use a gentle leg kick, up to pain tolerance

**7**
Bike routine (see p. 285). Do not use hamstring to pull through the pedal at the bottom of the cycle

**8**
Rowing and bike routines (see p. 285). Begin using hamstring to pull pedal through the bottom of the cycle. Start rowing, although coming forward may be painful; only work to discomfort

**9**
Start chair raises. Both legs together and move to one when 25–30 reps can be performed pain-free. Start isokinetic exercises in sitting and prone positions (see *Glossary*)

**10**
No pain? If walking and climbing do not produce pain, move to Hamstring top ladder

## Hamstring top ladder

**Use Achilles ladder** but switch stages 3 and 5. Add in the bean bag run after stage 10.

**Bean bag shuttle**. As for stage 10, but incorporate bending to touch or pick up an object, such as a bean bag, from the floor

Continue cross-training for fitness. Start each training session from the bottom of the ladder. Perform six of stage 1, then six of stage 2, etc., until pain or loss of rhythm halts the training. Early ladder steps may be reduced from six to two repetitions when working at the higher stages. Check that the leg rhythm is equal, and do not gallop. One way to avoid favouring an injured leg is to count from 1 to 9 whilst running, which sets a rhythm for the legs to follow. Match the feel of the bad leg to the good leg. Counting 1, 2; 1, 2; tends to stress any limp. Check heel pick up and knee lift are the same height. Stop if any pain lasts for more than 20–30 seconds, and do not progress up the ladders if there is loss of rhythm. Start using a ballistic stretch between each 100 metres by swinging the leg into a high kick, like a ballet dancer (see Stretching), slowly to the point of discomfort. As the injury improves, build up the speed of the leg swing, especially in kicking sports.

## Badminton ladder

This is for tennis elbow and shoulder injuries. Work with a willing partner for 5 minutes at each step, but start each training session from the beginning. Stop at the first sign of pain, but continue if the pain settles within 20 seconds. Otherwise stop, wait 24 hours then repeat from the first step (see How much training?). Concentrate grip on third, fourth and fifth fingers; relax second finger and thumb.

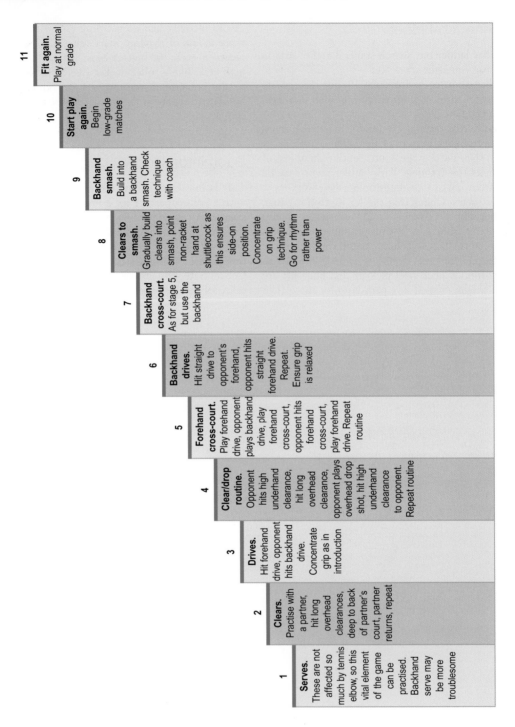

## Tennis ladder

This is good for a tennis elbow, which is mainly suffered by those using the standard grip and/or single-handed backhand grip. The semi-Western or Western grip is not often a cause of tennis elbow (see Figs 19.1–19.3). If it is, there may be too tight a grip with the thumb and second finger. Semi-Western grip is most likely to cause golfer's elbow.

Work with a willing partner or a tennis machine. Concentrate on footwork and technique. When playing a single-handed backhand, make sure that the racket head stays above the wrist level. Do not lead with the elbow (see Figs 18.7 and 18.8).

Work for 5 minutes at each level, stop at the first sign of pain. If the pain or ache goes away within 20 seconds, continue the exercises. If the ache or pain persists, stop, wait 24 hours, begin again from the first step (see How much training?). Do not grip the racket too tightly with the thumb and index finger.

## Standard grip

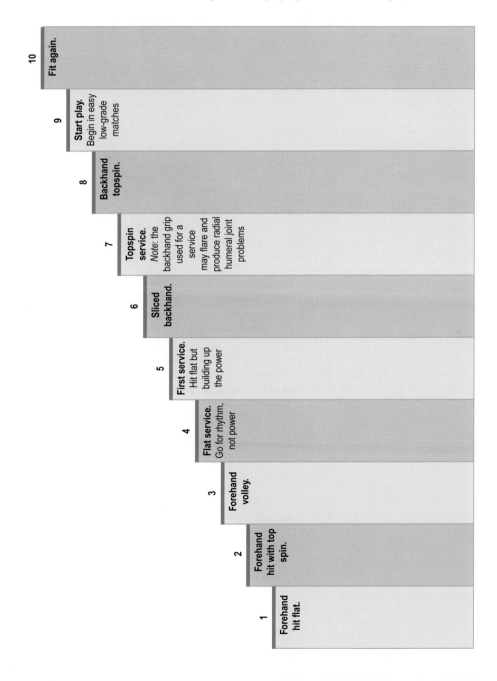

**10** Fit again.

**9** Start play. Begin in easy low-grade matches

**8** Backhand topspin.

**7** Topspin service. *Note:* the backhand grip used for a service may flare and produce radial humeral joint problems

**6** Sliced backhand.

**5** First service. Hit flat but building up the power

**4** Flat service. Go for rhythm, not power

**3** Forehand volley.

**2** Forehand hit with top spin.

**1** Forehand hit flat.

## Semi-Western grip and for golfer's elbow

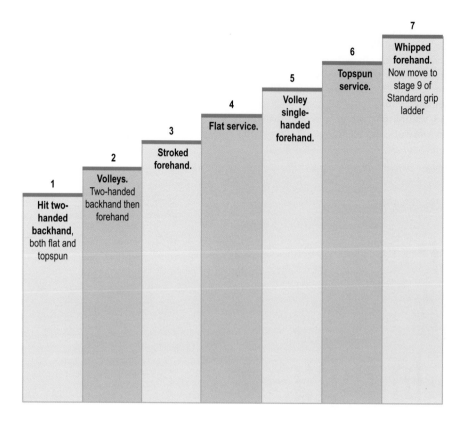

**7**
Whipped forehand.
Now move to stage 9 of Standard grip ladder

**6**
Topspun service.

**5**
Volley single-handed forehand.

**4**
Flat service.

**3**
Stroked forehand.

**2**
Volleys.
Two-handed backhand then forehand

**1**
Hit two-handed backhand, both flat and topspun

## Squash ladder

Useful for most squash injuries, legs and arms, and particularly tennis elbow, because the player can anticipate where the ball is going and will not be wrong footed. For golfer's elbow problems use the steps in a different order, as follows: 5, 7, 6, 2, 3, 4, 8, 9 and 10.

Practise with a willing partner, work for 2–3 minutes at each level. Start each training session from the lower steps. Stop at the first sign of pain, but, if the pain settles within 20 seconds, continue the exercises. Otherwise stop, wait 24 hours, begin from the first step (see How much training?). Concentrate on gripping with the third, fourth and fifth fingers, and releasing thumb and index finger.

**1 Serves.** These should be painless throughout training

**2 Forehand drives.** Play for length down the side wall

**3 Forehand boasts.** Hit forehand boast, partner hits backhand cross-court. Repeat. Do not hit any other type of shot

**4 Forehand cross-court.** Hit forehand cross-court, partner hits backhand boast. Repeat. Do not hit any other type of shot

**5 Backhand drives.** Practise drives for length down side wall

**6 Backhand cross-court.** Hit backhand cross-court, partner hits forehand boast. Do not hit any other type of shot

**7 Backhand boast.** Play backhand boast, partner plays forehand cross-court

**8 Paired boast and drive.** Hit forehand boast. Partner hits straight backhand drive. Hit backhand boast, partner hits straight forehand drive. Repeat. Swap position with partner

**9 Smash.** Concentrate on holding racket with third, fourth and fifth fingers. Relax thumb and index finger (Figure 18.1). Try to avoid face-on position

**10 The long game.** Use special rules, where the ball must bounce over the half-line, but a hard drive bouncing to a good length is permitted. The player forced into playing a drop shot loses the point

**11 Start play.** Begin in easy low-grade matches

**12 Fit again.** Play at normal grade

## Baseball or throwing ladder – for shoulder injuries

Work for 3–5 minutes at each level with a partner. Start each session from the bottom steps. At the first sign of pain, stop, but, if the pain settles within 20 seconds, continue. If the pain persists, stop, wait 24 hours, then begin again from the first step.

The shoulder muscles must build up strength, not only to throw but also to stop the arm following the ball! It is easy to overdo this ladder.

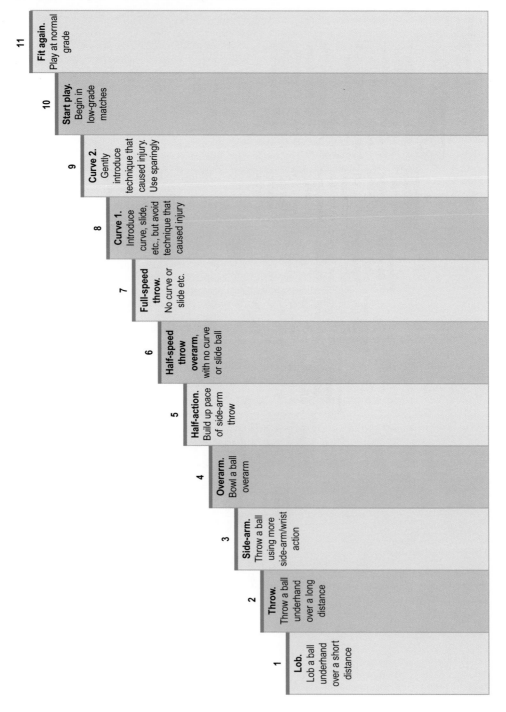

**11 Fit again.** Play at normal grade

**10 Start play.** Begin in low-grade matches

**9 Curve 2.** Gently introduce technique that caused injury. Use sparingly

**8 Curve 1.** Introduce curve, slide, etc., but avoid technique that caused injury

**7 Full-speed throw.** No curve or slide etc.

**6 Half-speed throw overarm,** with no curve or slide ball

**5 Half-action.** Build up pace of side-arm throw

**4 Overarm.** Bowl a ball overarm

**3 Side-arm.** Throw a ball using more side-arm/wrist action

**2 Throw.** Throw a ball underhand over a long distance

**1 Lob.** Lob a ball underhand over a short distance

# References

1 Grimby G. Progressive resistance exercise for injury rehabilitation. Special emphasis on isokinetic training. Sports Med 1985;2:309–315

2 Yack HJ, Collins CE, Wheildon TJ. Comparison of closed and open chain exercises in anterior cruciate ligament deficient knees. Am J Sports Med 1993;21(1):49–54

3 Wallin D, Ekblom B, Grah R, Nordenburg T. Improvement of muscle flexibility: a comparison between two techniques. Am J Sports Med 1985;13:263–268

4 Russell K. Increasing joint range of movement in young athletes. Paper to British Association of National Coaches, Birmingham; 1985

5 Osternig LJ, Hamill J, Lander JE, Robertson R. Co-activation of sprinter and distance runner muscles in isokinetic exercise. Med Sci Sports Exerc 1986;18:431–435

6 Smith CA. The warm-up procedure: to stretch or not to stretch. A brief review. J Orthop Sports Phys Ther 1994;19:12–17

7 Murphy DR. A critical look at static stretching: are we doing our patients harm? Chiro Sports Med 1991;5:67–70

8 Robbins S, Waked E, Rappel R. Ankle taping improves proprioception before and after exercise in young men. Br J Sports Med 1995;29:242–247

# Chapter Twenty-one

21

## Team doctoring

# Aerobic training

Trains the oxygen transport mechanism through the lungs, heart and cellular mitochondria. It requires low-intensity endurance work for 30 minutes, three to five times a week, and trains the red type 1 muscle fibres without producing much lactic acid.

# Aeroplanes

Neck supports are advised, especially when sleeping on an aeroplane, and the pillow provided should be used as a lumbar support. To avoid a deep vein thrombosis, walk around, perform heel raises, even when sitting, and do stretching exercises whenever possible. Keep well hydrated and use elastic compression stockings. One aspirin may have some benefit. Medical staff travelling with teams will have to carry all their own equipment and must not expect too much help from the team or other staff. Therefore, they should either plan on a crate-sized container, which is delivered to the venue, or use several smaller cases, as these stow more easily in the buses, and you will have to manage them all by yourself! Be patient, take a good book or writing pad to infill time, as travelling involves queuing and a big team cannot leave until the last person has collected his or her luggage off the travelator – and it may as well be you; keep reading the book! (See Team travel.)

# AIDS

Transmission during sport carries an extremely small risk. Transmission during sport is from blood, body fluids and other fluids containing blood. This weak virus is killed by soap and mild sterilizing solutions. Equipment, wrestling mats, diving boards, etc., should be wiped immediately with paper towels and can be cleaned with bleach, freshly prepared 1 : 10 with tap water. The dilution factor and chlorine of a swimming pool should prove sufficient to destroy the virus. Although those who sustain minor cuts or grazes may be left on the pitch, those who bleed must be removed from the pitch and blood-stained clothing changed. The wound should be sutured or steristripped, and covered, sufficient for the competition. Embucrylate, cyanoacrylate or superglue can seal the wound rapidly.

Latex or plastic gloves with appropriate receptacles should be provided for all carers, and disposal should be arranged for needles, syringes, surgical equipment, and soiled linen and uniforms. Post-event re-evaluation of the wound is required, and athletes should be responsible for proper treatment and covering of the wound before any competition. Confidentiality dictates that medical information is the property of the patient. Exceptions will include medical conditions that are reportable by regulation and statute. The physician is not liable for failure to warn the uninfected opponent because that legal responsibility lies with the HIV-infected athlete. The uninfected assume some risk in sports activities as it cannot be assumed that other competitors are HIV-negative, nor free of other blood-borne pathogens. Hepatitis B and C are more virulent, and the above recommendations should suffice, though vaccination is available for hepatitis B virus.

Exhaustive training regimens may compromise the immune system, and already compromised HIV sufferers should not exercise to exhaustion. After an appropriate physical examination, moderate exercise should be safe and beneficial to HIV sufferers. Education of athletes as to its infectivity should be undertaken, and this should be emphasized to touring teams.

This information was abstracted from FIMS position statement on AIDS 1997 and therefore may change.

# Alcohol

Alcohol causes peripheral dilatation and thus will hasten body cooling and should not be drunk to apparently warm a cold patient. Alcohol can calm a nervous tremor and is sometimes used with those who suffer from a familial idiopathic tremor, on account of beta-blockers being banned. Alcohol does decrease hand–eye coordination, accuracy and balance. It is also banned in several sports, such as modern pentathlon and shooting. The introduction of sports psychologists to teach stress management is more appropriate than knocking back the booze.

# Altitude sickness

This usually occurs above 10 000 feet (3000 metres). It presents with headache, fatigue and breathlessness. Increasing pulmonary oedema (HAPE) may be detected. Cerebral oedema (HACE), haemorrhage, thrombi and death may occur. Treatment consists of immediate oxygen, dexamethasone and diuretics, plus a descent immediately to 1000–2000 feet (300–600 metres) lower.

Acclimatize by going in slowly and climbing up, as opposed to flying straight in to a high base camp. Acet-azolamide may help to prevent the episode but does leave 'zingy pins and needles' in the fingers, toes and circumorally. A fit individual is just as likely to succumb as the unfit to altitude sickness.

# Altitude training

Generally known to increase the haematocrit, which takes about 2–3 weeks to reach significant levels. Athletes often feel a little enervated on return to sea level and race best 7–14 days after returning to sea level (see Erythropoietin).

# Amenorrhoea/oligomenorrhoea

See Bone density.

# Anabolic steroids

The use of anabolic steroids is banned by all sporting federations; however, they are available on the black market. Abusers tend to 'stack' drugs to avoid side effects, and thus take several different types, one after the other. Abuse should be suspected with the triad of increased acne, striae and increased aggressive personality, often known as 'roid rage'. Testicular atrophy and gynaecomastia may also be present. Premature fusion of the epiphyses produces a stunted growth. Females show increased androgenic effects, acne, male pattern hair growth, deepening voice, enlarged clitoris and suppression of menstruation, and both men and women may have skin abscesses from infected needle wounds.

Investigations should include blood pressure for hypertension, urine for diabetes, and blood for liver and renal function, as carcinomata are recorded. These drugs can be detected by gas chromatography and radioimmune assay. Testosterone is measured as a ratio to episterone. A positive test is a ratio of testosterone to episterone greater than 6 : 1. High testosterone levels inhibit the stimulating hormone episterone. Therefore, a high normal testosterone blood level should have a high stimulating episterone level, whereas extraneous testosterone will inhibit the episterone, increasing the normal ratio. Human growth hormone is abused in sport and requires blood tests to detect. Probenicid has been used as a masking agent and to delay the excretion of steroids in the urine, and diuretics are used to dilute any excreted steroids, in the hope of escaping detection, and both are banned. Testing for new substance abuse is invariably a few years behind its inception and its use in sport.

## Anaerobic training

Trains the white type 2 muscle fibres and requires high-intensity, short-duration work with longer recovery intervals (5 minutes); it produces lactic acid (see OBLA).

## Arthritis

Osteoarthritic joints are worse if totally rested or, conversely, overused. Ideally, the joints should be moved but not impacted; thus rowing, cycling and swimming are preferable to running. Osteoarthritis hurts at the limit of joint range, so a shortened walking pace, a thicker grip, etc., which places the joint movement into the middle range, can help. A thicker grip is not usually utilized by golfers, and yet it can make all the difference to the firmness of a pain-free grip. The explanation of a field surrounded by barbed wire, in which you can run around the field with no pain but, when you try to extend that run, you hit the barbed wire, can help patients to understand the pattern of arthritic pain.

Inflammatory arthritides require rest in the acute phase, isometrics for strength and mobilization when pain-free.

## Asthma

Atopics are naturally worse around their allergies (e.g. horses, grass pollen, tree pollen, etc.) so sports that avoid these contacts are recommended. However, note that high chlorine levels in a swimming pool can produce some surface chlorine gas, and thus irritation, in an apparently allergen-free climate. Even though the asthmatic lungs may still have a problem with oxygen transfer, if the transport system to the muscles is improved by general training, so overall fitness will improve. Cromoglycates, beta-agonists and cortisol insufflations are beneficial.

### Exercise-induced asthma (EIA)

EIA is worse in the cold, running long distances, and in dry conditions. It is better in warm, moist air and with interval games. Breathing warmer air through a mask or 'turbinator rebreather' may help. Interval games produce fewer problems because of the refractory period of EIA. A beta-agonist, with or without an alpha-antagonist, should be taken 15–20 minutes before exercise, plus standard maintenance therapy, such as sodium cromoglycate, is beneficial. Steroid insufflation is permitted but parenteral steroids are banned.

## Bending

Lifting increases intra-abdominal pressure, but, rather like the wall of a dam, the spine can resist this force by adopting a convex surface (lordosis), so that a neutral to lordotic spine is required for lifting. Strong abdominals and paravertebral muscles (see Chapter 2: Posture; Glossary: Core stability) will help to splint the spine in this position [1]. Too many types of abdominal exercise can harm the spine; for example, straight leg raises force extension of the spine, and flexion and rotation abdominal exercises may well stress the disc. So the bent position must have an extended or neutral back, locked by a core-stabilizing method, and the buttocks should be pushed backwards, feet wide apart, so that the forearms can be rested on the thighs (see Chapters 2 and 5). This is how weightlifters lift and how labourers in fields bend all day. This posture must be adopted for the slightest load, even cleaning the teeth, if the back is inclined towards flexion.

## Bends

Bends are caused by the release of nitrogen gas into the blood stream when decompression occurs too rapidly. Scuba divers should have diving guidelines from the British Sub Aqua Club (BSAC) or the Professional Association of Diving Instructors (PADI) for the depth and time of a dive and depressurization stops. However, divers presenting with joint pains, headaches, blurred vision and shortness of breath should be transferred immediately to the nearest depressurization chamber. Avascular necrosis from the 'bends', will show positive on bone scans and MRI, and lung perfusion studies can show bullae.

## Beta-blockers

Beta-blockers reduce stress. In many sports this is undesirable, but some sports do benefit; for example, shooters can also use the increased time of diastole, caused by the reduction in heart rate, in which to squeeze the trigger and obtain more accuracy! Familial idiopathic tremor is also helped by beta-blockers; however, as they are banned, these players may turn to alcohol, which is hardly a desirable substitute.

## Blood doping

Blood doping is illegal! Between 0.5 and 1 litres of autologous blood is packed and freeze-dried, and, about 4 weeks later, after the athlete has replenished his or her own haematocrit, prior to an event, the blood is retransfused. Even this illegal method has been reported to have been abused at an Olympic games, with the apparent transfusion, in a hotel bedroom, of heterologous blood.

## Bone bank

A phrase used to express the amount of bone, developed during growth, which is available to dissipate against the advances of senile osteoporosis.

## Bone density/osteoporosis

Exercises, even isometrics, improve bone density, and thus the 'bone bank'. Post-menopausal osteoporosis is therefore delayed by exercise. Equally, female hormones seem to be protective, so hormone replacement therapy may reduce post-menopausal osteoporosis, and bisphosphonates may delay or reverse this degradation [2]. Oligo/amenorrhoeic athletes may diminish their bone bank. This may be weight related, 7 stone (50 kg) being the critical weight below which amenorrhoea seems to occur. Many animals are oestrous and do not ovulate under stress, and it may be that humans alter from a menstrual to an oestral cycle if the stress is high, and therefore stop or delay their menstruation. Management should consist of:

(a) Checking dietary calcium intake, as this is often low.

(b) Beware of true anorexics using exercise as an excuse for their undernourished body image. Anorexics should be treated as athletes. They respond better to explanations of why athletes should eat rather than why medically they should eat. So explanations of carbohydrate loading, muscle glycogen replacement requiring carbohydrates within 2 hours post activity, and that muscles are heavier than fat seem to produce better results. They will then often listen if you prescribe an assessment by a sports dietician and the appropriate build up of food intake to handle their 'athletic requirements'.

(c) Beware of unusual stress fractures, such as the femur, pubic ramus or sacrum.

(d) Advise middle-distance runners that a power/weight ratio does not mean reducing the weight by dieting, because the subsequent reduction in muscle glycogen from the dieting will result in a reduction of muscle strength and endurance.

(e) Check pituitary and ovarian function.

## Bone growth

Children mature at different rates and should be matched in sport in both natal and developmental age. Monitoring of the Tanner scale for secondary sexual characteristics, though helpful, may be socially embarrassing [3]. Skeletal growth rates may be monitored radiologically but would be unethical. Parental morphology may indicate the child's future adult developmental status and the child's growth hormones may be monitored.

Children may be selected into sports by maturing early, but this maturation may be inappropriate for that sporting position at a later date or age. Reassessment of physical development, vis-à-vis the sport and position played, must be maintained throughout the teens. A 60 kg, 170 cm, 12-year-old may be ideal for the rugby scrum, but at 17 the child may still be 70 kg, 170 cm, and in fact should be playing in the backs (Fig. 21.1). During increased growth rate the epiphyses are most at risk, and flexibility is reduced because the muscle–tendon complex does not seem to lengthen at the same rate as the bone. Thus, avulsion apophysitides are common, and training should in fact be reduced during the growth phase. Broad-based training is required until apophyseal fusion, when specific event training and weight training may be increased. Management

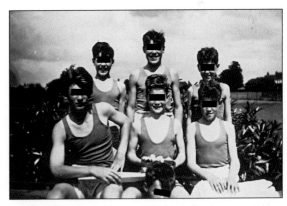

**Figure 21.1** • A group of 11- to 12-year-old schoolchildren showing different rates of growth. These may be even more diverse between 13 and 17 years.

should be directed towards a fit healthy adult, rather than a child prodigy (see Children).

## Brain damage

Although the 'punch drunk' syndrome, dementia pugilistica, is well recognized, there have been suggestions that heading a soccer ball can produce long-term damage to the brain. Evidence suggests that this might be more related to acute injuries rather than from repetitive heading [4]. Rapid rotational forces applied to the brain cause most of the damage. Pre-seasonal neuro-psychometric testing of players liable to head injury will give a base line with which testing after a head injury can be compared. This produces a more accurate assessment of the time to return to activities. However, brain injuries leave a secondary problem so that later, minor trauma may have an exaggerated effect.

## Breasts

Unsupported breasts may stretch and pull on the stroma and Cooper's ligaments and cause discomfort during exercise. Sports bras do provide the support and firmness for comfort. Protective plastic cups may be added in sports where trauma is expected. The nipples, of both males and females, can be chafed by a running vest, especially when it is roughened with sweat. This causes cracking and bleeding of the nipples. Cover the nipple with petroleum jelly, or preferably second skin gels or sleek plaster, to prevent this chafing. When traumatized, breast fat may become tender and lumpy for several weeks, raising the possibility of cancer – reassurance is required.

## Bunny hops

Hopping routines into a full squat position can produce meniscal tears – indeed the duck waddle (see Glossary) is used to test for meniscal tears. Virtually no sport requires strength in the full squat position and thus this training method should be abandoned.

## Calcium

Dietary assessment of oligo/amenorrhoeics shows a lack of calcium intake, either in the form of milk, with its supplementary calcium, or generally within the diet. Added calcium is advisable. Treatment of osteoporosis includes calcium supplements [1].

## Check-ups

These should include all the standard medical assessments, but for exercise must contain auscultation for cardiac murmurs and an exercise electrocardiogram (ECG). Pre- and post-exercise spirometry, or $FEV_1$, for asthma. Fainting or dizziness during exercise, requires further investigation, including an echocardiogram. An assessment of the back and the peripheral joints should be undertaken for biomechanical faults, and, particularly for runners, correction of overpronation with orthotics. Assessment of ligamentous laxity using the Beighton–Horan score (see Glossary) may suggest that some sports are best avoided, or that prophylactic bracing should be utilized. An indication of Marfan syndrome will not prevent activities but will raise the index of suspicion to any chest pains for aortic dissection. Routine scanning for hypertrophic cardiomyopathy, and spinal X-rays for congenital problems including spina bifida occulta, with its increased association with spondylolysis in gymnasts, is probably not cost-effective, although the previous East German regime would have excluded these congenital abnormalities from elite training squads [5]. However, there is a low yield per number of check-ups that makes routine scanning not very cost-effective for the standard athlete or child [6] (see Exercise prescription).

## Chewing gum

This can cause airway obstruction if inhaled, and should be discouraged during sporting activity.

## Children

Children should be trained on a broad basis, until epiphyseal fusion has occurred, when specialized event and weight training may be increased. During the growth spurt the bones grow faster and are weaker at the epiphyses than in the muscles and tendons. This promotes stiffness from the muscle–tendon complex trying to catch up, and stresses appear in the epiphysis rather than as a muscle or tendon lesion (see Bone growth). The child has a proportionately weaker torso to lower body strength and their strength develops by muscle hypertrophy rather than by an increase in muscle fibres. More time and information is required to guide coaches and doctors in developing the child into a high-earning potential sportsperson, and at the same time keeping the rest of the school population fit and actively enjoying sport. Young children are natural aerobes who develop their anaerobic capacity later. However, their energy costs are higher than adults' and they respire faster and shallower, thus wasting energy and water. They may suffer voluntary dehydration because of this high ventilatory rate, and their thirst is not equivalent to the amount of water they have lost. This can result in a raised temperature – 'thirst fever'. Their ability to balance heat is poor in that they produce more heat, sweat less, and they have a greater surface area, which makes them warm up in the heat and cool down faster in the cold. This latter element is exaggerated by their reduced amount of insulating fat. However, the obese are prone to overheat, raise their temperature and pulse and become dehydrated. The little 'fatties' who keep stopping and asking for a drink are expressing their true physiological needs, and are not just 'skiving off' [7]. Rutenfranz's [8] statement shows vision and understanding: 'Children involved in elite sport can be considered participants in an uncontrolled experiment. Ethics committees to control training procedures of gifted children, and to propose higher age limits for participants, especially in international sports events, seem to be needed. The basic ethical consideration is not to harm or alienate children, by using them as objects for sports organizations, spectators, or nationalists'. Think on the previous East German regime, which was shown to have systematically doped its developing athletes, and let us always watch the ethics of our behaviour during our involvement in sport.

## Circadian rhythm

Circadian rhythm is the body's natural basal metabolic rate, and it alters throughout the 24 hour cycle. This appears to adjust at approximately 1 hour per 24 hours of the time shift, and it is important to avoid participation in sport during time zones that are equivalent to the body's current basal metabolic rate running at its lowest level. Travel time should allow for this adjustment to take place. However, an alteration from, say, 10.00 a.m. to 10.00 p.m. is not likely to have an effect. Melatonin may help [9], and travelling westwards can have a faster adaptation time than travelling eastwards [10] (see Team travel).

## Claudication

A history of pain brought on by walking and relieved by rest suggests vascular or neurological claudication, and the older person, especially with a history of vas-

cular/cardiac problems, should be checked for abdominal aortic aneurysm and spinal stenosis. The young may have a peripheral vascular stenosis, such as popliteal artery entrapment, and their history is claudication with endurance running but not with interval exercises. Cyclists can produce an endofibrosis of their external iliac arteries [11].

## Coffee/caffeine

Caffeine helps the body metabolize fat and can therefore improve muscle endurance by delaying the utilization of muscle glycogen. Above 12 parts per million of caffeine is considered dope positive, but the average level in the normal population of coffee drinkers is only 2 parts per million, suggesting that anyone over the accepted level is definitely doping and not addicted to coffee!

## Collapse

Collapse during, as opposed to after, exercise should be taken very seriously. Look for temperature disturbance and cardiac or respiratory problems, and, in the slower runners or those who have drunk water excessively, hyponatraemia. Some suggest that, to avoid this problem, water stations in marathon events should not be closer than every 5 km. Collapse after an event is more likely to be from the cessation of the calf muscle pump in returning blood to the heart; in which case, keeping the athlete on the move or lying them with their legs elevated, and even possibly cycling their legs, will be of benefit.

## Corticosteroids

Oral and parenteral corticosteroids are banned but are permitted as a topical application, insufflation, and for local soft tissue or intra-articular injections, as long as this is reported in writing, pre-competition, to the doping control officer. Enteral steroids are permitted in special cases following permission from the governing body, e.g. in coeliac disease. A TUE (see this chapter) certificate should be applied for.

## Creatinine

Meat contains high levels of creatinine, but, on top of this, creatinine supplements do seem to aid anaerobic performance in some people.

## Dehydration

Warn athletes that, in the first 3–4 days before acclimatization, they do not have a thirst which is equivalent to their dehydration [12]; 5% dehydration can produce a 25% drop in performance. To ensure a team stays hydrated during both training and competition, an isotonic drink made up in a large container can be left out, near the exit to the team's accommodation. Also, scales can be stood nearby so that the athletes can weigh themselves before and after training. The athlete needs to be taught that most of the weight loss will be fluid. Athletes must also check the colour of their own urine, and, if it appears dark, they are dehydrated. Urine should be clear or straw coloured. Regular fluid replacement must be taken during performance. Sodium and potassium ions may be of benefit, but these ions also aid absorption of water. Five per cent glucose or glucose polymers increase water absorption, and if muscle energy is required at the same time then increase the glucose content of the replacement fluid. It is easier to drink from a squeeze bottle whilst running, but the athlete should practise this whilst training in order to find which technique suits them the best. Gassy drinks should be poured out early, and the addition of a sugar lump will decarbonate the drink, often violently. Alcohol causes dehydration.

### Caveat

The following pitfalls have been recorded in international competition:

(a) Officially supplied water for the marathon was gassy.

(b) Supplied water was put out too soon in the sun, so that, when the runners came to drink it, it was hot and undrinkable.

(c) Ice, to cool the bottled water, was found to be contaminated.

(d) The seals on the bottles were found to be broken, and the bottles had been filled from the local tap.

(e) Athletes have been known to drink too much. The urine is clear, but the athlete is passing water far too frequently and performance is thus also affected. This may be the early presentation of hyponatraemia.

## Diabetics

Diabetics must be advised to wear a MediAlert style disc, increase their glucose intake, and/or reduce their insulin before exercise, plus carry glucose and glucagons with them at competition. The team doctor and event doctor should be informed that they are diabetic. Type 2 diabetics, who are basically overweight, should have an exercise and dietary programme prescribed for them.

## Diarrhoea

### Travellers

Teams should be instructed and advised that, on going abroad:

(a) gassy drinks on aeroplanes cause gastric distension

(b) air conditioning causes dehydration

(c) they should beware of food outside the hotel, especially shellfish, reheated foods, ice and ice cream

(d) it is sensible to check that bottled water has a sealed cap, as the contents may be presented as 'bottled water' but have been filled from the nearest local tap. Note that bottled water may be stored in ice blocks, which have been known to be a source of contamination

(e) salad is to be avoided

(f) all fruit should be peeled

(g) teeth should be cleaned with bottled water.

### Treatment

Pre-check the prevalence of causative factors in the area, especially *Shigella* spp., *Giardia*, *Escherichia coli* and enteroviruses. It is generally thought that prophylactic antibiotics are unnecessary, unless in a particularly endemic area. Anti-diarrhoeal treatment is with Imodium, though at competition, and especially with bloody diarrhoea, ciprofloxin should be prescribed. (Note that atropine-containing drugs affect performance.) If possible, culture the stools and arrange microscopy, especially with bloody stools, when giardiasis can be expected. Prescribe an appropriate antibiotic, if required, and maintain fluid replacement.

### Runner's diarrhoea

Many sportspeople have pre-competition, gastric hurry, caused by anxiety, but long-distance runners may produce diarrhoea and even melaena, possibly from splanchnic ischaemia. Many a long-distance runner has to take toilet paper and spot the whereabouts of public toilets. It does appear to be runners, and rarely ball games players, rather than cyclists or swimmers who suffer, perhaps backing up the caecal slap theory. Appropriate fluid replacement is required later, but pre-competition 'gassy' drinks, available free at many venues, may also be causative [13]. Proton pump inhibiters given prophylactically can reduce the incidence of melaena in ultra-distance marathoners [14].

## Diet

### Carbohydrate loading

To increase muscle glycogen, light training only should be undertaken during the last week prior to an endurance event, and the diet switched to high carbohydrates, especially during the last 2 days when training should be suspended. Glycogen depletion beforehand, as originally described, is not required [15].

### Tournament diet

Muscle glycogen is replaced most rapidly when carbohydrate is taken within 30 minutes of the end of the game, and certainly within a 2 hour window, either as food or as a high-glucose drink. The evening meal may have steak, to add flavour to the meal and creatinine to the body, but the meal must have carbohydrates, such as potatoes and rice. The meal does not have to be pasta for the main course, as puddings may be used equally effectively as carbohydrate loaders. Gastronomic boredom is debilitating, especially on tour. Breakfast should be continental, with a high carbohydrate intake. Coffee may aid fat metabolism, but caffeine at high levels is banned (see Coffee/caffeine).

### Caveat

**Beware of the player who appears quite nervous and is noted not to be eating. High adrenaline levels will burn up the glucose and this athlete's performance will suffer. If the athlete cannot eat because of nervous tension, push high-glucose fluids or glucose polymer drinks, chocolate and fruit during the pre-match time available.**

## General diet

Many athletes eat badly and do not balance their fat and carbohydrate intake correctly. Fatigued athletes should have a dietary revue, and all athletes should be instructed on how a rest day can restore their muscle glycogen. Power/weight ratios are often misunderstood, athletes losing weight to improve the ratio, but forgetting that power (type 2) fibres are heavy and that their weight loss is often muscle bulk, which consequently reduces their power as well. Thus many one-paced, oligomenorrhoeic athletes will lose out on the sprint at the end of the race because they have not developed the muscle bulk of the fast twitch fibre. They require dietary advice, often to put on weight. Long-distance running has permitted the true anorexic to maintain their perceived body image without criticism, and as these athletes' performance improves so they are often prepared, with dietary advice, to accept the requirements of training rather than the requirements of body image. Body mass index (BMI; weight in kilograms/height in metres squared) is a useful guide to body fat content, but it is of less value when accurate measurements are required because of the variations between gender, race and athleticism [16]. An athlete whose weight is mainly made up of muscle requires skinfold thickness, or subcutaneous fat impedence, measurements [17].

## Diuretics

Diuretics have been used to dilute the urine, and hopefully escape the detection of banned substances, but they have also been used to 'make the weights'. In these weight category events, it can be particularly dangerous as dehydration reduces athletic performance and can promote hyperthermia and collapse under competition situations. Athletes self-medicating have the 'if one helps, four will help four times better' mentality. Diuretics can be responsible for gynaecomastia and are banned in sport.

## DOMS

Delayed onset of muscle soreness (DOMS) has been experienced by most of us as the tender aching muscle that appears 24 hours after unaccustomed activity. It is more apparent after eccentric exercise and after long endurance exercise, such as the marathon. It may be displayed on a bone scan, when the muscles show increased uptake. Creatinine phosphokinase will be raised for 3–5 days and T2-weighted or STIR sequence

MRI shows an increased signal. This increased signal has been recorded as lasting nearly 3 months after eccentric exercise – an important point when managing soft tissue pain [18].

# Drugs

Doctors prescribing for common illnesses must remember that some regularly prescribed medications contain drugs that are banned in a sporting situation. See the current WADA guidelines of banned drugs. The drug testing laboratories will probably be able to supply a list of drugs that can be used, as well as those that are banned.

## WADA list of doping classes and methods

Banned classes of drugs:

(a) Stimulants
(b) Narcotics
(c) Anabolic steroids
(d) Beta-blockers
(e) Diuretics
(f) Peptide hormones and analogues.

Banned doping methods:

(a) Blood doping
(b) Pharmacological, chemical and physical manipulation.

Classes of drugs subject to certain restrictions:

(a) Alcohol
(b) Marijuana
(c) Local anaesthetics
(d) Corticosteroids.

Some international federations test for marijuana, but not all, and snowboarding seems to permit its use.

Athletes not deliberately cheating are caught out by preparations in cough and cold mixtures, and by impure ginseng preparations that contain ephedrine or phenylpropanolamine, even though some labels of contents show only the permitted ingredients. Those athletes found positive on the 'A' test will have the 'B' sample tested by another technician, and are permitted to have their own expert present during the second test.

Many charges of drug abuse are defended, not against the presence of the drug but around the failure

to handle the sample procedures correctly (see Drug/dope testing).

# Drug/dope testing

## Who will be tested?

(1) An official decision will be made on the event or game to be tested by the body running the meeting. The testing laboratory should be notified of the date of this event and the turnaround time for results required, e.g. 24 hours, longer, shorter.
(2) An official decision on which place(s) in a race are to be tested, or whether a random draw of players from teams by numbers, will be required.
(3) Records will be ratified only after a negative dope test, done at the time.

## Notification

Athletes are notified by officials and given the appropriate documentation, indicating that their position or number has been randomly selected for dope testing. An official will fill in each athlete's name, in his or her presence. Athletes then sign to confirm that they are the relevant athletes and that they understand they must attend at the dope control centre within the specified time, which is usually in 30–45 minutes. Officials remain with the athletes until they enter the doping control centre. The time of notification is recorded. A copy of each athlete's document is kept by the officials and collected by the doping control officer. They need only be kept if an athlete does not attend on time and may be destroyed once the test is declared negative.

## Site

Signpost directions must be displayed, which are visible from all conceivable routes and at all conceivable corners, turns, etc. The use of lines on the floor to direct athletes to the testing centre can be helpful. There must be no possible reason for an excuse that the athlete could not find where to go. A map should be published in the official programme.

## Waiting area

Admit access to the athlete with a test form and one team official (doctor/manager), but all others should be excluded. The time of attendance at the centre should be recorded on the notification sheet, and the testing officer informed for recording on the documents. Seating and reading material are to be available. Drinks (non-alcoholic) must be available from sealed cans or bottles, and clean, disposable cups must be used. Athletes must take and pour their own drinks.

## Testing area

An official should check the identification of each athlete. The athlete will select a testing pack, and must always be offered a choice of at least two. The athlete opens the pack, breaking the seal. The official points out, but does not touch, sample A and sample B bottles that are engraved with a unique code. The official points out that, in the event of sample A being positive, sample B will be tested by another laboratory technician, and the athlete and professional representatives may be present. The athlete unscrews the top of the bottle and takes the top and bottle with him or her to the toilet. The athlete is accompanied to the toilet by an official of the same sex and is observed to pass, preferably, 100 mL of urine into bottle A. In practical terms 75 mL is acceptable.

Females may require a collecting slipper, which should be sterile, sealed in protective wrapping, and this again should be selected and opened by the athlete, from a choice of at least two. The athlete is observed by the official to decant 25 mL of urine from sample A into the sample B bottle. The athlete screws the tops on both bottles and places them in the testing pack. The athlete seals the testing pack and is offered a selection of coded sealant tags for this pack (some systems use a coded outer container, not a tag). This code is recorded on the athlete's form, and the athlete is required to check that this code is the same as that on the pack. The official will fill in the documentation.

Sheet 1 should contain:

- Name, sex, country, event
- Drugs currently being taken
- Time of notification, time of arrival at the testing centre, time of test
- Event code, pack sealant number
- Athlete's signature.

To be handed to the athlete.

Sheet 2 will be a copy of Sheet 1 and kept by the organizers, when it can be referred to in the event of a positive test to identify the individual from the pack number.

Sheet 3 will record only:

- Event code number and pack code number
- Drugs currently being taken.

Sheet 3 will be sent with the sample to the testing laboratory. The athlete signs the top form, which imprints the second, but not the third, and these facts are displayed to the athlete.

The pack is stored in a fridge until all the day's samples are collected, and then these packs are placed in a large container, sealed with a further coded sealant or a uniquely labelled outer bag, and transported to the testing laboratory within 24 hours.

## Problems

(a) Pack seal numbers are not recorded properly at the test site, or in the laboratory, or not checked by athlete – **double check!**

(b) The athlete cannot pass urine before the end of the meeting. As long as the official in charge approves, the athlete may leave, but always in the company of a test official, until the sample has been collected. Thus the athlete may return to the hotel.

## Random testing

This may be on a voluntary code, but many organizations will consider that an athlete is guilty of abusing the WADA codes of practice if he or she misses three tests in succession. The athlete's home, work, and training addresses are recorded, plus a photograph of the athlete. Notification should be given to all athletes that they will be banned if they fail the test under WADA laws, and if they are unavailable for testing on three successive occasions. Notification of testing within 24 hours is reasonable, when a convenient address (the athlete's home) may be agreed, plus a leaflet outlining the procedures for sample collection should be sent to the athlete. However, testing at training may be at short or no notice. The athlete signs to confirm the venue, date and time of collection, and the name of the athlete and the collector are printed out. The testing procedures that follow are the same as in competition.

## Some recorded or apocryphal methods of cheating

(a) A tube strapped to the penis, enabling urine to appear to be passed from the bladder, but in fact being squeezed from a bag hidden in the athlete's clothing. The athlete is asked to hold up their shirt and drop their shorts.

(b) Urine has been left by another source in the toilet, which the athlete has poured into the collecting container. The athlete must be observed, and the urine in the container must be warm, at body temperature.

(c) The athlete empties the bladder and is then catheterized, and someone else's urine is inserted into the bladder. Two athletes, after gas chromatographic testing, were found to have an exactly similar chemical make up of urine as each other.

(d) Most cases go to court on the technique of the testing procedure, not the drug analysis.

## ECG

Electrocardiograph (ECG) evidence of a large left ventricle and raised ST segments may be normal in an athlete, but ultrasound measurements, to include the ventricular wall thickness, must be undertaken to exclude hypertrophic obstructive cardiomyopathy (HOCUM).

## Epilepsy

Those sportspeople whose epilepsy is under control may take part in sport, avoiding contact games where the head is at risk and situations, such as climbing or sub aqua, where an epileptic fit may prove fatal. They should wear MediAlert discs and inform team doctors. Check with the relevant sports authorities, many of which will have their own guidelines.

## Erythropoietin

Erythropoietin is being abused to increase the haematocrit. Blood testing, as opposed to urine testing, has therefore become more common to detect this type of abuse.

## Ethics in sports medicine

Various countries have made some attempts to establish a code of ethics and some suggestions are made below. It is important that sports medics, with their lawyers, define the ethics of sports medicine and not so-called expert witnesses who have never faced the problems of elite sport.

For the purpose of this code, sports medicine shall mean medicine practised by a physician in the field of competitive and recreational sports, whether by advising on how to avoid illness and injury or by administering treatment.

## Medical practice

(1) The same rules that apply to general medical ethics shall apply to sports medicine.

(2) A physician who regularly treats or advises athletes shall possess the special knowledge of sports medicine, including the special physical and psychological demands of a sportsperson.

(3) Physicians shall not keep to themselves treatment methods for ill or injured athletes, nor restrict this knowledge to a select group.

(4) Physicians shall not keep to themselves any testing or training methods with a curative or injury preventative effect.

(5) Physicians shall not conceal harmful side effects of training or therapeutic strategies.

(6) Physicians must at all times consider the long-term health of the patient and the natural healing of the injury to be the prime objective, but recognize that sport practice has short-term goals. If these two requirements conflict then full and adequate explanation of possible risks and rewards shall be discussed between physician and athlete, and any other party of consequence to the decision. The physician shall apply no duress to influence the athlete's decision. For those under the legal age of consent, the physician shall take into consideration only long-term health and natural healing.

(7) The grounds for infusion therapy are no different for an athlete than for the general population.

(8) With the exception of the contraceptive hormones, hormone supplement is acceptable only if, compared with a norm, there is an abnormal decrease of hormone level, which in modern accepted practice is related to an increased threat to the athlete's health.

(9) A team physician has a duty to the team and the individual, but the prime concern is to the health and confidentiality of the individual. However, if this confidentiality is detrimental to the well-being and performance of the team, then the physician shall attempt to persuade the individual to inform team management. If this fails, the physician shall be permitted to advise

team management of the likely short- and long-term problems for the team. Notifiable diseases must be notified and the team management informed.

(10) If an athlete and/or team management wish the athlete to partake of activities that the physician considers deleterious to the athlete's health, the physician has a duty to point this out, but will respect the personal responsibility of the athlete to control his or her own destiny. An exception to this guideline occurs if health risks for third parties are involved, or the decision follows a medical emergency to the athlete.

(11) A team physician shall not prevent an athlete from taking a second opinion, but shall not be obliged to oversee, nor be held responsible for the practice of, this second opinion.

## Publicity

(12) Physicians shall refrain from publicly criticizing fellow professionals.

(13) Case studies may be presented in research papers, books and lectures, but the athlete should not be named without express permission from the athlete. Some athletes are so high profile that their case will still be recognizable, but the presentation should still not name the athlete and will confine itself to the medical and psychological incidents that have a direct bearing on the case.

(14) Physicians shall only release statements for publicity about an athlete's well-being in a format agreed with the athlete.

## Banned drugs

(15) Physicians who are approached by athletes to prescribe medication listed on the banned list, as defined by the national body for the participant's sport, and/or are confronted by the use of medication listed on the WADA banned list, which were prescribed by another physician on medical grounds, are obliged to advise the athlete and that medical advisor of non-banned therapies that will achieve the same therapeutic affect. Physicians confronted by the use of banned medication which the athlete is using on non-therapeutic grounds with the object of enhancing their performance shall advise against further use of this medication. If, after the

warning, the athlete continues, the physician shall advise the athlete that further persistence will be reported to the relevant governing body. If the transgression persists then the physician shall report the offender to the governing body.

(16) If the medication is listed on the banned list, there is no alternative medication, and its withdrawal will have a deleterious effect on the well-being of the athlete, then the physician shall inform the national governing body to request dispensation for this individual, and obtain a TUE (see this chapter).

(17) The physician will cooperate in performing, or arranging to be performed, compulsory anti-doping tests for athletes, as laid down in the sports regulations.

(18) The physician may express an opinion on doping problems, regardless as to whether this opinion is for or against the medication on the banned list.

## Children

(19) Physicians responsible for the medical supervision of athletes under the legal age of consent will take due regard of problems that can arise from the excesses of sports practice on the well-being of the developing child, and the possibility of child abuse.

(20) Physicians will not artificially alter the growing rate of a child.

## Third parties

(21) Physicians who perform examinations at the request of a third party will, on request, show the results to the athlete before sending them to the third party. The objections of the athlete to release of this information shall be respected, but the physician shall inform the athlete of an obligation to advise the third party as to the fitness, unfitness, or fitness under certain defined conditions of this athlete.

## Monies

(22) Physicians shall not falsify their findings by omission or deception. They may accept financial reward or gifts.

## Records

(23) Physicians will record medical notes of consultations, and these records will be kept for the required legal duration.

(24) These records will be kept in the usual confidential filing system accepted for standard medical practice. If, for the sake of continuity, the records are housed at team headquarters, then due diligence to security and confidentiality shall be ensured.

## Exercise prescription

It is important to consider that advice on exercise is the same as a prescription. The advice should be given only after a diagnosis of the problems has been made and the requirements of the patient understood. The type of exercise, the dose of exercise and the frequency of exercise must be defined. Many taking exercise, after a long lay off, will in fact break down their musculoskeletal system before they overstress their cardiovascular system. Arbitrary exercise targets should not be set, rather the exercise programme should be adjusted regularly to match the physiological and musculoskeletal progress of the individual. Start slowly, at a speed where the patient can talk, but has a catch in the breath. Weights should be low, building to 25–30 repetitions before incrementing the weight. Stop if the muscles feel fatigued or ache. Build to a distance slowly and then increase the speed, in gentle increments, until the desired running speed has been obtained. Step up the distance, but slow down the speed again. Once the increased distance has been obtained without muscle discomfort, gradually increase the speed until the desired distance and speed are reached. An easy guideline is:

(a) No reaction to exercise on two occasions – increase the amount of exercise.

(b) Ache after exercise, but better by the morning – maintain but do not increase.

(c) Ache after exercise, and lasting through the next morning to midday – reduce by 10%.

(d) Ache after exercise and all the next day – rest that day and reduce by 50%.

## Fainting

See Collapse and Fatigue.

## Fatigue

(a) **Anaemia**. Sportspeople may have a physiological anaemia, from a greater circulating volume, and therefore serum ferritin should also be measured if anaemia is suspected.

(b) **Post-infective**. The ubiquitous virus that is never proven may exist. Investigations should include viral antibodies, monospot and Epstein–Barr, but, as the athlete usually presents some weeks after the problem, there will be no rising titre to establish the diagnosis.

(c) **Diet.** Carbohydrate stores, muscle glycogen, are depleted by a poor diet, but more usually because a rest day to replenish glycogen stores is not programmed into the training. The glycogen stores are gradually used up until muscle fatigue results (see Diet).

(d) **Muscle damage**. Muscle breakdown is shown by a highly raised creatinine phosphokinase. The muscles are tender to palpation, and a history of direct muscle trauma, eccentric exercises, DOMS or extreme endurance exercise is obtained. This normally settles in 3–5 days but MRI suggests that after nearly 3 months an increased signal on STIR sequences may be obtained [18].

(e) **Overtraining/underperformance syndrome**. Physiologically not well understood, but the immune mechanism may show alterations in T cell ratios, and viral antibodies show titres for Coxsackie B, *Toxoplasma gondii*, cytomegalovirus, Epstein–Barr, etc., but they are not suggestive of a current infection [19]. The athlete seems to underperform and OBLA shows a shift to the left (see this chapter). Branched chain amino acids [20] may be altered, and some athletes have thicker tenuous bronchial mucus and altered hormonal ratios. Three weeks' rest in the early stage is curative [21], but, when underperformance is established, the symptoms are similar to a chronic fatigue state, when exercise must be severely curtailed to the patient's tolerance; 100 metres may be tolerated but 101 metres produces 4 days' fatigue. Short distances with rest are required. Viral protein one (VP1) may be positive. During incremental training, 'runners' should be moved onto ball games and exercises that they have not done before, because they have a tendency to try to monitor themselves on a previous training diary, which of course bears no relation to their current fitness. Their failure to achieve previous goals often provokes a reactive depression, complicating the whole assessment of the situation. Thus many symptoms have been reported, fatigue and a sense of effort during training, a history of heavy training and competition, frequent minor infections, stiff and sore muscles, mood disturbances, altered sleep patterns, loss of energy, appetite, competitive drive and libido, and excessive sweating [22].

## Femininity check

It appears that the current thinking defines men's events as open events, so women may be seen playing in men's golf tournaments. Entry to women's events is restricted. At one stage entry was open to those who had external anatomical features of females, and these females were screened by a panel of doctors. Then entry was restricted to those who possessed a double X chromosome, confirmed by finding Barr bodies in the buccal cells. Athletes possessing the testicular feminization syndrome [23] were therefore banned from entry. Once again, possession of the external anatomical features of a female are recognized for entry, whether they be natural or surgically produced, and no official confirmation is required. A protest can initiate a formal medical examination by a panel of doctors.

## Flexibility

See Chapter 20: Stretching; Glossary: Beighton–Horan score.

## Growth rate

See Bone growth; Children.

## Gumshields

Gumshields can be made from moulds, but really should be cast-made for the upper teeth. Gumshields mainly prevent fractures of the teeth, and perhaps reduce some impaction to the skull from a blow through the jaw. Trimming of the palateal portion of the gumshield may be required, for easier respiration.

## HACE

High-altitude cerebral oedema. See Altitude sickness.

## Haematuria

Frank haematuria may occur after marathon or ultra-marathon runs, and is often associated with melaena. There may be some association with splanchnic and renal ischaemia, and dehydration. The haematuria settles with appropriate rest from activities, but further investigation should be undertaken to exclude any underlying disease. The urine should be tested with a haemastick, as haemoglobinuria or myoglobinuria may occur, which test negative to blood.

## Haemoglobinuria

Haemoglobinuria produces red urine, but is negative to tests for blood when tested with haemasticks. It is caused, in sensitive people, by fragility of the blood vessels, particularly in the inferior calcaneal fat pad, and may be prevented by a shock absorbent sole inserted in the shoes.

## HAPE

High-altitude pulmonary oedema. See Altitude sickness.

## Hay fever

Systemic corticosteroids are banned, and antihistamines can be too sedative, so cromoglyconate and/or nasal steroid insufflation, plus menthol-containing drops (such as Synex), are permitted. Great care should be taken to establish whether proprietary menthol drops contain any ephedrine, as the formulation for the same proprietary drug may differ between various countries.

## Headaches

The standard infective causes and referred cervical pain (see Chapter 3) must be excluded. Exercise-induced migraines are reported, but are difficult to diagnose, and a neurological opinion should be sought. Acute post-traumatic headaches must be examined urgently (see Chapter 1).

## Head colds

Menthol crystals, or nasal sprays such as Synex, are permitted. Anything containing ephedrine or pseudo-ephedrine is banned, and great care should be taken to establish whether proprietary formulations of the same drug differ between countries and ensure that they do not contain banned drugs. However, do not allow training or competition if:

(a) the temperature is raised
(b) there is a generalized myositis
(c) the resting pulse is raised 10 beats per minute. However, if the resting pulse is raised 5–10 beats per minute, complete a medical examination before making a decision.

## Headguards

Headguards are designed to prevent cuts, as in boxing, or to decelerate impact, as in motorcycling, ice hockey, etc. The hard outer shell of a motor cycle helmet may appear intact after an accident, but the polystyrene inside can be damaged and the helmet is thus defective. These types of helmet must be changed after each accident. There is an argument that the face guards in boxing, and also the mandibular extension in motor cycle helmets, prevent cuts and lacerations but increase the rotational force of head blows, and thus the likelihood of concussion or a tentorial tear.

## Hepatitis

See AIDS.

## Hyperthermia

Hyperthermia at rest and pre-exercise is a contraindication to exercise. The temperature should be monitored rectally after exercise (aural/oral thermometers can read low). If the athlete is hyperthermic then cool with a spray or ice pack, particularly over the groin and neck. If the mental state is normal and the athlete is sweating, observation is the best management and there is probably no problem. If the athlete is confused and dry, then oral rehydration and external cooling are required, but the temperature should be taken regularly, as, if treatment is proving successful, this should return to 40°C in 10 minutes. If not, or the patient remains confused and rigors, admission for intravenous rehydration is necessary. Beware that the onset of neurological signs is indicative of severe problems. Early rehydration is essential – usually orally, but many require intravenous fluids.

## Hypothermia

Prevention is better than cure! Be prepared – take waterproofs on mountains, even in fine weather, and carry a thermal blanket or a plastic bag to act as a whole body protector. People should be aware that the effect of wind chill on top of being wet can cool the body even faster than normal. Heat loss occurs, particularly from the head, hands, feet and the legs, and especially in those who wear jeans. Alcohol should not be taken to 'warm' the body as it dilates the periphery and increases temperature loss. Anyone caught in the cold should curl into a ball to reduce the exposed surface area, stay still in water and, if possible, float rather than swim. The body core should be reheated with warm drinks and body blankets, and the periphery should not be massaged or exercised until the core temperature is above 35°C. Those who are mentally confused or have a temperature below 35°C should be admitted to hospital.

## Isotonic drinks

Quite what they are isotonic to is debatable, but the principle is for the drinks to contain sodium, potassium and chloride, to replace loss in sweat, and also glucose or glucose polymers for energy, whilst at the same time attempting to be iso-osmolar to normal plasma. If dehydration is the problem then water must be replaced, and these solutions may be diluted. If glycogen depletion accompanies the dehydration, the proportion of glucose or glucose polymer is increased. Pure glucose, in high concentrations, can be sickly and can be absorbed so rapidly that it produces an insulin oversecretion and subsequent hypoglycaemia – possibly this is more experimental than practical. If no commercial replacements are available then a pinch of salt and a tablespoon of sugar in a pint of water will be suitable.

## Jet lag

See Team travel.

## Jogger's nipple

See Breasts.

## Melaena

See Haematuria.

## Menstruation

It is generally accepted that normal athletic performance can be achieved during menstruation, but some females have perimenstrual problems of water retention, which cannot be controlled with diuretics because they are banned in sport. Hormonal adjustment (contraceptive pill) can be of benefit, and menstrual bleeding during competition can be prevented by shortening or lengthening the menstrual cycle, as a planned exercise. Regular, heavy exercise seems to delay menarche and can produce oligo/amenorrhoea in the heavily exercising adolescent. Some athletes have low weight-induced oligo/amenorrhoea, but those athletes who weigh above 50–55 kg are unlikely to fall into this category and should have a hormonal assay. The bone density may be lowered (see Bone density).

## Muscle fibre

Type 1  Aerobic, oxidative metabolism of glycogen, with $CO_2$ as a waste product.
Type 2b Anaerobic, glycolytic metabolism, with lactate as a waste product.
Type 2a Perhaps an intermediate between types 1 and 2, with some aerobic capacity.

Type 2b is called 2x in some circles. Training does not alter the genetic balance between type 1 and type 2 muscle fibres, but it can alter the balance between type 2a and type 2b/x

## Muscle imbalance

Muscle function requires a balance of strength between agonist and antagonist, and this balance may alter with speed. When the muscle balance is upset, muscle damage may occur. However, it must also be noted that one side of the body should have a balanced relationship to the other side. Frequently the weak side is the side to be damaged. However, the damaged side is not necessarily the weak side, as the strong side may have to work disproportionately hard to make up for the weak side, and thus become damaged. This can be found whilst testing hamstring strength with an isokinetic dynamometer [24]. Racket sports may produce disproportionate shoulder strength from the dominant arm

and this can induce a dorsal scoliosis. Exercises should be given to the non-dominant side to maintain muscle balance.

## Myoglobinuria

Local trauma or excessive exercise may produce muscle breakdown, with the appearance of myoglobin in the urine.

## OBLA

Onset of blood lactic acid (OBLA). This is monitored during exercise, and standard fitness levels are recorded by monitoring the amount of work performed against a blood lactate of 2 or 4 mmol/L. The fitter an athlete gets the more work the athlete can do before reaching these levels of blood lactic acid, and the curve is said to move to the right. Loss of fitness shows by levels of blood lactic acid reaching 2 or 4 at lower work levels, and moves the curve to the left.

## Physical maturity

See Bone growth.

## Psychology

Sporting performance can be influenced by many psychological aspects, some of which are positive but many of which are negative; fear of failure, loss of concentration, loss of rhythm and technique under pressure, to name but a few. Many coaches have skills that incorporate a psychological approach for their athlete. However, specialist advice and help is available from sports psychiatrists and should be used when required.

Athletes can have a different mental picture of the damage that has been caused by their injury, which does not relate to their actual problems. If athletes are failing to progress as fast as their clinical findings would indicate that they should, asking the athletes to explain their picture of the problem can be quite revealing and enables an accurate, clear picture to be given to them. This will usually resolve the problem.

## Resting pulse

The resting pulse should be taken first thing in the morning, on wakening and before rising. The athlete should be taught to take this pulse, as it may be used as a rough and ready guide to fitness for competition or training. It can be used to monitor an aerobic training effect, when the improved fitness will show as a slowing of the resting pulse. It may also be used to monitor stress and illness, where a pulse raised 10 beats per minute probably reflects illness or an incipient illness, and suggests physical activity should be curtailed. Athletes with pulse increases of 5–10 beats per minute should see the doctor, who should check for illness and signs of stress. This player should be watched. If the cause is anxiety then it may prevent the athlete from eating, and the adrenaline surge will also deplete muscle glycogen. Invariably it is this player who is substituted or performs badly. High-glucose energy drinks can be a way to top up the muscle glycogen in this type of player.

## Sunburn

Many athletes enjoy bronzing whilst on tour but they must be warned against sunburn, especially of the head, neck, nose, ears and tops of feet and knees, as well as the usual torso, shoulders and arms. Sunglasses should always be worn around water and snow, because they reflect the sun's rays, and protective sun creams or blocks applied.

## Tanner scale

An assessment of physical maturity based on the development of secondary sexual characters: breast buds, pubic hair, etc. (see Bone growth and Children).

## Team talk

The 'team talk' will be given by the coach, and the doctor may have to spend long nights listening to the coach rehearsing this talk. Some coaches will deliberately raise the level of stress. However, to some players, who are already tense, this is not to the best advantage, and during the talk the doctor should observe the team for individual signs of stress and anxiety that may inhibit the player from eating and thus from loading the pre-match carbohydrates. Glucose energy drinks may be the best substitute for food for these players.

## Team travel

A pre-tour medical, or questionnaire, should be obtained to establish each individual's basic medical history and inoculation requirement. Both the 'proba-bles' and 'possibles' should be inoculated in case of any last-minute substitutes. Check time zone differences and allow approximately 24 hours per hour of time zone difference for an adjustment in circadian rhythm:

(a) Advise management of the optimum acclimatization time.

(b) Start adjusting sleep routines at home, or on the plane, to fit with the host country. Sleeping tablets and melatonin can help.

(c) Plan training times as near to match times as can be obtained, but training abroad at the home time equivalent to a low body biorhythm should be light until biorhythm adjustments have been made.

If uniform is worn then loose clothes and shoes should be taken to change into on the plane. Security permitting, analgesia, antacids, antiemetics, antihistamines, antidiarrhoeals and sleeping tablets should be carried by the team physician within the cabin baggage, rather than being left in a bag that will be stored in the hold. Most countries do not require a licence to practise if the physician is treating only team members, and will allow the relevant drugs to be carried whilst travelling with the team, but this should be cleared with the appropriate embassy. Advice should be given to team members on dehydration from alcohol, coffee and the air-conditioning, plus gastric distension from decompression and from gassy drinks. This is important if flying out to compete that same day. Administer sleeping tablets if appropriate – not to the physician! Recommend regular walks, compression stockings and exercises for the calves during long journeys.

## At the accommodation

Take the largest room available, as it will have to be both a consulting room and a bedroom. Post the doctor's room number on the team notice board and leave a notice on your door indicating when you are out and when you are expected back, and where you are. Arrange surgery times – but you will still end up consulting ad hoc as well. Obtain a print-out of competition times and travelling times to and from the venue, on the grounds that:

(a) management often forgets to inform the medical staff about these details

(b) in track and field, for instance, one can prioritize consultations to those still in the competition.

Arrange to review your patients at the training ground, or to be with those who have a known problem during their event. Arrange and organize training for the injured, as the coach has too much to think about with the fit team, and those left out through injury get depressed unless they are physically worked and rehabilitated. Liaise daily with the physiotherapist over all injury problems, and inform the coach of injury problems, actual and potential. Put out scales in the team corridor to monitor:

(a) Weight gain. Food on tour can be fantastic, and, when the athlete is bored, eating becomes a communal habit.

(b) Weight loss. This is especially suggestive of dehydration, or stress.

Make available daily fluid drinks in the team corridor as this encourages athletes to drink and observe their urine colour for dehydration (see Dehydration).

Know the location of the polyclinic in the village and what other medical services are available, as they may be of value. Record telephone numbers of the venue and village in your medical case. Do not forget your pass – hang it on the door handle at night. If appropriate, have at least two pairs of spectacles – leave one at the venue and one at the village. Make accurate notes and arrange with management about where they will be kept for the intervening legally required years.

## At the venue (Fig. 21.2)

Reconnoitre as soon as possible to find:

(a) the shortest distance from the team changing or warm-up area to the competition area and finishing line

(b) the stadium medical room, and meet the stadium medical officers if possible

(c) the source of ice

(d) the source of drinks

(e) the dope testing room.

Try and meet the stadium manager to discuss:

(a) medical track clearance – to where will sports people be taken, especially in events such as the marathon, time trials, walks and triathlon

(b) the nearest stretcher and type of stretcher

(c) the nearest first aid team, and where others are stationed

(d) the nearest hospital and its telephone number.

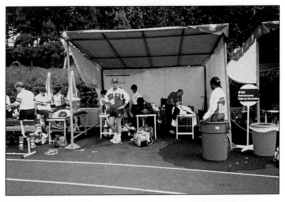

**Figure 21.2** • Millions are spent on Olympic games, but facilities for medical care are often appalling. Pictured are the facilities for two Olympic track and field squads. Note the sprinter standing in the water butt is having a post-race ice bath to reduce muscle oedema from minor trauma, especially from eccentric muscle work.

Take down a sticky label with the team name on it and put it on the best changing room you can find; however, you may have to get up early on the day of competition to bag this room, but, once you have it, most other teams will treat it as sacrosanct.

## Medical requirements at a venue

The following people are needed: team doctor, crowd doctor with advanced life-saving training, ambulance/St John's/paramedics stationed around the venue, drug testing team, track or playing area clearance team who are trained in first aid and the proper use of stretchers. Some events, golf and 3 day eventing for instance, require a map, split into designated grid areas, so that the site of the problem can be located easily and coordinated between the medical staff. Golf requires a communication system, where a vibrating as opposed to ringing call system ensures no distraction to the players. Fluorescent jackets, with the job title inscribed, aid communication in an emergency. The major hospital, especially the accident and emergency consultant, close to the event should be informed of the date and type of event. The accident and emergency telephone numbers of this hospital and the names of the relevant hospital doctors should be recorded, and visible in the event medical room.

## TUE

WADA, the controlling organization for recognizing or banning drugs that are used by athletes, has recognized that some athletes will suffer from medical disorders that require treatment and has decided that, though these drugs are on the banned list, their use will be permitted under these strict medical circumstances, if applied for as a **treatment under exemption.**

## WADA

The World Anti-Doping Agency, which controls which drugs will be recognized for doping and non-doping treatments of athletes.

## References

1 Mottram S, Comerford M. Stability dysfunction and lower back pain. J Orthop Med 1998;20:13–18

2 O'Brien M. Osteoporosis and exercise. Editorial. Br J Sports Med 1996;30:191

3 Caine DJ, Broekhoff J. Maturity assessment: a viable preventative measure against physical and psychological insult in the young athlete? Physician Sports Med 1987;15:67–80

4 Jordan SE, Green GA, Galanty HL, Mandelbaum BR, Jabour BA. Acute and chronic brain injury to United States National Team soccer players. Am J Sports Med 1996;24:205–210

5 Donath R. GDR sports-medical care for walkers. Abstract from lecture to the Amateur Athletics Association seminar for coaches in walking. Birmingham; 1985

6 Rowland TH. Preparticipation sports examination of the child and adolescent athlete: changing views of an old ritual. Pediatrician 1986;13:3–9

7 Caine DJ, Lindner K. Preventing injury to young athletes. Parts 1 and 2. J. de l'ACSEPL 1990;Part I, pp. 30–35; Part II, pp. 24–30

8 Rutenfranz J. Ethical considerations: the participation of children in elite sports. Pediatrician 1986;13:14–17

9 Arendt J, Marks V. Physiological changes underlying jet lag. BMJ 1982;284:144–146

10 Winget CM, DiRoshia CW, Holley DC. Circadian rhythms and athletic performance. Med Sci Sports Exerc 1985;17:498–516

11 Wijesinghe LD, Coughlin PA, Robertson I, Kessel D, Kent PJ, Kester RC. Cyclist's iliac syndrome: temporary relief by balloon angioplasty. Br J Sports Med 2001;35(1):70–71

12 Greenleaf JE. Exercise and water electrolyte balance. Special Publication, 1966;110:47–58

13 Brouns F, Saris WHM, Rehrer NJ. Abdominal complaints and gastrointestinal function during long lasting exercise. Int J Sports Med 1987;8:175–189

14 Thalmann M, Sodeck GH, Kavouras DS, Matalas A, Skenderi K, Yannikouris N, Domanovits H. Proton pump inhibition prevents gastrointestinal bleeding in ultramarathon runners: a randomised, double blinded, placebo controlled study. Br J Sports Med 2006;40:359–362

15 Fogelholm GM, Tikkanen HD, Näveri HK, Näveri LS, Härkönen MHA. Carbohydrate loading in practice: high muscle glycogen concentration is not certain. Br J Sports Med 1991;25:41–44

16 Gallagher D, Visser M, Sepúlveda D, Pierson RN, Harris T, Heymsfield SB. How useful is BMI for comparison of body fatness across age, sex and ethnic groups? Am J Epidemiol 1996;143:228–239

17 Prentice AM, Jebb SA, Beyond body mass index. Obesity Rev 2001;2(3):141–147

18 Stoller DW. Magnetic resonance imaging in orthopaedic and sports medicine, 2nd edn. California: Lippincott Williams & Wilkins; 1994. p. 1352

19 Shephard RJ, Sheck PN. Potential impact of physical activity and sport on the immune system: a brief review. Br J Sports Med 1994;28:247–255

20 Blomstrand E, Cesling F, Newsholme E. Changes in plasma concentrations of aromatic and branched chain amino acids during sustained exercise in man and their possible role in fatigue. Acta Physiol Scand 1988;133:115–121

21 Koutedakis Y, Budgett R, Faulmann L. Rest in underperforming elite competitors. Br J Sports Med 1990;24:248–252

22 Budgett R, Newsholme E, Lehmann M, et al. Redefining the overtraining syndrome as the unexplained underperformance syndrome. Br J Sports Med 2000;34(1):67–68

23 Fox JS. Gender verification – what purpose? what price? Br J Sports Med 1993;27:148–149

24 MTF Read. Unpublished results

## Further reading

Bruckner P, Khan K. Clinical sports medicine, 3rd edn. New York: McGraw-Hill; 2006

# Glossary

# Glossary

## Accessory navicular or os tibialis externum

An accessory ossification centre of the navicular, which, when fixed and large, is referred to as a cornuated navicular. About 10% of the young have an accessory ossification centre, but only about 2% remain uncoalesced in adults. It may produce symptoms due to its prominence, when the skin over the area is rubbed on by the shoes, or because of its tibialis posterior attachment, which produces stress across the fibrous attachment (see Chapter 13; Fig. 13.12).

## Acromioclavicular joint

| | |
|---|---|
| **Grade 1** | Superior ligament damage or sprain. |
| **Grade 2** | Superior and inferior ligament tear. |
| **Grade 3** | Superior and inferior ligament tear with disruption of the conoid and trapezoid ligaments. |
| **Grades 4 and 5** | Show severe instability and require surgical fixation. |

A more chronic onset causes degenerative changes within the joint and shows osteophytic lipping (see Chapter 17).

## Active compression test

A test to display **intra-articular shoulder lesions or acromioclavicular joint** problems. The standing patient forward flexes the arm to 90°, with the elbow in full extension, and then adducts the arm 10–15° medial to the sagittal plane of the body and internally rotates it to point the thumb downwards. The examiner applies uniform downward pressure on the arm. The manoeuvre is repeated with the palm upwards. The test is positive if pain is elicited in the first manoeuvre and reduced in the second. The acromioclavicular joint sufferer 'points' to the top of the shoulder and the labral tear produces pain and clicking 'inside' the shoulder [1].

## Adson's manoeuvre

**For arm pain.** Abduct the elbow to 90° with the shoulder and add external rotation of the arm. Pain reproduced on looking towards the painful arm equals a possible disc. Pain on looking away, or a decrease in pulse volume, equals a possible thoracic outlet syndrome.

## Adverse neural tensioning

**Nerves** must be capable of moving and to adapt to the altered length required of the neurovascular bundle as a joint is flexed and extended. The spinal cord similarly moves within the spine. If the nerve is trapped by a disc, adhesions, or tumour, then free movement cannot occur and pain is produced. The classic example would be the straight leg raise test, made worse by stretching the sciatic nerve (Lasègue's) and then adding a stretch of the spinal cord (Kernig's). This is the mechanism of the slump test, which becomes the combination of these two tests. Gently stretching, just into pain, over a long time may free up these adhesions, or possibly encourage growth of the neurovascular bundle to produce adequate length. Therapeutic, adverse neural tension uses gentle stretching techniques to stretch the nerve, perhaps releasing the fixation and restraint applied by the compressive areas. However, the Iliserov technique to lengthen bone has to be accompanied by lengthening of the neurovascular bundle. The technique cannot be forced beyond an increase in length of 2 mm per day, and it is possible that adverse neural tension techniques do not free up the adhesions but encourage a lengthening of the neurovascular bundle so that the nerve develops enough length to cope with the functional movement required [2]. Adverse neural tension is used clinically for nerve root adhesions in the arm and leg, and peripheral adhesions such as the piriformis and hamstring syndrome (see Chapter 9).

## Alexander technique

A technique to improve posture, but particularly using pelvic tilt.

## Allen's test

Pressure is applied at the wrist on both the radial and ulnar arteries to exclude the blood flow and, with the release of one at a time, a flush of the hand occurs as the blood flow returns and indicates whether each **artery is patent**.

## Anderson's test

A grinding test for **meniscal lesions**.

## Anterior apprehension test of the shoulder

The patient faces a mirror. The clinician stands behind the patient, flexes the shoulder to 90° and externally rotates the shoulder as fully as possible. The clinician then applies pressure on the posterior aspect of the humeral head to increase anterior translation. Apprehension or pain, which can be seen in the reflection of the patient's face in the mirror, is a positive test for a **subluxing** or **unstable shoulder**.

## Anterior draw test

The knee is flexed to 90° and the tibia rotated internally. The clinician sits on the patient's foot so that the distal tibia is fixed. The proximal tibia is then drawn anteriorly. Increased translation is permitted by a torn or ruptured **anterior cruciate ligament**. The starting position must be noted, as any sag caused by a posterior cruciate rupture will then allow an increased, apparent anterior gliding, and a false positive. Comparison must be made with the other leg.

**Anterior translation of the talus** can be produced by the clinician restraining the tibia with one hand and then forcing the calcaneum forward with the other hand. Ligamentous strains and talar osteochondral defects produce pain. The amount of anterior draw can be visualized on X-ray by supporting the heel on a block and applying a weight over the tibia. The upper limit of normal translation is 6 mm.

**Shoulder instability** can display increased movement, when the humerus is translated forwards.

## Apley's test

For the **knee**. Compression and distraction manoeuvres of the tibia are performed on a flexed knee at 90° through to 180°, with the patient lying prone. Pain only on distraction suggests a **ligamentous** cause, whereas pain and grinding on compression and rotation suggests **meniscal** or **articular surface** damage.

## Apprehension test

See Anterior apprehension test of the shoulder and Patella apprehension test in the **knee**.

## Arcade of Frohse

A ligamentous band over the posterior interosseous nerve as it enters between the two heads of the supinator. A tight band can cause **radial nerve entrapment** and is released by surgery.

## Babcock's triangle

A triangle that can be imagined on the superior surface of the femoral neck and which lies between the femoral head, the greater trochanter and the inferior surface

## Ballottement

A fluid-filled space will transmit a pressure wave from one side to the other. Ballottement is the creation and palpation of this wave. See Bulge test.

## Bankart lesion

This is a bony fracture defect in the inferior glenoid caused by **shoulder** dislocation. Visible on X-ray, but an MRI may show an inferior labral defect with no bony lesion (see Chapter 17; Fig. 17.16).

## Bankart's repair

Surgical repair of the glenoid labrum and reattachment of the Bankart lesion in a dislocated or recurrent **dislocating shoulder**.

## Bayonet sign

A sign indicative of possible **patellar maltracking**. The patella tendon insertion lies well lateral on the tibia, thus producing a valgus alignment of the patella tendon from the lower patellar pole to its insertion on the tibia, giving the appearance of a bayonet on a rifle.

## Beighton–Horan score

A score for **ligamentous laxity**. Score 1 point for right side and 1 point for left side:

- Little finger extending to 90°.
- Hyperextension of the elbow beyond 15°.
- Hyperextension of the knee.
- An ability to touch the back of the thumb onto the front of the forearm.

Score 1 point for:

- Touching the flat of the hands onto the floor.

Total score = 9.

## Bennett's fracture

For the **thumb**. Fracture dislocation of the proximal end of the first metacarpal (see Chapter 19; Fig. 19.5).

## Blocked movement

It is easiest to consider this in a kick of the football. The kicker subconsciously prepares the whole movement pattern, to conclude with the 'follow through', but if an opponent stops the ball from moving then the kicker's movement is 'blocked' and does not reach the 'follow through'. Because the programmed musculoskeletal action was completion of the kick, there is no preparatory deceleration and the muscle contraction continues on after the leg has been stopped from moving, and this produces an acute **resistance to the contraction**, which often ruptures the muscle. Clinically the expression can be used for describing a resisted muscle test, e.g. 'block external rotation'.

# Bone scan

Radioactive technetium-99, given intravenously, is taken up by active bone, and, when this radioactivity is counted, early stress lesions in bone will be displayed. When these are accompanied by pain they are defined as stress fractures. Increased blood supply will be displayed by an increased radioactivity count, but only during the phase when technetium is in the blood. A count taken during the injection phase, and monitored over 2 minutes, will display areas of poor **blood supply** (reflex sympathetic dystrophy) (see Fig. 12.8) and increased blood supply, as in an inflammatory lesion (Fig. 22.1). The three-phase bone scan reports the early and late blood phase and then, 2–4 hours later, the bone phase (Fig. 22.2). Muscle damage, as in **DOMS**, can show as a hot muscle scan in the blood phase.

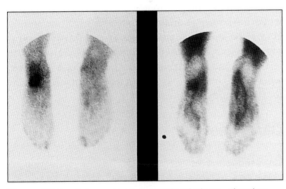

**Figure 22.1** • A bone scan, in its blood phase, showing increased uptake in the right ankle with soft tissue inflammation.

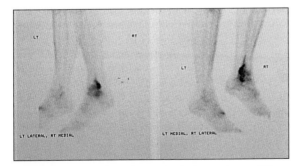

**Figure 22.2** • Increased uptake in the bone phase of the right ankle.

# Bowstring sign

The bowstring sign attempts to differentiate between a **hamstring lesion** and **sciatica**. The straight leg raise is taken up to the onset of pain, then the knee is allowed to flex until the pain disappears, at which stage pressure is applied to the popliteal fossa to restretch the sciatic nerve. A recurrence of pain suggests sciatica.

# Brachial nerve tensioning tests

**Neural stretch tests** for the brachial, ulnar, median and radial nerves, respectively. See Adverse neural tensioning.

# Bristow repair

For recurrent **dislocation of the shoulder**. The tip of the coracoid containing its attachments, short head of biceps and coracobrachialis is screwed to the neck of the scapula and produces a dynamic sling anteroinferiorly.

# Brostrom repair

Surgical repair of ruptured **lateral ligaments of the ankle** – resuturing the ruptured ligaments.

# Bulge test

A small amount of **fluid in the knee** may be displayed by compressing one side of the knee to move all the fluid to the other side. The suprapatellar pouch is compressed during this manoeuvre. The opposite side of the knee is then compressed with a stroking movement. Fluid will return again to the first side and is seen as an increasing bulge. Too much fluid, 20 mL or so, will not empty from one side to the other and is palpated by **ballotting** the fluid with one hand and feeling the impulse with the other. A volume of 30 mL or more will show as a **patellar tap**, because increased fluid lifts the patella off the femur, from where it may be pressed down onto the femur but springs out again when the pressure is removed.

# Burner/stinger

Transient irritation of a **cervical nerve root** with temporary paralysis, often C6 distribution, plus lancinating pain into shoulder and arm, which may last only 10–15 minutes. Traces of a neurological deficit may last for months.

## Calcaneotibial compression test

Because standing on tiptoe can load the Achilles or compress the posterior structures of the ankle, this test is used to differentiate **Achilles lesions** from **posterior ankle and talar/subtalar lesions**. With the patient lying prone, the foot is whipped into passive plantar flexion to impinge the superior surface of the calcaneum against the posterior structures of the ankle. No pain occurs with Achilles lesions as the Achilles is shortened, but does occur if structures at the back of the ankle are damaged (see Chapter 13, Part 5; Fig. 13.10).

## Camber running

Many **roads are domed**, to run water off to the sides, and this produces a slope or camber. Running on the same side of the road all the time will produce a functional long and short leg. This functional inequality may stress ligaments throughout the lower limb, especially in the knees and ankles. Runners must vary the side of the road on which they run.

## Chair test

The patient lies on their back with their feet resting on the seat of a chair. Without help from their arms, they raise their buttocks as high as they can off the ground. A damaged hamstring will cause pain or be weak. The test may be repeated, using one leg at a time or by increasing the number of repetitions. This is also a very good method of strengthening the hamstring without expensive equipment.

## Checking shoes

The most important aspect of a shoe is the **integrity of the uppers**. The heel cups must be capable of holding the heel stable and must not be warped inwards or outwards. Their attachment must be solid to hold the calcaneum, the heel tag must be soft so as not to compress the Achilles, and the sides not so high as to rub on the peroneals or tibialis posterior (see Chapter 16: Oddities caused by the sports shoe).

## Clarke's test

This is a compression test of the patella to display **patello-femoral pain**. The clinician compresses the patella in a distal direction and then the patient contracts the quadriceps. This may produce total inhibition of quadriceps contraction, pain and/or grating under the patella. Clarke's test is an indicative test, rather than an absolutely positive test, and the test on one side should be compared with the other side as a normal knee may produce positive signs.

## Claw hand

When the **median nerve** is involved as well as the **ulna**, all the fingers claw.

## Closed chain exercises

Muscle exercises can be performed with the more proximal joints held stable and the periphery moved, which are known as **open chain exercises**, or the periphery can be stabilized and the body and proximal joints moved, which are **closed chain exercises**. Balancing on one foot and squatting is a closed chain exercise, whereas sitting and swinging a weight attached to the foot is an open chain exercise.

## Clunk test

Circumduction of the **shoulder** in full abduction. A clunk or grinding suggests internal derangement.

## Compartment pressures

These can be measured by a split catheter with a pressure transducer, which is inserted into a **muscle compartment**. These pressures are read before and after exercise or monitored continuously. A rise in pressure beyond a certain level, either at rest or after exercise, may be pathological. Various levels are recorded as abnormal in the calf, such as with continuous monitoring, when readings above 30 mmHg in the relaxation phase and above 50 mmHg in the contraction phase are considered positive, although some accept above 85 mmHg in the contraction phase. Although controversy exists regarding what pressure should require intervention, pressures of >15 mmHg before exercise, >30 mmHg 1 minute post exercise, or prolonged pressures of >20 mmHg after 5 minutes' post exercise rest, in the anterior compartment, are considered abnormal [3]. Chronic exertional compartment syndrome responds better to surgery when the problem lies within the anterior compartment rather than the posterior compartments. Patients should be tested by repeating the exercise that brings on their pain, as purely 'test running' a patient may not do this [4]. Sometimes, if a patient has rested for some weeks before the test, his or her pressures recordings may be normal because the chronic increase in pressure of the compartment only builds up with repeated exercises, where the effects of one training session are not allowed to settle before the next is started.

## Concentric muscle contraction

The muscle force elongates the stretch elastic component before shortening occurs. The mechanical force is positive and the muscle contraction occurs together with shortening, such as the biceps lifting a weight up towards the shoulder. It is an acceleratory force. See Eccentric muscle contraction.

## Congruence angles

These are the angles, measured on X-ray, between the patellar and femoral condyles at 45° of flexion that are used to assess **malalignment of the patella**.

## Core stability [5]

Various techniques – Alexander [6] and active alert [7] – have been around for many years, and the early 21st century prefers the 70-year-old Pilates techniques. Essentially, the lumbar spine is held in the patient's neutral position, though the Alexander technique encourages pelvic tilt, and is then splinted by the transversus abdominis and multifidis muscles. Pelvic stabilizers, which are the external rotators of the hip, are strengthened to control pelvic rotations and functional protruberance of the greater trochanter.

## Cortisone in soft tissues

Methylprednisolone (Depo-medrone) should not be used with epidurals, particularly translumbar, as the dilutant/preservative is irritable to the meninges if the dura is penetrated. Hydrocortisone acetate produces less subcutaneous atrophy and may be preferred in superficial injections, such as for the Achilles peritendon and tennis elbow. Triamcinolone remains active

locally for longer. Cortisone should be used to treat only inflammatory conditions.

## Cram test

Pressure is applied by the clinician on the **sciatic nerve** at the popliteal fossa to exacerbate the tensioning of the sciatic nerve, produced by the straight leg raise test. See Bowstring sign.

## Crank test

The circumducted arm is moved backwards and forwards between external and internal rotation, and pressure is exerted axially through the arm towards the joint. Pain and clunking suggest possible internal ligamentous disruption, such as a 'SLAP' lesion.

## CRP

C-reactive protein. A rise in its level can be an early blood marker of some systemic diseases.

## CT

**Computed tomography** of X-rays, to produce 'slices' through body tissues, displaying both soft tissue and bone. Spiral CT can produce excellent views of vascular structures and the colon.

## Depth jumping

See Pliometrics.

## Disc probe

The annulus of the disc has nerve ends, and some annular discs lesions probably present only as increased nucleus pulposus pressure on the annulus, without herniation. Some show on MRI as an annular tear. They may be treated by an intradiscal injection of cortisone. The disc can be destroyed with chymopapaine, but the occasional complication of transverse myelitis makes intradiscal radiofrequency, or microdiscectomy, a safer procedure [8]. With neuroleptanalgesia [9] the stimulation from an intradiscal injection may be used for the **diagnosis of vertebral** pain when the facet and sacroiliac joints can also be injected to register the site of pain.

## DISH

**Disseminated idiopathic skeletal hypertrophy** has a tendency to produce traction spurs at many apophyses. Known also as Forestier's disease.

## DOMS

**Delayed-onset muscle soreness.** Endurance events, eccentric muscle work and muscle overtraining cause muscle stiffness and pain some 24–48 hours after the exercise, which may last 5–7 days. During this time creatinine kinase is raised, the technetium bone scan may be positive and T2-weighted and STIR imaging MRI scans show an increased signal over the muscle concerned. At its severest the pain may even last 2–3 months, with the changes visible on T2-weighted MRI (Fig. 22.3).

## Downing's sign

The supine leg is flexed at the hip, externally rotated and then straightened. An apparent leg lengthening,

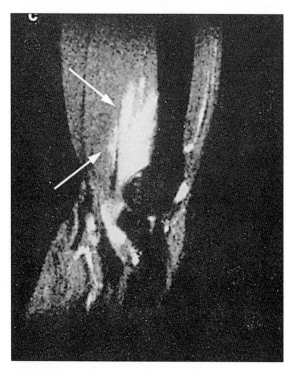

**Figure 22.3** • T2-weighted MRI sequence showing increased signal in the biceps following eccentric muscle exercise.

registered by the medial maleolus, indicates the **sacroiliac joint** is mobile. This apparent lengthening reduces with hip flexion, adduction and straightening of the leg. It is not an accurate test but may help to decide whether a sacroiliac joint should be manipulated or sclerosed. The mobile joint does not need manipulating. The signs may be associated with T12 problems [10]. However intra-examiner reliability is poor [11].

## Drop jumping

See Pliometrics.

## Drop tests for the shoulder

The examiner passively abducts the humerus 20° and supports it. The humerus is then passively rotated to 5° less than maximum and the support removed from the arm. Damage to the **supra- and/or infraspinatus** will not allow the patient to hold this position actively.

The examiner supports the elbow with the shoulder in 90° of abduction and almost full external rotation, with the elbow flexed. The support at the wrist is released, but not that at the elbow. Damage to the **infraspinatus** is shown by the inability of the patient to hold external rotation.

The humerus is passively extended behind the back to 20° and is 20° abducted away from the body, with nearly full internal rotation. Inability to hold this position is shown by **subscapularis** weakness.

## Duck waddle

This is a test used for subtle **meniscal** pathology. Moving forward in a full squat position is painful, but an effusion, lack of full extension, pain on full flexion and patellofemoral problems may complicate this test (Fig. 22.4).

## Dural stress tests

Straight leg raise, slump, Kernig's, prone lying knee flexion and femoral nerve stretch tests for the leg, and brachial nerve tensioning and arm raising for the arms, plus the general tests Valsalva and Lhermitte's, can all stress the dura, and, if the dura is prevented from moving, it will produce pain. The straight leg raise and slump tests will be variably positive with herniated

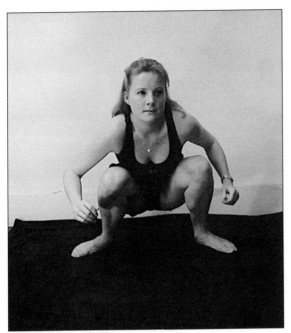

**Figure 22.4** • The 'duck waddle'.

discs and adhesions of the nerve root or dura, whilst blowing a Valsalva may also produce lumbar pain in the presence of acute dural irritation. See Adverse neural tensioning.

## Dye strapping

The subcutaneous fat pad of the heel is separated into separate compartments by fibrous stromal bands that run vertically. The fat globules sit in the compartments created by these bands. On impact the fat spreads out sideways, but is held by the stroma, and thus acts as a shock absorber. Dye strapping is a strapping technique to squeeze the subcutaneous fat pad of the heel, preventing it from spreading sideways on heel impact. The strapping thus maintains the thickness of the heel pad and adds support to the stroma. This is the mechanism that has been copied by the 'air soles' in running shoes. Used for type 1 **plantar fasciitis**.

## Eburnation

A description relating to degenerative joints when the articular cartilage is destroyed and bone is articulating with bone.

## Eccentric muscle contraction

The load lengthens the stretch elastic component first, and then the muscle lengthens during contraction. The mechanical force is negative and is a deceleratory force. Fewer motor fibres per Newton are required than for concentric muscle contraction. This movement is more prone to muscle damage, and a raised creatinine phosphokinase may be measured for 3–5 days after heavy eccentric work, e.g. the biceps lowering a weight onto a table (see Fig. 22.3). See Concentric muscle contraction.

## ECG

**Electrocardiogram** recording of the heart's electrical activity. A large left ventricle and raised ST segment may be normal in athletes but should evoke an ultrasound scan to measure ventricular wall thickness, to establish whether it is a physiological enlargement or some other problem, such as HOCUM, hypertrophic cardiomyopathy.

## Effort thrombosis

**Paget–von Schroetter syndrome**, with distended veins and oedema, which is usually found in the arm and requires a venogram and possible anticoagulation. It is a rare syndrome.

## EMG

**Electromyogram.** Checks how well a nerve muscle complex is working by measuring conduction rate of peripheral nerves.

## Enthesis/enthesopathy

The enthesis is the cellular transition zone where the **tendon becomes bone**, i.e. the attachment of tendon to bone. An enthesopathy is an inflammation or damage of this area.

## Epidural injections

May be given by the caudal or translumbar approach. The caudal, with 0.5% procaine, allows the patient to walk away and be treated as an outpatient. A stronger solution may be given for intense pain, giving some short-term analgesia, but the motor effects of this must be considered when releasing the patient as a day case. The 'caine anaesthetics, possibly, may close the S or H gates within the myelin sheath so that a continued sodium ion leak, which produces a continued ionic-induced noci stimulus, is aborted. Certainly, there appears to be a desensitization occurring over a few days, rather than a short-term analgesic effect, from epidural therapy. In the acute prolapsed disc there will be accompanying oedema, which increases the pressure on the dura and nerve root. This increases the damage and neuropraxia so that the addition of a steroid to the epidural solution will reduce the increased inflammation and swelling, and, therefore, reduce the subsequent pressure and pain. It may also help to prevent long-term adhesions. The epidural does not reduce a herniated disc, and in the presence of increasing disc herniation, when a nerve palsy is developing, will not appear to help, as the mechanical pressure from the disc is too great for the reduction in swelling to make any difference. The **reasons for epidural therapy** are:

(a) Night pain

(b) Neurological signs. Note S3 and S4 require immediate surgery

(c) Too intense a pain to give any other treatment, bar rest

(d) Sciatica uncontrolled by other analgesics

(e) Chronic sciatica, when the cause is ionic root irritation

(f) As a diagnostic test, when there is a suggestion of dural irritation

(g) Chronic hamstring injury with a positive slump test.

## ESR

Erythrocyte sedimentation rate is raised in the older person, but particularly with systemic disease. The rise in ESR is slower than the elevation of the CRP. Polymyalgia rheumatica and temporal arteritis, which usually but not invariably have a very raised ESR, must be considered in the 55 plus age group, if mechanical signs are not found to back up the symptoms of shoulder girdle (with sometimes pelvic girdle) and headaches.

## Faber's test

Flexion, abduction and external rotation of the **hip**, while the ankle is placed on the opposite knee. Groin pain and limited abduction suggest hip or iliopsoas

problems. Back pain may be from the **sacroiliac joint**. This test is very similar to the figure-of-four test.

## Facet joint and sacroiliac joint stress tests

Tests for the facet joint and sacroiliac joint dysfunction are only indicative rather than absolutely diagnostic, as stress tests almost certainly impinge on both elements. One must also remember that, with even a minor disc disturbance, there may well be associated disturbance of the other articular structures, such as the facet joints:

(a) **Facet joint rocking.** With the patient lying prone, the ilium is pulled posteriorly, whilst the butt of the other hand holds down the transverse process of L5, thus forcing the facet of the sacrum to be impinged onto the facet of the adjacent L5. This is repeated by rocking L5 into L4, etc. The examiner tests each segment at a time, and then the other side.

(b) **Facet joint rolling.** If there are no signs of dural tensioning then rolling the supine patient into a ball, and taking both legs towards first one shoulder and then the other will gap the facet joints – if there is capsular irritation then this will produce pain.

(c) **Local palpation.** The facet joints lie level with the gaps between the spinous processes, and local pressure about 2 cm out may be tender. Rocking the spinous process only shows the dysfunctional level, not the underlying cause.

## Facet joint injections

Perifacetal injections of corticosteroid will relieve the acute episode and may, when combined with local anaesthetic, provide for earlier manipulation. Chronic osteoarthritis of the facet joints will be improved on the same basis as injections of any osteoarthritic joint, i.e. if there is capsular inflammation then there will be benefit but if the source of the pain is bony then there is less improvement. In these cases it is important to know that the facet joint has been injected, and facetal injections should be done under image control.

## Femoral stretch

A dural tensioning test for the **femoral nerve** where the patient is laid on their side with legs held straight. The upper straight leg is taken backwards to extend the hip; however, as this movement can also extend the lumbar spine, pain produced at this stage may be from the spine and not the nerve. Then the knee is flexed to stretch the femoral nerve, and pain produced in the back or down the front of the thigh that is similar to the patient's pain is a positive test. See Adverse neural tensioning and Prone lying knee flexion.

## 'Figure-of-four' sign

For **popliteal muscle strain**. Flex the knee and externally rotate the hip, whilst resting the ankle on the contralateral thigh. The appearance is of a figure '4' (Fig. 22.5).

## Finklestein's test

For extensor **tenosynovitis of the thumb** (de Quervain's), where the wrist is ulnar flexed and the thumb passively flexed across the palm. Pain on this manoeuvre, over the dorsum of the wrist, is a positive test.

## Fitch catch

The patient leans backwards, trying to grab the back of one Achilles with the opposite hand. This test provokes greater lumbar extension with some rotation and, plus the one-legged hyperextension test, may be the only tests to hurt with **facet joint** or **pars interarticularis lesions** (Fig. 22.6).

## Flamingo view

See Stork view.

## Forestier's disease

See DISH.

## Fowler's position

See Traction.

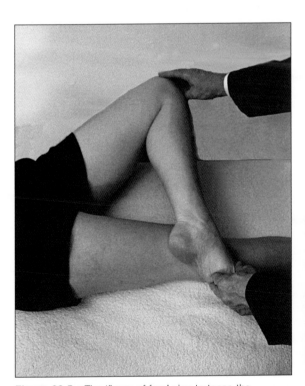

**Figure 22.5** • The 'figure-of-four' sign to tense the popliteus is very similar to Faber's test.

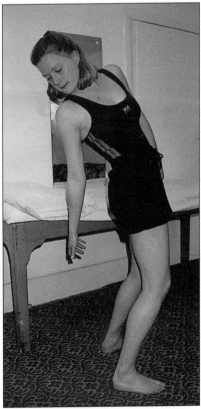

**Figure 22.6** • Fitch catch.

# Freiberg's infraction/infarction (Köhler's second disease)

Osteochondral necrosis of, usually, the second or third **metatarsal head** of the metatarsophalangeal joint (see Fig. 16.2).

# Freiberg's sign

Passive internal rotation of the **hip** causes pain. Possibly diagnostic for piriformis syndrome; however, the hip joint, sacroiliac joint and trochanteric bursa may also cause pain.

# Froment's sign

A test for **ulnar nerve** damage where a piece of paper is gripped between the straight thumb and index finger – if the adductor pollicis does not work then the long flexors help and the thumb bends at the proximal inter-phalangeal joint to maintain grip. The damage must be proximal to Guyon's canal to involve the motor branches. Damage at Guyon's canal at the wrist (sensory branch) will not produce this sign.

# Gadolinium

A contrast dye used with **MRI** to differentiate scar or fibrous tissue, especially from a disc lesion.

# Gerdy's tubercle

The insertion of the lateral collateral ligament and iliotibial tract on to the **tibia**.

# Gilmore's groin

(See Chapter 8: Conjoined tendon.)

# Glasgow coma scale or coma score

A standardized chart to record levels of consciousness. To be repeated over time. A score under 10 requires immediate admission to hospital.

| Condition | Response | Score |
|---|---|---|
| Eye opening | Spontaneous | 4 |
| | To verbal commands | 3 |
| | To pain | 2 |
| | None | 1 |
| Best motor response | Follows commands | 6 |
| | Localizes stimuli | 5 |
| | Withdraws | 4 |
| | Flexion posturing | 3 |
| | Extension posturing | 2 |
| | No movement | 1 |
| Verbal response | Orientated | 5 |
| | Confused | 4 |
| | Inappropriate words | 3 |
| | Incomprehensible sounds | 2 |
| | No verbal response | 1 |
| **Total maximum** | | **15** |

# Godfrey test

See Sag sign.

# Golfer's elbow

A medial epicondylitis of the **elbow**.

# Guyon's canal

The pisohamate tunnel, at the wrist, through which passes the sensory branch of the ulnar nerve.

# Haembursitis

Bleeding within a bursa, from trauma or a bleeding diathesis. This can be aspirated in the early stages but if deep may require ultrasound control, and a pressure bandage should be applied. It tends to recur and frequently the aspiration needs repeating several times. An injection of cortisone into the bursa probably does not reduce the recurrence. It is theoretically a potent site for infection, so it may be judicious to cover the aspiration with antibiotics for 48 hours.

# Haglund's syndrome

**Heel pain.** Superficial Achilles bursa, retro Achilles bursa and enlarged posterior calcaneal boss. Large 'pump bumps' (see Chapter 13, Part 5).

## Half squat test

Gives an indication as to whether there is a functional **valgus of the knees** and functional **overpronation of the feet** (see Figs 11.10 and 11.11).

## Haswell's lesion

Defect of the **patella**, typically superior lateral quadrant, of either necrotic or vascular fibrous tissue. Benign progressive lesion – observe. A biopsy may be required if the lesion is hot on the bone scan or gives an increased signal on T2-weighted MRI.

## Hawkins' sign

An impingement sign for the subacromial bursa. The arm is circumducted and internally rotated (Fig. 22.7). See Impingement test for the shoulder.

## Hill–Sachs lesion

**Recurrent dislocation of the shoulder**. X-ray, CT or MRI changes in the superior humeral articular surface from chronic subluxation, caused by impingement of the posterior superior humeral head into the acromion (see Fig. 17.17).

## Hoffa's fat pads

Extra-articular fat at the front of the **knee** that function as shock absorbers.

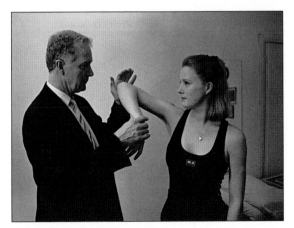

**Figure 22.7** • Hawkins' impingement test for the subacromial space.

## Homans' test

Homans' test is a test for deep vein thrombosis in the calf. The gastrocnemius is relaxed by flexing the knee, and then the soleus and to some extent the gastrocnemius are stretched by the examiner dorsiflexing the ankle. Thrombosed deep veins will cause pain.

## Hoover's test

A test to check whether a patient is positively, or volitionally, showing **rectus femoris** weakness. Resisted contraction of the rectus femoris will provoke downward pressure onto the couch or testing hand of the contralateral leg.

## Hughston's jerk test

See Jerk test and Reverse pivot shift.

## Hypermobility

This is usually recorded as a **Beighton–Horan** score and usually has a congenital link. These hypermobile people are more prone to ligamentous injuries. Elastic supports, taping and commercial supports may help, but these should be reinforced with postural exercises that set the gamma efferents to balance between agonist and antagonists, so that joint control is maintained. This applies particularly to anterior knee pain, sway back knees and elbows. Suppleness has advantages but may not take the heavy strain of some sports, so that four-piece gymnasts, with sway back elbows, are most unlikely to make the grade and may have to be pushed towards rhythmic gymnastics instead. Congenital problems, such as Marfan syndrome and Erb–Duchenne syndrome, are particularly prone to these problems and may have added complications, e.g. aortic dissection.

## Impingement test

For **subacromial space inflammation** and **rotator cuff injuries**. Shoulder pain on internally rotating the circumducted humerus (see Fig. 22.7). See Hawkins' sign and Neer's sign.

## Interferential

Slow electromagnetic waves are therapeutic but do not penetrate body tissues. Two fast waves, say 1045 Hz and 1050 Hz, will penetrate and can be made to interfere with one another, thus leaving a residual slow wave of 5 Hz, which is therapeutic. Various wave lengths are said to heat muscles and joints, and can also stimulate muscles and control pain.

## Iselin's disease

This is a traction apophysitis of the proximal **fifth metatarsal**.

## Isokinetic muscle contraction

A test of muscle strength, which can be made at a constant speed through angular rotation. The force can be eccentric or concentric. Peak torque occurs at different angles. It is used both in rehabilitation and in testing to record muscle balance, such as between quadriceps and hamstrings. The strength diminishes with increased speed.

## Isometric/isostatic muscle contraction

This produces a force without movement, by blocking the movement or working the antagonist against the agonist muscle. Therefore the mechanical movement is zero. The training effect is angle specific and is a differential training method for type 2 muscle fibres (white).

## Isotonic muscle contraction

A contraction involving the same muscle tone throughout its length of contraction. Cam pulleys are required, as otherwise peak torque changes through the angles of movement. The mechanical force may be positive or negative, concentric or eccentric.

## Jerk test

For **anterior cruciate ligament tear**, where the patient lies supine with the hip flexed to 60°, the tibia in internal rotation, and a valgus stress is applied across the knee. Slowly extend the knee. Tibial subluxation and relocation is felt as a jerk. This fails in subtle anterior cruciate ligament tears.

## Jobe's test

See Relocation test.

## Jones' fracture

Fracture of the proximal shaft of the fifth **metatarsal**. Prone to non-union (see Chapter 16).

## Jump sign

For **anterior cruciate ligaments** when, during movement of extension and flexion, the femur may ride up on the posterior horn of the meniscus and then 'jump' back into place. This suggests anterior cruciate ligament instability.

## Kager's triangle

The area of fat subtended between the anterior surface of the **Achilles** and soleus, the posterior surface of the tibia and flexor hallucis longus, and the calcaneum inferiorly. Soft tissue swellings that distort this area may be visualized on ultrasound, X ray, CT or MRI.

## Keinbock's disease

Idiopathic, avascular necrosis of the **lunate**. Initially the bone is cold on a bone scan, hot during revascularization (see Fig. 19.4).

## Kernig's test

Neck flexion will stretch the proximal elements of the **dura** and produce pain if the dura is tethered. This test is often added to the straight leg raise and Lasègue's to constitute the slump test. It is also used to diagnose meningism. See Adverse neural tensioning and Dural stress tests.

## Köhler's disease

Idiopathic osteochondrosis or avascular necrosis of the **tarsal navicular**. The average age of the child at diagnosis is 6 years. The child walks on the outside of the foot and it is symptomatic for 3–9 months. Scan and X-ray changes evolve over 2–4 years but it is not associated with long-term osteoarthritis. Also known as

Köhler's second disease is Freiberg's infraction/infarction (see Chapter 16: Freiberg's osteochondritis/infraction/infarction).

## Lachman's test

A test for **anterior cruciate ligament** instability where the basic principle is to relax the restraining, posterior pull of the hamstrings on the tibia, thus allowing easier anterior translation. This test may be done by holding and supporting the patient's femur, either on your own leg or on the edge of the examination couch [12], and then drawing the tibia anteriorly whilst holding the femur down (Figs 22.8 and 22.9).

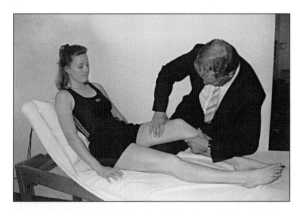

**Figure 22.8** • Lachman's test with the hamstring relaxed and supported on the examiner's thigh.

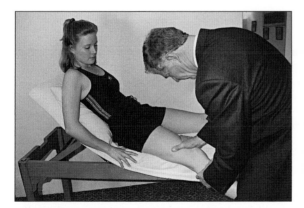

**Figure 22.9** • The femur is supported on the couch, the ankle between the examiner's legs. Then with the femur stabilized by one hand, anterior draw is applied to the lower leg.

## Lasègue's test

Dorsiflexion of the foot is added to the straight leg raise to stretch the sciatic nerve further. This is a **nerve root or sciatic nerve test**, rather than a dural stress test. Thus hamstring and piriformis entrapment of the sciatic nerve has a positive straight leg raise and Lasègue's, but a negative slump test (Fig. 22.10). See Adverse neural tensioning.

## Laser

(a) **Surgical**: higher frequency laser light is used as a surgical tool to vaporize and cauterize.

(b) **Medical**: laser is applied to soft tissues where it seems to have a similar effect to **ultrasound**. However, its effect does seem to reach a maximum over four sessions, and an increase in intensity and length of treatment does not produce further benefit. The higher wavelengths, over 800 Hz, do not seem to be effective, and variations in wavelength may benefit different types of tissue. Laser light is no longer columnated after contact with the skin and it may be that multiple light wavelengths are of similar benefit, though not so accurately directed at the tissue [13].

## Leg length

Osteopaths are taught to call rotations of the ilium (anterior spine – anterior or posterior) as leg length discrepancies, so that often their phrase of a 'short leg'

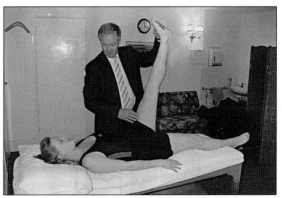

**Figure 22.10** • Lasègue's test. The straight leg raise tensions the sciatic nerve, and this pull is increased by adding dorsiflexion of the ankle in this position.

does not reflect a true short leg but a possible functional short leg. The only true measurement of bony leg length is by X-raying the patient standing against a graded screen. Clinically, assessing the levels of the iliac crests to check leg length is usually sufficient, and, by getting the patient to stand with supinated feet, the inequality caused by pronation will be eliminated. Most patients have adjusted to 1–2 cm of shortening and do not require treatment. However, larger discrepancies may cause back problems, which will benefit from a shoe raise for partial correction. In this case, measurements from the umbilicus and anterior superior iliac spine to the inferior border of the medial malleolus and checks that the medial malleoli remain the same length when the patient sits from lying and when the pelvis is raised and dropped on the couch must all register the same leg as being shorter before a leg length discrepancy should be diagnosed. Less than 2 cm is within tolerance. However, if symptoms persist then correction with a heel raise, at first inside the shoe, may help. If this helps, the raise may be moved to the exterior of the shoe heel and, if necessary, a further raise introduced inside the shoe as a trial, which again would be attached to the exterior of the shoe heel, if successful. Note camber running and pronation can produce an apparent short leg.

## Lhermitte's sign

A **dural stress test**, where neck flexion or extension produce symptoms in the back and legs. See Dural stress tests.

## Lisfranc joint

The **second tarsometatarsal** joint, which may be inflamed or fractured, particularly in dancers.

## Lombard's paradox

A **muscle that crosses two joints** may have to contract at one end whilst relaxing at the other, i.e. contraction of the hamstring should flex the knee and extend the hip, but some movements produce a paradoxical flexion at the hip and a flexion at the knee.

## Losee's subluxation test

See Reverse pivot shift.

## Ludloff's sign

An inability to actively flex the hip whilst sitting is indicative of **psoas** weakness.

## Magnuson–Stack procedure

Repair of **anterior dislocation of the shoulder** – strengthening of the anterior inferior margin with subscapularis, capsule and rotator cuff.

## Manipulation of the spine

There are various manipulative techniques, e.g. Cyriax, Maitland, osteopathic, chiropractic, Mulligan's, etc., all of which may prove successful with some problems, but only some of them will prove useful in others. However, a disc lesion will probably not respond well to manipulation, whereas a facet joint or the facetal element of a disc problem will. Sacroiliac joint manipulation can also be successful. There is discussion as to when mobilization, which is a gentle rocking of a joint, finishes, and manipulation, which has an end-point thrust, begins. In practical terms this will inevitably depend on the patient, who will either be too sensitive to allow the joints to reach end point, and thus only permit mobilization, or will relax enough to permit manipulation. Treatment of the soft tissues can be given at the same time, by massage [14] and heat, and the improved healing time with ultrasound or laser [15] treatment may also be beneficial.

## March fracture

Stress fracture of the **metatarsal** bone, usually the second, third, or fourth (see Chapter 16; Fig. 16.1).

## Massage

A variety of stroking, rubbing, pummelling or slapping techniques to remove oedema, encourage an increased blood supply, organize scar tissue and prevent adhesions [14].

## McConnell strapping regimen

Used for **anterior knee pain**. An assessment of patellar glide, tilt and rotation is made by the clinician, who then uses the appropriate strapping techniques to control the diagnosed patellar maltracking. Vastus medialis obliquus coordinated work, with biofeedback and coordinated control of external rotation of the hip, is also trained.

## McKenzie extension exercises

These may be done whilst lying or standing, straight in line or with a side flexion. They should be used for **flexion-orientated disc** problems but not for extension-orientated problems. A trial of extension exercises should be undertaken to see if the pain peripheralizes down the leg, or leg pain is produced. If this occurs, then extension exercise should not be utilized. If the leg pain centralizes then the exercise is safe. This exercise can make the collar stud L5/S1 disc positively worse, but as the disc improves, and the collar stud deformity settles into the more normal hernial configuration of the disc, so extension exercises may be added. Facet joint, sacroiliac joint and lateral canal entrapments will be made worse (Fig. 22.11) (see Chapter 2).

## McKenzie flexion exercises

Pulling the knees to the chest and stretching the low back into flexion will aid extension-orientated spinal problems, such as facet joints and the L5/S1 collar stud. The addition of gapping rotations (rolling the knees to one side, or hanging one leg over the other) will help the facet joint, lateral canal and sacroiliac joint. Creeping, unstable, flexion-orientated discs will be made worse (Fig. 22.12) (see Chapter 2).

## McMurray's test

A test for **meniscal lesions**, but impossible to perform with moderately tense effusions as this prevents the full knee flexion required for the test. It is a grinding test of the tibia onto the femur, with the patient lying supine. Forced internal and external rotation of the knee, through flexion into extension, with varus and valgus stress, is then applied via axial compression of the tibia. Results show about 60% positive, 5% false positives. A clunk and pain is the classical positive sign, whereas the deep fibres of the medial collateral ligament are painful without the clunk.

## Meniscal cyst

The lateral **meniscus** is more frequently involved than the medial. The cyst is usually accompanied by a radial tear of the meniscus. Clinically, the swelling becomes more prominent to palpation in extension of the knee. An anterior cyst can less commonly occur (Fig. 11.27).

## Mills' manipulation

For chronic **tennis elbow** to free up adhesions on the lateral condyle, but the radiohumeral joint must be exculpated first. The wrist is fully pronated and then flexed, at which stage the elbow is jerked into full extension (Fig. 22.13).

## MJO

Milne J. Ongley's stress test for the **sacroiliac joint**. See Sacroiliac stress tests.

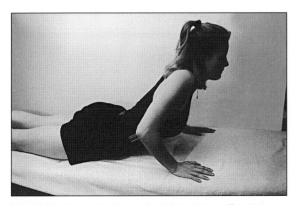

**Figure 22.11 •** McKenzie extension exercises. Breathing out allows the muscle tension to relax and the extension to be applied more directly to the vertebrae. Its acute angle should be directed towards the problem level.

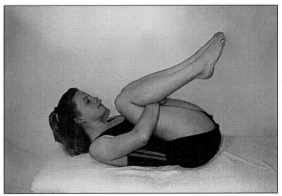

**Figure 22.12 •** McKenzie flexion exercises. Good for extension-orientated problems.

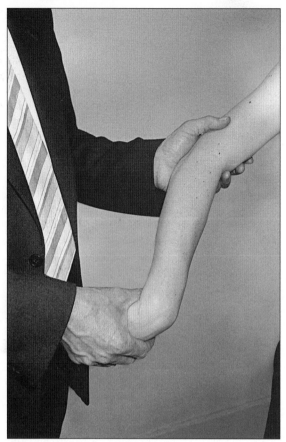

**Figure 22.13** • Mills' manipulation position.

## Morton's foot

Present in about 50% of the population. The first metatarsal is shorter than the second, giving a longer second toe.

## Morton's neuroma

**Interdigital neuroma** of the foot, which classically lies adjacent to the third or fourth metatarsophalangeal joints. It can produce interdigital neuritis, but all interdigital neuritis is not produced by a neuroma. It may be visualized with ultrasound or MRI. There is a tendency for the neuroma to recur on the resected nerve end after surgery.

## MRI

**Magnetic resonance imaging**. A body scan. The body tissues' ionic charges can be polarized along magnetic lines, and the relative rates of return to normal, after the magnetic field is changed, differentiates various tissues, giving good but not perfect pictures of body parts.

## Mumford procedure

Operation for chronic **acromioclavicular joint** arthrosis, or arthritis, which removes the distal clavicle and, sometimes, part of the acromion. Good results in sport, although 3 months' healing are required before increasing the loads. Weightlifters may still have problems.

## Myofascial pain

The fascia extends in its own planes throughout the body and yet its function is least well understood. Fascia coats all muscles and is the plane in which the neurovascular bundles run. In the dissecting room it is discarded without further examination. Some inflammatory diseases seem to affect the fascia. In musculoskeletal medicine, trigger points of pain are detected that ease with acupressure, wet and dry needling and massage. Whether these are the sites of spindle cells, which control the gamma efferents and thus muscle tension, is debated. Certainly muscle tension and tender trigger points are associated. Chronic neuropathic pain may be associated with the neurovascular bundles within the fascia but has many parameters (see Further reading).

## Myositis ossificans

Myositis ossificans is the development of ossification within connective tissue of muscle. The quadriceps and the rectus femoris origin are particularly prone. Increase in pain, or decrease in range of movement, that occurs over the first 5 days is indicative of impending myositis. Stretching, massage and heat promulgate the problem and must be avoided. An NSAID such as indomethacin should be tried, as may bisphosphonates (e.g. pamidronate). Activities should be severely restricted until the bone scan shows reduced or no activity. Surgery of a large mass should not be undertaken until the bone scan is negative, as recurrence is high.

## Nage's test

Another test for assessment of **anterior cruciate ligament** instability.

## Neer's sign

An impingement test for the **shoulder**, which is passively flexed and internally rotated. See Impingement test.

## Noble's sign

For **iliotibial tract syndrome**. The iliotibial band flicks over the lateral femoral condyle at about 30° of knee flexion, and this may be palpated. Pressure over this condyle whilst the knee is moved through flexion and extension produces pain at about 30° of flexion.

## Noye's flexion rotation draw test

A test for **anterior cruciate ligament** tears. This is a gentle pivot shift. The 10–15° flexed knee is supported at the tibia. This allows the femur to drop back and externally rotate. Increased flexion with downward pressure on the tibia, to drop the knee backwards, reduces the subluxation.

## NSAIDs

**Non-steroidal anti-inflammatory drugs** to counter and inhibit inflammatory prostaglandins.

## Ober's test

To display tightness of the **iliotibial band**. The patient lies on his or her side, knee slightly flexed; the hip is flexed, abducted and externally rotated, and then taken into extension. A tight iliotibial tract does not allow the knee to drop down level with, or below, the hip.

## Obesity

Obesity is defined at various levels of a body mass index over 25: 25–30, overweight; 30–40, obese; 40+, morbidly obese. However, for athletes the BMI has cardinal errors (see Chapter 21: Diet).

Management for the obese requires a lifestyle change to be truly successful. Control of diet will contribute 90%, whilst exercise only adds some 10% to weight loss. Commitment to an exercise regime will help, especially in the early evening after work. Exercise at this time should take the place of a gin and tonic and three packets of crisps that are often used to unwind from the stress of the day.

The extra weight creates problems. Weight-bearing joints have a heavier load and the extra fat mechanically creates tracking problems at the knees and feet, leading to earlier osteoarthritis, which needs to be corrected, and the cardiovascular system is compromised. Non-weight-bearing exercise is therefore preferable, but it is difficult to persuade the obese to exercise hard enough. A five times a week tennis player may only serve and stand at the net, getting no cardiovascular fitness at all. During cardiovascular exercise they should be able to talk but have a catch to their breath. Urine should be tested for type 2 diabetes.

## O'Donoghue's triad

**Trauma to the knee**, resulting in damage to the medial collateral ligament, the meniscus (usually medial) and the anterior cruciate ligament.

## One-legged hyperextension test

A test for **spondylolysis** and **extension-orientated back pain**, in which the patient stands on one leg, raises the contralateral knee towards the chest, and leans backwards (Fig. 22.14). See Fitch catch.

## Open chain exercise

See Closed chain exercise.

## Orthotics

By definition, this would include any addition to the inside of a shoe that alters foot mechanics. However, the term is generally used to describe formal inserts that are often purpose made for the individual.

## Os acetabulare

An accessory ossicle of the **hip**, from the acetabulum, which may limit the range of hip movement and thus become a problem in gymnastics, dancing, martial arts, etc. (see Chapter 8; Fig. 8.2).

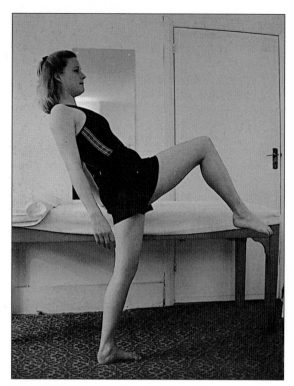

**Figure 22.14** • The one-legged hyperextension test.

## Osgood–Schlatter disease

Apophysitis of the patellar tendon attachment, at the **tibial tubercle** (see Chapter 11; Fig. 11.17).

## Osteoarthritis

A degenerative condition of articular cartilage, which may follow trauma and attrition through age and wear and tear. Articular cartilage is nourished by synovial fluid, but movement is required to massage the fluid into the nutrient cannaliculi. Thus, total rest in a cast brace makes osteoarthritis worse, but equally too much impact stresses the subchondral bone, because the protective thickness of the articular cartilage is reduced. Therefore, non-impact exercise of low loads, high repetitions are the best exercises for osteoarthritis.

## Os trigonum

This is the separate ossification centre of the **talus**, which may impinge between the calcaneum and poste-

rior surface of the tibia during plantar flexion (see Chapter 13, Part 5; Fig. 13.23). See Calcaneotibial compression test and Stieda process.

## Overpronation

The pronated foot is a soft foot that can adapt to the ground contours. A firm, supinated foot is required for impact and to make a firm platform for lift-off. The overpronated foot cannot move back from its excessively pronated position to achieve supination in time for impact or lift-off. This may come from calcaneovalgus, a collapsed mid-foot, forefoot varus, posterior tibialis weakness or ligamentous laxity. See Supination/pronation.

## Paget–von Schroetter syndrome

See Effort thrombosis and Chapter 12.

## Panner's disease

An osteochondritis of the capitulum in the **elbow joint**, possibly from an avascular or traumatic cause. The incidence is 90% males and 5% bilateral. Loose bodies are more frequent over the age of 8, and pain from the joint locking, clicking, and swelling are found clinically.

## Paravertebral blocks/root blocks

**Lateral canal entrapment** of the nerve root, by enlarged facets or synovial cysts, narrowed lateral canal from disc collapse, and lateral disc prolapse may irritate the nerve. Patients often have discomfort standing and walking around, and may relieve the discomfort by sitting, squatting or drawing the knees up to the chest. They tend to perch on table edges and may be eased by using a shooting stick if they are on their feet for a long time. An epidural may not reach the root, as the canal is blocked mechanically; however, an injection of hydrocortisone and local anaesthetic into the lateral canal may be achieved by a paravertebral approach.

## Patella alta

**High-riding patella**, which may have the camel sign of two lumps – one the patella and the other from the fat pads. Patella alta is associated with patellar maltracking.

## Patellar apprehension test

Whilst the patient is sitting, knees extended and relaxed, the patella is pulled laterally by the clinician. The patient with the **dislocating or subluxing patella** will be worried that it might dislocate, or the patient may experience discomfort if the patella has been mal-tracking, and this fear shows on the patient's face, which should be watched throughout this test.

## Patella baja

**Low-placed patella**. At 30° angle of flexion, the patella to patella tendon length ratio should be 1. More than 20% is abnormal. Patella baja is associated with mal-tracking problems of the patella, causing anterior knee pain.

## Patellar tap

See Bulge test.

## Patrick's test

See Faber test.

## Pellegrini–Stieda syndrome

This is a type of myositis ossificans, or bone formation, that may complicate medial (tibial) collateral ligament or adductor tendon lesions over the **medial femoral condyle** (see Chapter 11; Fig. 11.22).

## Pelvic spring

A test for the **sacroiliac joint** stability. See Sacroiliac stress tests.

## Perthes' disease (Legg–Perthes)

Avascular necrosis of the **femoral head**, which appears between the ages of 5 and 10 years, with disturbance of the bone structure and flattening of the femoral head. This deformity and a restricted hip range remain into adult life. May be more prone to eventual osteoarthritis (Fig. 22.15).

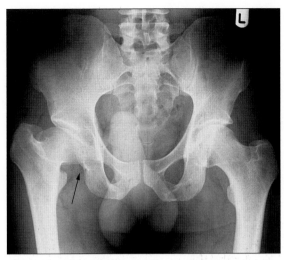

**Figure 22.15** • Old Perthes' disease of the hip.

## Pes anserine bursa

The bursa lying on the medial side of **the knee**, beneath the semitendinosus and semimembranosus, as these extend to their insertions (see Fig. 11.26).

## Phalen's test

Tingling, within the first, second, and third fingers, with the wrist held in flexion for 60 seconds, is produced with a **carpal tunnel syndrome**. Phalen's and Tinel's sign have a good specificity but not a high sensitivity [16].

## Piedallu's sign

The examiner places the thumbs on the posterior inferior iliac spines (PIIS) and asks the patient to raise a knee towards the chest. The PIIS should move downwards on that side and, in the abnormal fixed sacroiliac joint, may elevate. Fixation and elevation of the PIIS may indicate **sacroiliac joint** dysfunction. However, one must be careful when assuming that we humans are absolutely symmetrical creatures, as too many manipulations to correct a non-painful, probably non-pathological asymmetry can produce ligamentous laxity and further problems. Intra-examiner agreement is only fair in this test [11].

## Pivot shift

A test for **cruciate ligament** instability. The 20° flexed knee is internally rotated and a valgus force is applied. In the cruciate-deficient knee, the lateral side of the tibial plateau subluxes anteriorly and this is increased by thumb pressure over the proximal fibular head. As the knee is extended, the iliotibial band pulls the sub-luxed tibia backwards into place with an appreciable jump [17]. A patient who has pain with this movement may resist the test, in which case this sign can be exposed only under general anaesthetic (Fig. 22.16).

## Pliometrics

A **training method** that involves landing and taking off again immediately so that eccentric and concentric muscle work is cycled, as would occur whilst running. It is usually trained by depth jumping. Jumping down from a maximum height of 20–40 cm and then jumping as high as one can. Hop step jump routines, and bounding, are pliometrics [18,19] (see Chapter 20).

## Point sign

When the acromioclavicular joint is involved, the patient points directly at the joint to indicate the source of pain (Fig. 22.17).

## Pope's sign

Flexion contracture of fourth and fifth fingers due to **ulnar nerve palsy**.

## Posterior apprehension test

For **posterior subluxation of the shoulder** when, with the patient lying supine, the humerus is flexed to 90° and axial pressure is added through the elbow to force the humeral head posteriorly. If this produces a click, or apprehension, and is relieved by external rotation of the humerus, and a feeling of anterior shift of the

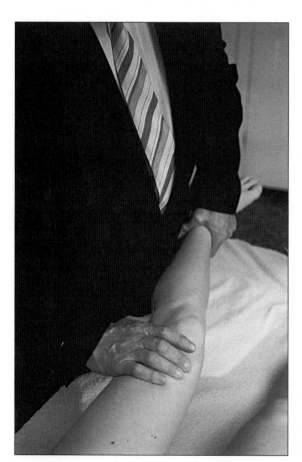

**Figure 22.16** • The pivot shift.

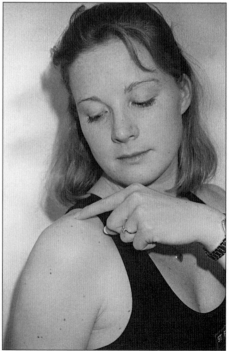

**Figure 22.17** • Point sign.

humeral head when the posterior aspect of the joint is palpated, it is a positive test.

## Posterior calcaneal compression test

See Calcaneotibial compression test.

## Power

Power is **speed × strength**. Slow speeds generate more strength, high speeds less strength, but the power may be equal. This principle may be seen in the karate chop, or in the rugby scrum where the slow application of more force is less effective than the concerted, timed shove, when force is applied with speed. The essence of power is timing.

## Prolotherapy

See Sclerosant injections.

## Pronation

See Overpronation and Supination/pronation.

## Prone-lying knee flexion (PLKF)

A **femoral nerve** stretch test, where the patient lies prone and the knee is bent passively. Increased pain in the thigh or the back is a positive test, whilst flexing the hip as well will increase any neural tension. Extension of the hip can produce facetal discomfort, so the knee movement, which stretches the femoral nerve, is the important indicator. See Adverse neural tensioning and Dural stress tests.

## Pulled elbow

Swinging a child by the arm can sublux the proximal **radial head**. Flexion and rotation of the forearm usually reduces this subluxation.

## Putti–Platt procedure

A type of repair for recurrent **shoulder dislocation**, which shortens and plicates the subscapularis. Repaired shoulders have limited external rotation.

## Pyramids

This is a method of resistance training, which may start, for instance, with a light resistance and 30 repetitions, then medium resistance and 20 repetitions, reaching a high resistance and 5 repetitions. The schedule then moves out, through the 20 repetitions, to the '30 repetition' stage. This may be performed in the reverse order.

## Q angle

Relates to the **knee**. The Q angle is the angle, whilst standing or lying supine, that is subtended by a line drawn from the femoral head to the centre of the patella, and a line from the central patella to the tibial tuberosity. It is generally accepted that 15° or less of valgus is normal (see Fig. 11.10, Chapter 11).

## Referred pain

This is generally thought of as nerve in origin, and the somatomal, dermatomal or myotomal distribution may suggest the level of the problem. However, referred pain may also be from other structures and is not necessarily of nerve origin. Injections into facet joints, the sacroiliac joint, myofascial trigger points, ligaments and joints have displayed referred pain. Various organs, the heart to the arms and neck, the diaphragm to the top of the shoulder, etc., refer pain. Thus, not all pain referred down the leg is sciatic nerve in origin. Experimental evidence, and clinical experience of injecting various sites, will produce referred pain as well. Sciatica is leg pain from the sciatic nerve but not all leg pain is sciatica. Elbow pain may be a brachialgia or referred from the subacromial space.

## Reflex sympathetic dystrophy/ regional pain syndrome

The cause is not fully known, but guanethidine works on the sympathetic sites within the arterioles and may have a curative effect.

| | |
|---|---|
| Stage 1 | Raised circulation. Oedema. Hot dry skin. Livid colour. Burning, everlasting pain that is worse to touch and not in a dermatomal distribution. |
| Treatment | is intravascular, sympathetic blockade with guanethidine. Sympathetic ganglion block, peripheral nerve block and |

epidural or spinal block with an indwelling catheter should all be tried, if required. Elevate the limb. NSAIDs. Exercise but no massage. Neuroleptics (see Fig. 12.8).

Stage 2    Pale, cold, cyanotic skin. Vasospasms. Sweating. Atrophy of the skin and muscle. Contraction of the joint.

Treatment    is to treat the pain as in stage 1, but the therapy is less effective.

Stage 3    Irreversible atrophy of bone, muscle, and connective tissue. Joint contractures. The skin is cold, pale and dry. X-ray shows osteoporosis, particularly around the joint. The pain may ease at rest but movements cause terrible pain. Sympathetic blockade may not work.

Treatment    is with an epidural or plexus block to try and obtain movement, TENS and neuroleptics.

## Reiter's syndrome

Urethritis, arthritis and conjunctivitis. There may be a venereal link but it is also part of the inflammatory spondylarthropathies.

## Relocation test/Jobe's test

For the **anterior subluxing shoulder**. Whilst lying supine, the arm is taken into 90° circumduction, the elbow is flexed to 90° and the shoulder taken into increasing external rotation. If the pain produced by this manoeuvre is reduced by pressure on the anterior humeral head, but worse on release of this pressure, then this is a positive test for anterior subluxation of the shoulder. If the pain is relieved by the anterior pressure then the shoulder may be taken a little further into external rotation and, on release of the restraining hand on the humeral head, will sublux forward, producing sudden pain (Fig. 22.18).

## Renne's test

For **iliotibial tract syndrome**. Stand on the painful leg, with the knee bent to 30–40°. Pain at the lateral femoral condyle is indicative. Hopping may accentuate the problem. It should be noted that the external rotators of the hip will be affected by this manoeuvre as well and can also refer pain towards the knee.

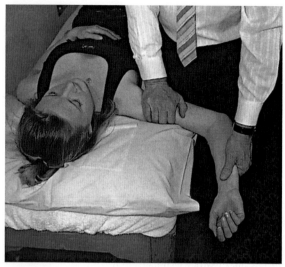

**Figure 22.18** • The relocation test.

## Resting pulse

The pulse rate taken first thing in the morning, before getting out of bed (see Chapter 21).

## Reverse pivot shift

For the **anterior cruciate ligament**. Start with the patient lying supine and relaxed, the knee bent and tibia externally rotated. Straightening takes the knee into subluxation (near the end of extension) and back to location, in full extension. This movement can be appreciated.

## Rhizotomy

Chronic, facetal osteoarthritic pains may be helped by ablation of the **sinuvertebral nerve**. The ablation may be via a cryo- or radiorhizotomy (see Chapters 2 and 5).

## RICE

**Rest, Ice, Compression, Elevation**
The first-line principle for treating an acute injury:

(a) Rest for 24–48 hours to prevent the clot spreading and an increase of inflammatory exudate. Mobilization too soon produces thicker scar tissue, which is not easily penetrated by fibroblasts and it may provoke continued bleeding.

(b) Ice will cool the periphery and shut down local vessels to decrease bleeding. Ice straight from the fridge may be less than 0°C and will produce an ice burn, unless separated from the skin by a cloth. Melting ice (wet ice) will be at 0°C and may be used as a bath for 20 minutes, but locally applied ice, for 5–10 minutes can have an effect [20]. Reusable cold packs, which may be stored in the fridge, are available, as are some chemicals that freeze on mixing. Frozen packets of peas, which mould to the shape of the body, may prove most cost-effective. Care must be taken with ice placed around nerves, as they can suffer a cold-induced neuropraxia.

(c) Compression is again designed to reduce inflammatory exudates, and the spread of haemorrhage.

(d) Elevation prevents tracking of inflammatory products to the periphery, thus requiring less effort to return these products centrally.

## Rock onto heels test

An individual displays an inability to perform this manoeuvre when weakness of the tibialis anterior, extensor hallucis and extensor digitorum exist, usually from an L4 or L5 **nerve root palsy** (see Chapter 5).

## Roos' test

For **thoracic outlet syndrome**. The patient sits or stands with the arms abducted to 90° and externally rotated, at which stage the elbows are flexed to 90°, with the shoulders slightly braced. The patient opens and closes the fingers slowly and steadily for 3 minutes. Drooping of the shoulders, decreasing rate of finger contraction or reproduction of the symptoms is considered positive [21].

## Sacroiliac joint

The sacroiliac joint has an auricular shape and, although it has articular cartilage, it has an irregular surface and ligamentous attachments within its joint. It moves, in an anteroposterior plane, by a few millimetres. The movement of the sacrum within the iliac wings is called nutation, a nodding movement. In particular, it transmits impact loads, up from the legs to the spine, and is

crossed by only the psoas muscle. Sacroiliac dysfunction is often seen during pregnancy, and around menstruation, perhaps because the hormone relaxin levels, which increase ligament laxity, are higher. Dysfunction can often be reduced by sacral manipulative techniques, and sclerosant/prolotherapy (see Chapters 2 and 5).

## Sacroiliac stress tests

(a) Pelvic spring. Distracting, or compressing the anterior wing of the ilium will produce the opposite effect on the posterior structures. This is thought to be a test for the sacroiliac joint but, quite obviously, when one can reduce some types of pain from this test by supporting the L4/5 segments on the patient's hand, then other structures must be involved as well.

(b) MJO. With the patient supine, the hip is flexed and a posterior compression and internal rotation force is applied, in an axial direction, through the femur, by downward pressure through the knee. Pain over the sacroiliac joint is indicative. With the hip in full flexion and the force directed from the region of the contralateral shoulder, the stress is thought to be across the sacrotuberous ligament; mid-range, across the sacroiliac ligaments; and with the knee being tensioned from the direction of the mid-opposite thigh, across the iliolumbar ligaments.

(c) Direct compression of the sacroiliac joint may be painful.

See Piedallu's sign and Facet joint and sacroiliac joint stress tests.

## Sag sign

When the knee is flexed at 90° and the patient is lying supine, the tibia gives the appearance of sliding backwards under the femur. This indicates a **posterior cruciate ligament tear**. Note that this starting position, therefore, may produce a false-positive anterior draw sign (see Fig. 22.8).

## Salter's classification of epiphyseal fracture

**Type 1** Through the zone of hypertrophy; it is treated by closed reduction, with good results.

**Type 2** As type 1, but with metaphyseal involvement; treated by closed reduction, with a few complications.

**Type 3** A fracture through the zone of hypertrophy and epiphyseal plate, where open reduction is complicated by joint incongruity.

**Type 4** A fracture through the epiphysis and metaphyseal plate, which is treated by open reduction but has a high complication rate.

**Type 5** Crushing of the zone of hypertrophy; treated by closed reduction, with a high complication rate.

## Scheuermann's disease

Osteochondritis of the ring epiphysis of the **vertebrae**, which can produce altered growth in the thoracic spine of adolescents, especially in 12- to 13-year-olds. It is less commonly seen in the lumbar spine. These changes may allow herniation of the disc into the vertebral body. There is a boy–girl ratio of 2:1. Treat by modifying activity until bony maturity. There may possibly be an increased incidence in gymnasts (see Chapter 2; Fig. 2.2).

## Schmorl's nodes

Herniation of a disc into the **vertebral body**, which is usually pain-free. Diagnosed on X-ray and scans.

## Schober's test

For **ankylosis of the spine**.

(a) **Dorsal vertebrae**. A measuring tape is placed on the vertebral prominence and 30 cm measured off and marked on the skin; full vertebral flexion should increase this distance by 3 cm.

(b) **Lumbar vertebrae**. Mark up 10 cm from the spinal dimples. Full flexion should increase this distance by 5 cm, or mark up 10 cm and down 5 cm from the dimples, when full flexion should be 20 cm plus.

## Sclerosant injections (back)

A solution of dextrose sclerosant, diluted with equal parts anaesthetic, may be injected into the posterior lumbar ligaments and sacroiliac joint. It is particularly useful for ligamentous pain and the unstable pelvis with pelvic spring positive, and has a lesser but definite benefit in helping to stabilize the spondylolisthesis and unstable vertebral segment. It is known in the USA as prolotherapy, as it has a fibro-proliferative effect. Sclerosants may be used for ligamentous laxity, pelvic spring-positive patients, patients testing positive for sacroiliac joint stress, and the unstable disc, plus spondylolisthesis, chronic facet joint dysfunction and post surgery to the posterior lumbar ligaments. It may well have a long-term, beneficial effect on myofascial tissue.

## Scoliosis

Primary scoliosis does not correct when the patient bends forward, so that the asymmetry and fullness in the paravertebral muscles remains. The anterior chest wall may also show this asymmetry. Progressive increase in the distortion of a scoliosis should be referred on to a specialist scoliosis clinic, for possible surgical correction. Secondary scoliosis does correct with forward bending. It may be due to leg length difference and can later promote facet joint dysfunction, but it does not require surgery.

## Segond's sign

Avulsion of the lateral or medial collateral ligament of the **knee**; leaves a small flake of avulsed bone visible on X-ray and scans (see Chapter 11; Fig. 11.23).

## Shaving test

An **anterior interosseus nerve neuropathy** where the individual cannot put the tips of the first and second fingers together, only pulps, owing to weak flexor digitoris profundus and flexor pollicis longus.

## Shoes

What to look for:

(a) A curved last is for supinated feet.
(b) A straight last is for pronated feet.
(c) Thick soles with shock absorbency are for 'straight line' sports.
(d) Lower soles are required for twisting, turning sports, as the high sole is too unstable.
(e) The first indicators of a broken shoe are distorted or loose heel cups rather than worn soles (Figs 22.19 and 22.20).

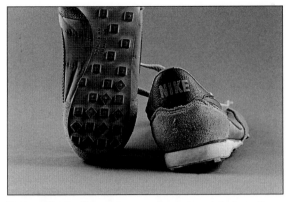

**Figure 22.19** • These shoes are new enough to have the nipples on the studs, but the right shoe is rolling into pronation by itself and will cause the foot to follow.

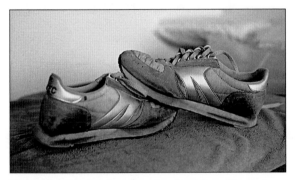

**Figure 22.20** • The line of mud on the soles with a clear area above shows that during use the heel cups crush over the sole and are in fact broken.

(f) The so-called 'Achilles protector' is just for appearance and, if anything, may cause Achilles peritendinitis (Fig. 22.21). In some shoes, the apparent cut down part of the Achilles tag is as high as a plain Achilles tag, and the side elements of the tag even higher. These high side elements may sometimes rub under the malleoli, causing pain. The tag should be soft and pull easily away from the Achilles with light finger pressure. At the slightest indication of Achilles problems, or before, the heel tags should be cut off, or cuts made wide out on either side, down to the heel cup.

(g) Eye holes for laces that are placed further back along the shoe tighten the Achilles tag.

(h) Cut away arches remove support from the foot and can precipitate overpronation (see Fig. 22.19).

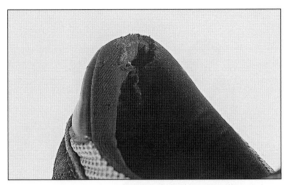

**Figure 22.21** • This stiff Achilles protector has been worn away by rubbing on the Achilles, causing Achilles peritendinitis.

(i) Sprint spikes, with no heel raise, should not be used for endurance training. Middle distance spikes with a heel raise are required.

(j) Worn studs alter foot balance.

(k) Track spikes, with spikes that come over the outside of the ball of the foot, can produce a Ben Hur effect and lacerate other runners. These shoes have largely disappeared today.

## Short-wave diathermy

An electromagnetic wave length, which produces deep tissue heating.

## Shoulder–hand syndrome

The hand and wrist on the ipsilateral side of a **frozen shoulder** may swell, possibly from postural disuse oedema or possibly from a reflex sympathetic dystrophy.

## Simmonds' test

For **Achilles rupture**. Simmonds reported this test first, but it seems to be known generally as Thompson's test. See Thompson's test.

## Sinding–Larsen–Johansson syndrome

Apophysitis of the inferior pole of the **patella** in those with an accessory ossification centre at the lower pole (see Chapter 11; Fig. 11.15).

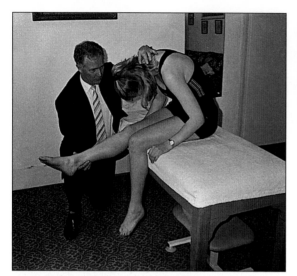

Figure 22.22 • The slump test. If thought to be positive, then extension of the neck in this position should relieve the symptoms.

## Slipped capital femoral epiphysis

This may follow trauma, be found in an immature Frohlich type, and a tall-for-age group. The injury presents between the ages of 10 and 15 years, often as thigh and knee pain rather than hip pain, and as such is often missed unless the **hip** is examined in all cases of knee pain.

## Slocum's test

A test for rotatory instability of the **knee** in patients with large heavy legs. Positive anterior draw fails to tighten in 25° of external rotation.

## Slump test

The slump test is **a dural and neural stress test**. Flexion of the neck and spine, added to a straight leg raise and Lasègue's test, is performed in the sitting position. The test is positive if the pain is relieved by neck extension. The interpretation of a positive test, and no relief of pain by reduction of neck flexion, is open to interpretation (Fig. 22.22) See Adverse neural tensioning and Dural stress tests.

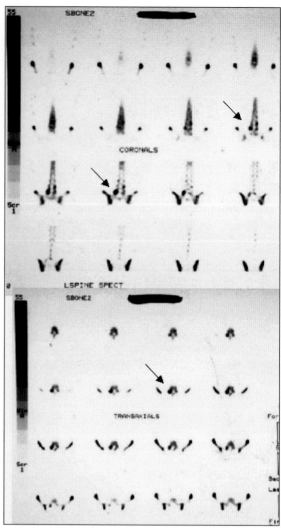

Figure 22.23 • The SPECT scan shows an increased uptake of technetium 99 by the stress fracture in coronal and transaxial sections.

## Sodium hyaluronate

Hyaluronic acid is a constituent of synovial fluid, and injections of hyaluronate have been accepted by the US Food and Drugs Agency as a prosthetic aid but not as a drug. It is used in cases of osteoarthritis.

## SPECT

**Single photon emission computed tomography**. An extremely sensitive bone scan (Fig. 22.23). See Computed tomography.

## Speed's test

For **bicipital** impingement and tendinitis. Resisted flexion, adduction and supination of the humerus, with the elbow extended, produces pain at the shoulder. See Yergason's test.

## Spinal probe

If the exact cause of back pain is undiagnosed then under a neuroleptanalgesia, which allows the patient to respond to pain but leaves him or her with no memory of the incident, the disc, facet joint and sacroiliac joint may be injected to establish which causes concordant pain. See Disc probe.

## Spurling's manoeuvre

For **cervical root entrapment**, where extension and rotation of the neck pinches the nerve in the lateral canal of the neck, producing nerve root symptoms.

## Steinmann's test

Similar to McMurray, but the object is to record pain rather than clunks over the joint line. Pain that moves posteriorly with increasing degrees of flexion suggests **meniscal** pathology. See McMurray's test.

## Step down test

The patient stands on a bench or raised dais and steps slowly forwards to the ground. Higher loads can be achieved by jumping down. The clinician compares the left with the right side and observes the **tracking of the knee**, and also whether the leg can hold the movement. Failure to control the movement indicates weakness, maltracking or pain and will produce an increased force of foot impact. This can be heard as well as seen.

## Stieda process

Posterior protrusion from the back of the **talus**, which may be impinged in a similar way to an os trigonum. See Os trigonum.

## Stork view

For the **pelvis**. The pelvis is X-rayed with the patient standing on one leg and then on the other. A shift in the pubic symphysis of over 2 mm is significant.

## Straight leg raise (SLR)

A **neural stress test** for the lumbar disc and sciatic nerve, but by itself represents tensioning of the nerve roots or sciatic nerve. See Adverse neural tensioning.

## Sudeck's dystrophy

A **reflex sympathetic response**, usually following trauma, such as a Colle's fracture, but it may be represented in an early stage as the shoulder–hand syndrome. See Reflex sympathetic dystrophy/regional pain syndrome.

## Sulcus sign

For **shoulder instability**. If **inferior subluxation** is present, a sulcus shows between the humeral head and the acromion when there is downward traction of the humerus.

## Supination/pronation

At **foot** strike, the foot needs to be firm to meet the impact, the weight being on the outside of the heel, and the mid-foot is lifted upwards to produce a high arch (supination). During mid-stance the foot has to adapt to the ground, and to do this it rolls inwards and becomes soft, so that it can seek the ground (pronation). To push forwards, the foot, at the lift-off, must go hard to give a solid base, and once again supinates, although the centre of the load is through the first and second toes. This is normal. Failure to resupinate at lift-off is referred to as overpronation and produces a soft foot (like running off jelly), maltracking and overload problems at the knee.

## Surgery for the spine

Loss of bowel and bladder control or altered perineal sensation indicates an S3/4/5 root compression, and must be relieved surgically as an emergency. Surgery for the spine is becoming more definitive to the problem

– discectomy for the disc; X stop insertion, laminectomy or foramenotomy for spinal or lateral canal stenosis; fusion for spondylolisthesis, and disc replacement, etc. When should a back have surgery? Most backs get better with conservative management, and repeat scans invariably show the reduction in size of a prolapsed disc over time [22], or reduction in symptoms despite the ongoing disc. Probably, the best guide is failure to progress, either with pain or mechanical signs over 1 month, in spite of the correct conservative therapy. The unstable back, with repeat episodes of severe to moderately severe problems, may earn its surgery on the recurrent history alone.

## Syndesmotic (syndesmal) stress test

For syndesmotic disruption between the tibia and fibula, at the **ankle**. One hand prevents the tibia and fibula from rotating whilst the other forces dorsiflexion of the foot, and then external and internal rotation of the foot.

## Tarsal coalition

Calcaneonavicular and talonavicular joints can have a congenital fibrocartilaginous or osseous union of the **two tarsal bones** (see Chapter 14).

## Tennis elbow

**Lateral epicondylitis** of the elbow.

## TENS

**Transcutaneous electrical nerve stimulation**. This uses the 'gate principle' of spinal nerve conduction to stimulate or irritate a new area, thus interrupting the noci stimulus from the painful area. It may be used to provide a gentle faradic twitch to a damaged muscle.

## Terry Thomas sign

The wrist, with widening of the **scaphoid lunate gap** on X-ray, shows ligamentous damage.

## Thomas's test

For **hip contraction**. Flex the hip until the lumbar lordosis reduces and the back is flat on the couch. If the

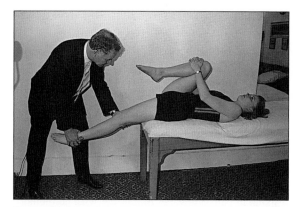

**Figure 22.24** • Modified Thomas's test for psoas tightness.

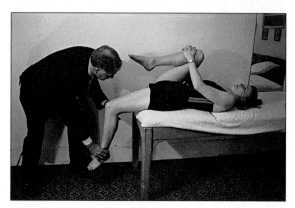

**Figure 22.25** • Modified Thomas's test for rectus femoris tightness.

contralateral hip is tight, it will have lifted off the couch.

## Thomas's test, modified

This extends the contralateral hip, as in the Thomas's test, with a straight knee to test psoas contracture (Fig. 22.24). Then, with the hip extended, the knee is flexed as far as it will go to assess **rectus femoris** tightness (Fig. 22.25). If both have a full range, but the knee moves laterally, it is because the **tensor fasciae latae** is tight (Figs 22.26 and 22.27).

## Thompson's test

For **ruptured Achilles**. First described by Simmonds. With the patient lying prone, squeezing the calf muscle produces a plantar flexion of the foot if the Achilles

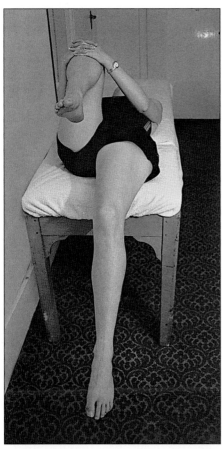

**Figure 22.26** • Modified Thomas's test with a normal tensor fasciae latae, and normal psoas and rectus femoris.

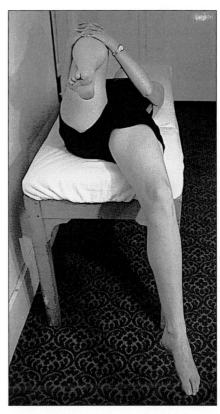

**Figure 22.27** • Modified Thomas's test with a tight tensor fasciae latae and iliotibial band, which pulls the leg into abduction.

tendon is intact, and no movement with an Achilles rupture. Note, however, that too wide a grip of the calf muscle may squeeze the posterior tibialis and produce some plantar flexion movement.

## Three-phase bone scan

See Bone scan.

## Tinel's sign

**Tapping over a nerve** produces pain and tingling, or paraesthesia, distal to the point of pressure. This test is used particularly for the median nerve at the wrist (carpal tunnel) and the posterior tibial nerve (tarsal tunnel).

## Tiptoe stand

**Nerve weakness**. To test for weakness from the calf muscle. If no muscular or tendinous damage exists then the cause is usually from a S1 root palsy.

## Torg ratio

An X-ray investigation to assess the **functional size of the spinal canal**, which is calculated by dividing the shortest distance between the posterior vertebral body and the spinolaminar line by the anterior posterior distance of the vertebral body.

## Traction

The idea is to pull the vertebrae apart so that a negative pressure effect is exerted on the disc, trying to reduce disc herniation. Though this technique has fallen out of vogue, it is especially useful when an 'arc' of pain exists with the straight leg test. Traction does seem to slide the cranial vertebra posteriorly and can influence spondylolyses. It reduces disc herniation whilst it is applied [23]. Traction may be performed in:

(a) Fowler's position – hips bent, calves resting up on a stool. Good for L5/S1 collar stud disc, the early stage of L2/3, 3/4 discs.

(b) Supine or prone. Good for discs improved with extension or worse with flexion. L4/5, later L5/S1, when extension does not make the pain worse. L2/3, 3/4 discs, which no longer irritate the dura (can straighten and do extension manoeuvres without pain). Traction can be given daily, or every other day, the kilo-pull will be increased as required by the therapist. Beware of a history of shooting pains and/or sudden stabs of pain into the leg, because the patient is wonderful on traction but may need an epidural to get them off traction.

(c) Home traction, either by lying flexed over a bar or hanging by the feet on a tipping bed, 'back swing' (see Chapters 2 and 5).

## Trendelenburg gait

Whilst standing, the abductors of the **hip** tighten to support the pelvis. When the contralateral leg is raised, the pelvis should remain parallel or rise on the contralateral side. Lowering or excessive side flexion to the ipsilateral side is positive. The sign occurs with an osteoarthritic hip, stress fracture of the hip and trauma to the abductors.

## Ultrasound

(a) **Diagnostic**. Ultrasound is very useful for soft tissue injuries, and particularly so for displaying haematomas and intratendinous cysts. Tendinous tears, scar tissue and abnormal muscular contraction can also be shown. Scanning can aid the accurate placement of injections. Doppler scanning displays neovascularization around tendons, and vascular problems.

(b) **Therapeutic**. Ultrasound appears to be of value to treat scar tissue, as an adjunct to mobilization and stretching regimens. In particular, it has been shown to advance the migration of mast cells to, and their action at, the site of tissue damage. This is often degradative during the

first 24–48 hours, which indicates that ultrasound should be applied around (but not on the site of) an acute lesion, but, after the 48 hours, the reparative function of mast cells is enhanced and serial observations of tissue fractions show an advance in healing by about 4 days. The problems created by penetration depth, standing waves and cavitation should be appreciated by practitioners using therapeutic ultrasound [13].

## Valsalva

A **dural stress test**. Exhalation against a closed glottis, or 'popping an ear', increases intraspinal pressure. See Dural stress tests.

## Vastus medialis obliquus (VMO)

Part of the **quadriceps muscle**; it attaches to the medial aspect of the patella and can therefore help to pull the patella medially and control maltracking (see Chapter 11).

## Ward's triangle

An area of weakness, noted in the trabecular lines in the inferior neck of the femur, that may be the site of a stress fracture – the compression stress fracture.

## Watson Jones

Operation for **an unstable ankle**, using the peroneals to strengthen the lateral complex.

## Watson test

When the wrist is moved into ulnar deviation, the scaphoid bone flexes. Watson's positive pivot test is performed by holding the poles of the scaphoid between the fingers and then ulnar deviating the wrist. In the normal wrist, the scaphoid can be felt pressing into the finger, but with scapholunate dissociation the scaphoid subluxes with a click and some pain.

## Weiberg score

Defined from 1 to 4, with a Jagerhut variety, this is a **classification of patellar shapes** and how they relate to the femoral sulcus. The higher the score, the more likely that patellar incongruity will be the cause of the tracking problem in anterior knee pain.

## Wright's manoeuvre

The pulse of the abducted and externally rotated arm disappears when the neck is rotated to the opposite side, the shoulders depressed, and a deep breath taken. This may be positive for **thoracic outlet syndrome**. False positives occur.

## Yergason's test

For bicipital tendinitis, where resisted flexion and supination in the neutral position of the arm are painful over the biceps. See Speed's test.

## References

1 O'Brien SJ, Pagnani MJ, Fealy S, McGlynn SR, Wilson JB. The active compression test: a new and effective test for diagnosing labral tears and acromio clavicular joint abnormality. Am J Sports Med 1998;26:610–613

2 Butler D, Gifford L. The concept of adverse mechanical tension in the nervous system. Physiotherapy 1989;75:622–636

3 Pedowitz RA, Hargens AR, Mubarak SJ, Gershuni DH. Modified criteria for the objective diagnosis of chronic compartment syndrome of the leg. Am J Sports Med 1990;18:35–40

4 Padhair N, King JB. Exercise induced leg pain – chronic compartment syndrome. Is the increase in intra-compartment pressure exercise specific? Br J Sports Med 1996;30:360–362

5 Motram S, Comerford M. Exercise therapy; spine. In: Hutson M, Ellis R (eds). Textbook of musculoskeletal medicine. Oxford: Oxford University Press; 2006, Ch. 4.3.12

6 STAT and PAAT. Injury in sport. Society of Teachers of Alexander technique and Professional Association of Alexander teachers.

7 Tucker WE, Armstrong JR. Injury in sport. Staples Press; 1964

8 Brock M. Chemonucleolysis – has it come and gone? J Orthop Med 1987;2:31

9 Crosse MM. Neuroleptanalgesia during discolyisis. J Orthop Med 1987;2:32–35

10 Sweetman BJ. Low back pain and the leg twist test. J Orthop Med 1998;20(2):3–9

11 Bowman C, Gribble R. The value of the forward flexion test and three tests of leg length changes in the clinical assessment of movement of the sacroiliac joint. J Orthop Med 1995;17(2):66–67

12 Adler GG, Hoekman RA, Beach DM. Drop leg Lachman test: new test for anterior knee laxity. Am J Sports Med 1995;23:320–323

13 Dyson M. Mechanisms involved in therapeutic ultra sound. Physiotherapy 1987;73:116–120; and lecture series and personal communication, Mary Dyson, Guy's Hospital, London

14 Coates GC, Keir KA. Connective tissue massage. Br J Sports Med 1991;25:131–133

15 Coates GC. Massage – the scientific basis of an ancient art: part 2. Physiological and therapeutic effects. Br J Sports Med 1994;28:153–156

16 Rayegani SM, Adybeik D, Kia MA. Sensitivity and specificity of two provocative tests (Phalen's teat and Hoffman-Tinel's sign) in the diagnosis of carpal tunnel syndrome. J Orthop Med 2004;26(2):51–55

17 Noyes FR, Grood ES, Cummings JF, Wroble RR. An analysis of the pivot shift phenomenon. The knee motions and subluxations produced by different examiners. Am J Sports Med 1991;19:148–155

18 Bobbert MF, Huijing P, van Ingen Schenau GJ. Drop jumping. 1. The influence of jumping technique on the biomechanics of jumping. Med Sci Sports Exerc 1987;19:332–338

19 Bobbert MF, Huijing PA, van Ingen Schenau GJ. Drop jumping. 2. The influence of dropping height on the biomechanics of drop jumping. Med Sci Sports Exerc 1987;19:339–346

20 Ho SSW, Illgen RL, Meyer RW, Torok PJ, Cooper MD, Reider B. Comparison of various icing times in decreasing bone metabolism and blood flow in the knee. Am J Sports Med 1995;23:74–76

21 Roos DB. Congenital abnormalities associated with thoracic outlet syndrome. Am J Surg 1976;132 771–777

22 Bush K, Cowan N, Katz DE, Gishen P. The natural history of sciatica associated with disc pathology. A prospective study with clinical and independent radiological follow up. J Orthop Med 1993;15(2):31–38

23 Onel D, Tuzlaci M, Sari H, Demir K. Computed tomographic investigation of the effect of traction on lumbar disc herniations. J Orthop Med 1990;12(1):6–14

## Further reading

Hutson M, Ellis R (eds). Textbook of musculoskeletal medicine. Oxford: Oxford University Press; 2006

# Index